THE HARVEY LECTURES

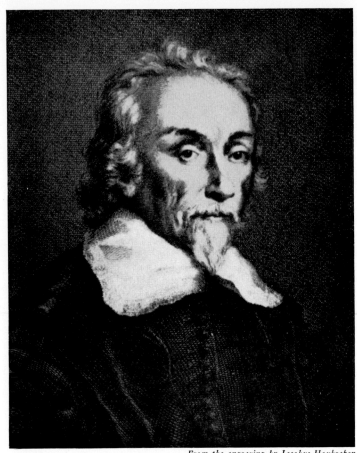

WILLIAM HARVEY

BORN APRIL 1, 1578 - DIED JUNE 3, 1657

THE HARVEY LECTURES

DELIVERED UNDER THE AUSPICES OF

The HARVEY SOCIETY of NEW YORK

1971–1972

———

UNDER THE PATRONAGE OF THE NEW YORK
ACADEMY OF MEDICINE

———

BY

JULIUS AXELROD
BARUJ BENACERRAF
PAUL BERG
EDWARD A. BOYSE

VINCENT P. DOLE
ROBERT A. GOOD
BRUCE MERRIFIELD
LLOYD J. OLD

MICHAEL SELA

SERIES 67

1973

ACADEMIC PRESS, New York and London

ACADEMIC PRESS, INC.
111 Fifth Avenue, New York, New York 10003

United Kingdom Edition published by
ACADEMIC PRESS, INC. (LONDON) LTD.
24/28 Oval Road, London NW1

LIBRARY OF CONGRESS CATALOG CARD NUMBER: 7-2726

PRINTED IN THE UNITED STATES OF AMERICA

CONTENTS

HARVEY LECTURES 1971–1972

THE HARVEY SOCIETY*

A SOCIETY FOR THE DIFFUSION OF KNOWLEDGE
OF THE MEDICAL SCIENCES

CONSTITUTION

I

This Society shall be named the Harvey Society.

II

The object of this Society shall be the diffusion of scientific knowledge in selected chapters in anatomy, physiology, pathology, bacteriology, pharmacology, and physiological and pathological chemistry, through the medium of public lectures by men who are workers in the subjects presented.

III

The members of the Society shall constitute three classes: Active, Associate, and Honorary members. Active members shall be laboratory workers in the medical or biological sciences, residing in the City of New York, who have personally contributed to the advancement of these sciences. Associate members shall be meritorious physicians who are in sympathy with the objects of the Society, residing in the City of New York. Members who leave New York to reside elsewhere may retain their membership. Honorary members shall be those who have delivered lectures before the Society and who are neither Active nor Associate members. Associate and Honorary members shall not be eligible to office, nor shall they be entitled to a vote.

Members shall be elected by ballot. They shall be nominated to the Executive Committee and the names of the nominees shall accompany

* The Constitution is reprinted here for historical interest only; its essential features have been included in the Articles of Incorporation and By-Laws.

the notice of the meeting at which the vote for their election will be taken.

IV

The management of the Society shall be vested in an Executive Committee to consist of a President, a Vice-President, a Secretary, a Treasurer, and three other members, these officers to be elected by ballot at each annual meeting of the Society to serve one year.

V

The Annual Meeting of the Society shall be held at a stated date in January of each year at a time and place to be determined by the Executive Committee. Special meetings may be held at such times and places as the Executive Committee may determine. At all meetings ten members shall constitute a quorum.

VI

Changes in the Constitution may be made at any meeting of the Society by a majority vote of those present after previous notification to the members in writing.

THE HARVEY SOCIETY, INC.

A SOCIETY FOR THE DIFFUSION OF KNOWLEDGE OF THE MEDICAL SCIENCES

BY-LAWS

ARTICLE I

Name and Purposes of the Society

SECTION 1. The name of the Society as recorded in the Constitution at the time of its founding in 1905 was the Harvey Society. In 1955, it was incorporated in the State of New York as The Harvey Society, Inc.

SECTION 2. The purposes for which this Society is formed are those set forth in its original Constitution and modified in its Certificate of Incorporation as from time to time amended. The purposes of the Society shall be to foster the diffusion of scientific knowledge in selected chapters of the biological sciences and related areas of knowledge through the medium of public delivery and printed publication of lectures by men and women who are workers in the subjects presented, and to promote the development of these sciences.

It is not organized for pecuniary profit, and no part of the net earnings, contributions, or other corporate funds of the Society shall inure to the benefit of any private member or individual, and no substantial part of its activities shall be carrying on propaganda, or otherwise attempting, to influence legislation.

ARTICLE II

Offices of the Society

SECTION 1. The main office and place of business of the Society shall be in the City and County of New York. The Board of Directors may designate additional offices.

Article III

Members

Section 1.   The members of the Society shall consist of the
incorporators, members of the hitherto unincorporated Harvey
Society, and persons elected from time to time. The members of the
Society shall constitute three classes: Active, Associate, and Honorary members. Active members shall be individuals with either the
Ph.D. or the M.D. degree or its equivalent, residing or carrying on a
major part of their work in the New York metropolitan area at the
time of their election, who are personally making original contributions to the literature of the medical or biological sciences. Associate
members shall be meritorious individuals with either the Ph.D. or
M.D. degree or its equivalent, residing or carrying on a major part of
their work in the New York metropolitan area at the time of their
election, who are in sympathy with the objectives of the Society.
Honorary members shall be those who have delivered a lecture before
the Society and who are neither Active nor Associate members.
Honorary members shall be exempted from the payment of dues.
Active and Associate members who have remained in good standing
for 35 years or who have reached the age of 65 and have remained in
good standing for 25 years shall be designated Life members. They
shall retain all the privileges of their class of membership without
further payment of dues. Associate and Honorary members shall not
be eligible to office, nor shall they be entitled to participate by voting
in the affairs of the Society. Volumes of The Harvey Lectures will be
circulated only to Active, Associate, and Life members. Honorary
members will receive only the volume containing their lecture. New
Active and Associate members shall be nominated in writing to the
Board of Directors by an Active or Associate member and seconded
by another Active or Associate member. They shall be elected at the
Annual Meeting of the Society by a vote of the majority of the Active
members present at the meeting. Members who leave New York to
reside elsewhere may retain their membership. Active and Associate
members who have given a Harvey Lecture and who have moved
out of the New York metropolitan area may, if they wish, become
Honorary members. Membership in the Society shall terminate on
the death, resignation, or removal of the member.

Section 2.   Members may be suspended or expelled from the Society by the vote of a majority of the members present at any meeting of members at which a quorum is present, for refusing or failing to comply with the By-Laws, or for other good and sufficient cause.

Section 3.   Members may resign from the Society by written declaration, which shall take effect upon the filing thereof with the Secretary.

Article IV

Meetings of the Members of the Society

Section 1.   The Society shall hold its annual meeting of Active members for the election of officers and directors, and for the transaction of such other business as may come before the meeting in the month of January or February in each year, at a place within the City of New York, and on a date and at an hour to be specified in the notice of such meeting.

Section 2.   Special meetings of members shall be called by the Secretary upon the request of the President or Vice-President or of the Board of Directors, or on written request of twenty-five of the Active members.

Section 3.   Notice of all meetings of Active members shall be mailed or delivered personally to each member not less than ten nor more than sixty days before the meeting. Like notice shall be given with respect to lectures.

Section 4.   At all meetings of Active members of the Society ten Active members, present in person, shall constitute a quorum, but less than a quorum shall have power to adjourn from time to time until a quorum be present.

Article V

Board of Directors

Section 1.   The number of directors constituting The Board of Directors shall be seven: the President, the Vice-President, the Secretary, and the Treasurer of the Society, and the three members of the Council. The number of directors may be increased or reduced

by amendments of the By-Laws as hereinafter provided, within the
maximum and minimum numbers fixed in the Certificate of Incorporation or any amendment thereto.

SECTION 2. The Board of Directors shall hold an annual meeting
shortly before the annual meeting of the Society.

Special meetings of the Board of Directors shall be called at any
time by the Secretary upon the request of the President or Vice-
President or of one fourth of the directors then in office.

SECTION 3. Notice of all regular annual meetings of the Board shall
be given to each director at least seven days before the meeting and
notice of special meetings, at least one day before. Meetings may be
held at any place within the City of New York designated in the
notice of the meeting.

SECTION 4. The Board of Directors shall have the immediate
charge, management, and control of the activities and affairs of the
Society, and it shall have full power, in the intervals between the
annual meetings of the active members, to do any and all things in
relation to the affairs of the Society.

SECTION 5. Council members shall be elected by the members of
the Society at the Annual Meeting. One Council member is elected
each year to serve for three years, there being three Council members
at all times. Vacancies occurring on the Council for any cause may be
filled for the unexpired term by the majority vote of the directors
present at any meeting at which a quorum is present. Only Active
members of the Society shall be eligible for membership on the
Council.

SECTION 6. A majority of the Board as from time to time consti-
tuted shall be necessary to constitute a quorum, but less than a
quorum shall have power to adjourn from time to time until a
quorum be present.

SECTION 7. The board shall have power to appoint individual or
corporate trustees and their successors of any or all of the property of
the Society, and to confer upon them such of the powers, duties, or
obligations of the directors in relation to the care, custody, or
management of such property as may be deemed advisable.

SECTION 8. The directors shall present at the annual meeting a
report, verified by the President and Treasurer, or by a majority of
the directors, showing the whole amount of real and personal

property owned by the Society, where located, and where and how invested, the amount and nature of the property acquired during the year immediately preceding the date of the report and the manner of the acquisition; the amount applied, appropriated, or expended during the year immediately preceding such date, and the purposes, objects, or persons to or for which such applications, appropriations, or expenditures have been made; and the names of the persons who have been admitted to membership in the Society during such year, which report shall be filed with the records of the Society and an abstract thereof entered in the minutes of the proceedings of the annual meeting.

ARTICLE VI

Committees

SECTION 1. The Board of Directors may appoint from time to time such committees as it deems advisable, and each such committee shall exercise such powers and perform such duties as may be conferred upon it by the Board of Directors subject to its continuing direction and control.

ARTICLE VII

Officers

SECTION 1. The officers of the Society shall consist of a President, a Vice-President, a Secretary, and a Treasurer, and such other officers as the Board of Directors may from time to time determine. All of the officers of the Society shall be members of the Board of Directors.

SECTION 2. The President shall be the chief executive officer of the Society and shall be in charge of the direction of its affairs, acting with the advice of the Board of Directors. The other officers of the Society shall have the powers and perform the duties that usually pertain to their respective offices, or as may from time to time be prescribed by the Board of Directors.

SECTION 3. The officers and the directors shall not receive, directly or indirectly, any salary or other compensation from the Society, unless authorized by the concurring vote of two thirds of all the directors.

Section 4. The officers shall be elected at the annual meeting of the Active members. All officers shall hold office until the next annual meeting and until their successors are elected or until removed by vote of a majority vote of the directors. Vacancies occurring among the officers for any cause may be filled for the unexpired term by the majority vote of the directors present at any meeting at which a quorum is present. Officers must be Active members of the Society.

Article VIII

Fiscal Year—Seal

Section 1. The fiscal year of the Society shall be the calendar year.

Section 2. The seal of the Society shall be circular in form and shall bear the words "The Harvey Society, Inc., New York, New York, Corporate Seal."

Article IX

Amendments

Section 1. These By-Laws may be added to, amended, or repealed, in whole or in part, by the Active members or by the Board of Directors, in each case by a majority vote at any meeting at which a quorum is present, provided that notice of the proposed addition, amendment, or repeal has been given to each member or director, as the case may be, in the notice of such meeting.

IMMUNODEFICIENCY IN DEVELOPMENTAL PERSPECTIVE*†

ROBERT A. GOOD‡

*Pathology and Pediatric Research Laboratories,
University of Minnesota Hospitals, Minneapolis, Minnesota*

I. INTRODUCTION

A T the outset I must make clear that much of the work I will report reflects collaborative effort with my fellows and students through the years. Consequently, my use of the word "we" throughout this lecture will represent not mere rhetorical convention, but my recognition of the contributions of my many younger associates in development of our views and perspectives. Because of its pertinence to the philosophy guiding our studies I would like to begin my address by quoting from Harvey's letter to John Vlackveld, distinguished physician at Harlem. Harvey wrote:

> Learned Sir,—Your much esteemed letter reached me safely in which you not only exhibit your kind consideration of me, but display a singular zeal in the cultivation of our art.
>
> It is even so. Nature is nowhere accustomed more openly to display her secret mysteries than in cases where she shows traces of her workings apart from the beaten path; nor is there any better way to advance the proper practice of medicine than to give our minds to the discovery of the usual law of nature, by the careful investigation of cases of rarer forms of disease. For it has been found in almost all things, that what they contain of useful or applicable, is hardly perceived unless we are deprived of them, or they become deranged in some way.
>
> The case of the plasterer to which you refer is indeed a curious one, and might supply a text for a lengthened commentary by way of illustration. But it is in vain that you apply the spur to urge me, at my present age, not mature merely but declining, to gird myself for any new investigation. For I now consider myself entitled to my discharge from duty. It will, however, always be a pleasant sight for me to

* Lecture delivered September 23, 1971.

† This work was supported by The National Foundation-March of Dimes, American Heart Association, American Cancer Society, U.S. Public Health Service (AI-08677, NS-02042, HE-06314), and NIH contract (22-761).

‡ Present address: Memorial Sloan-Kettering Cancer Center, New York, New York.

see distinguished men like yourself engaged in this honorable arena. Farewell, most learned sir, and whatever you do, still love.

Yours most respectfully, William Harvey

In his beautiful and simple prose, quoted at least once before in a Harveian oration (Garrod, 1924), Harvey states clearly a philosophy which has guided our efforts over the 30 years during which we have struggled to gain understanding of the relations between structure and function in the lymphoid system. As I try to share with you our experiences spanning nearly a third of a century, I will show over and over again how Experiments of Nature (McQuarrie, 1944) have guided our inquiry. These natural experiments have been particularly useful as a source for incisive questions which can be taken from the clinic to the laboratory for definitive analysis. Experiments of Nature function in another way: Information from the laboratory can often be returned to the clinic, and when manipulations derived from the laboratory insights are useful in correcting abnormal functions and treating or preventing disease, the correctness of their predictions are verified in a most relevant way.

Several of the Experiments of Nature we consider to have been especially useful to us in developing our approaches to immunobiology. These are listed on Table I.

When we began our work in 1942–1943, little was known of the (1) cellular, (2) organ, or (3) molecular basis of immunity. It has been a privilege to work during the third of a century when major understanding has been developed in each of these important areas. For us the first of these major insights was focused by the audacious interpretation in 1937 of an Experiment of Nature in hematology. Bing and Plum (1937) had encountered 13 cases of agranulocytosis. In three, hyperglobulinemia and plasmacytosis were striking features, an association which prompted the Danish investigators to suggest that globulin synthesis may be the work of the plasma cells. The publication of this work found consonance in Minneapolis because at exactly the same time, 1938, Fred Kolouch, a medical student then working also for a Master's degree, was interpreting another Experiment of Nature. He had been studying the bone marrow taken at postmortem from a patient who had died of sub-

TABLE I

EXPERIMENTS OF NATURE

1. Bing and Plum—agranulocytosis, plasmacytosis and hypergammaglobulinemia (1937)
2. Kolouch (1938)—association of streptococcal SBE, and bone marrow plasma cells with antigenic stimulation and antibody production
3. Multiple myeloma—wellspring for analysis of molecular basis of B-cell immunity. Waldenstrom's macroglobulinemia and Bennich and Johansson and McIntyre IgE myeloma are special instances of this influence
4. Myeloma—defective resistance to encapsulated bacterial pathogens, e.g., pneumococci. Vigorous cell-mediated and allograft immunity and defective antibody production
5. Bruton agammaglobulinemia, X-linked infantile agammaglobulinemia, defective resistance to same pathogens as troubled patients with myeloma, absence of plasma cells, germinal centers. Presence of abundant lymphocytes especially in deep cortical regions of nodes. Humoral immunities lacking. Cell-mediated immunities vigorous
6. Hodgkin's disease—counterpoint to agammaglobulinemia and myeloma. Defective cellular immunities, progressive with disease progression, immunoglobulins and antibody production vigorous
7. Thymoma-immunodeficiency syndrome. Deficiency of lymphocytes, cellular immunity and humoral immunity. Raised question of role of thymus in immunobiology
8. Glick's chance discovery that bursa is essential to development of antibody-producing ability. Conjunction of teaching assignment and study of influence of extirpation of bursa
9. DiGeorge syndrome—counterpoint to X-linked infantile agammaglobulinemia. Correctable by thymic transplant
10. Nude mice—genetically determined counterpart of DiGeorge syndrome. Correctable by thymic transplant
11. Swiss type agammaglobulinemia, a dual system immunodeficiency correctable by bone marrow transplantation but not by thymus transplantation
12. Chronic lymphatic leukemia—immunoglobulin deficiencies associated with monoclonal expansion of B-cells
13. Lymphoid malignancy occurring in patients lacking B-cells—began in the thymus
14. High frequency of autoimmunity in immunodeficiency
15. High frequency of autoimmune phenomena in patients lacking IgA system
16. High frequency of malignancy in all genetically determined immunodeficiencies of man
17. High frequency of malignancies in iatrogenic immunodeficiency diseases

acute bacterial endocarditis. Kolouch had noted an extraordinary plasma cell accumulation in both marrow and spleen. Since both his teacher of hematology, Downey, and his teacher in pathology, Clawson, suggested that the plasmacytosis might be attributable to the continuing bacterial infection, Kolouch had carried out laboratory experiments which associated the plasma cell accumulation with repeated antigenic stimulation (Kolouch, 1938). He speculated that the plasma cells which he observed to accumulate after repeated antigenic stimulation and anaphylactic shock might be producing antibodies. Several years after his initial studies Kolouch, then a surgical resident persuaded me, a freshman medical and graduate student in Berry Campbell's laboratory, to do something important, namely, to help him with his experiments on the relationship of plasma cells to antigenic stimulation and anaphylactic shock. From our experiments with Kolouch, it was clear that the physiological perturbations associated with passively induced anaphylactic shock did not lead to the plasmacytosis (Good, 1948). Further we found that secondary stimulation with simple protein antigens like hen's egg albumin and serum proteins, just as with bacterial antigens, could induce the plasmacytosis (Kolouch et al., 1947). Kolouch's studies led directly to the exciting investigations of Bjoerneboe and Gormsen (1943), who associated extreme hypergammaglobulinemia with extremes of plasmacytosis. These studies in turn led to Fagraeus' (1948) classical investigation, stimulated independently by an encounter with myeloma, which showed that plasma cell-rich but not lymphocyte-rich populations of lymphoid cells produced and released antibodies in vitro. Fagraeus' investigations further culminated in the demonstration by Coons and associates (Coons et al., 1955; Leduc et al., 1955; White et al., 1955) that plasma cells, and not lymphocytes, are the major producers of gamma globulins as well as antibodies after antigenic stimulation. Thus, in my earliest work on the immune system I had the privilege of participating in a small way in the resolution of what at that time seemed to be almost violent controversy. This resolution came from experimental studies set in motion by the interpretation of an Experiment of Nature.

When I came to the Rockefeller Institute in 1949 I was still among a minority—those plasma cell hunters who believed that plasma cells, not lymphocytes, produce antibody. Here I encountered two additional Experiments of Nature which influenced immensely our subsequent work. Since I had come to study in Maclyn McCarty's rheumatic fever division, I continued to search for and even to try to quantitate my favorite cells in children with acute rheumatic fever. Using simple morphological tools, and relatively crude methods for quantitating gamma globulins, I was able to correlate the *absolute* numbers of plasma cells in hematopoietic tissues with the slope of the curve of gamma globulin accumulation in the serum (Good and Campbell, 1950). Further, first with Kunkel and later on my own with my students (Page and Good, 1960), I found that in the Kunkel–Eisenmenger (Kunkel *et al.*, 1951a) girls with chronic active hepatitis and extreme hypergammaglobulinemia (Bearn *et al.*, 1956), I could associate extremes of gamma globulin elevation with extremes of plasmacytosis, especially in the liver. Some of our collaborative findings in the latter realm were not viewed with favor by editors who considered our attempts to quantitate plasma cells in tissues to be inadequate and so were only published later when I had accumulated more material. Henry Kunkel in those days was most anxious to carry out immunochemical studies on the proteins from patients with multiple myeloma. As I recall, he was having some little difficulties getting serums from myeloma patients as a point of departure for his studies. Largely, because I was then known to be a plasma cell hunter, even in certain centers in New York, I was able to collect several such serums which Kunkel then studied with his student Robert Slater. From generosity and perhaps because the serums came at a most propitious moment in a competition with other investigators who were hot on the myeloma problem, Kunkel included my name on what I consider to be a most important publication–a little note in *Proceedings of the Society for Experimental Biology and Medicine* (Kunkel *et al.*, 1951b). In this paper, Kunkel and Slater showed that each of the myeloma proteins was unique immunochemically. Yet, each was related immunochemically to all the others. Further, each was both related to and immunochemically different from the purest γ_2-globulin Kunkel could prepare from normal serum. For me, this experience with myeloma was most crucial. Again the interpretation of an Experiment of Nature seemed to cut through much confusion. Indeed, the interpretation of this one could be taken as the opening of a Pandora's box which has led to the entire modern understanding of the molecular basis of humoral immunity through study of the myeloma proteins by such giants as Kunkel, Edelman, and Putman (Slater *et al.*, 1955; Edelman and Poulik, 1961; Edelman and Gall, 1969; Putman *et al.*, 1967) using immunochemical, chemical, and physicochemical techniques. To be sure, prior studies had linked myeloma with accumulations of globulin and gamma globulin (reviewed by Good, 1957), but Kunkel's insights had derived from addressing this Experiment of Nature with the improving methods of immunochemistry and protein-physical chemistry. The legacy of this approach can be witnessed each day as we routinely work with immunoglobulins and analyze both disease and bodily defense in precise terms based on the potentialities of the molecular analysis made possible by these vital studies.

Because to obtain the serum specimens from the myeloma cases, I saw and talked to myeloma patients, sometimes at great length, I became much more interested in an aspect of myeloma other than the immunochemistry of their myeloma proteins. It had been known from writings dating to the early 1930's that patients with myeloma are very susceptible to infection. Not all kinds of infection seemed to cause trouble for these unfortunate victims of a plasma cell malignancy. Pneumonia and septicemia, due especially to *Pneumococcus* or *Hemophilus influenzae* bacilli, seemed to be diseases that were repeatedly encountered. By contrast, viral and fungal infections and infections with most of the enteric pathogens did not seem to be a major problem. It was known also from earlier clinical experiences that patients with certain forms of lymphoma, especially Hodgkin's disease, who likewise had frequent infections, had major trouble with fungi, acid-fast bacilli, herpes viruses, and other pathogens that we considered to be of a lower grade of virulence. In those early days we recognized clearly this counterpoint relationship between myeloma on the one hand and Hodgkin's disease on the other and were puzzled by it. The meaning of these Experiments of Nature began to emerge from four separate directions: (1) Bruton's discovery of agammaglobulinemia (1952); (2) Zinneman and Hall's (1954) immunologic studies of patients with myeloma; (3) Schier's description of anergy in Hodgkin's disease (Schier *et al.*, 1956); and (4) our

own analysis of the kinds of immunological deficiency and histo-
logical abnormalities that characterize patients with certain forms
of agammaglobulinemia, myeloma, and Hodgkin's disease (Good,
1957; Kelly *et al.*, 1960).

Immediately after Bruton's description of the association of
immunodeficiency with agammaglobulinemia in a single patient in
1952; both Janeway's group in Boston (Janeway *et al.*, 1953; Gitlin
et al., 1956, 1959) and our group in Minneapolis (Good and Varco,
1955; Good and Zak, 1956; Good *et al.*, 1962b) launched studies on
a substantial series of patients with agammaglobulinemia. We
encountered a small group with an X-linked agammaglobulinemia
who showed an extreme deficiency of gamma globulins. We and
others found them likewise to lack all of the subsequently described
immunoglobulins (Bridges and Good, 1960; Gitlin *et al.*, 1956).
These patients revealed no plasma cells or germinal centers in their
hematopoietic and lymphoid tissues, but possessed circulating
lymphocytes in normal numbers. They sometimes could not form
antibody in amounts demonstrable by even the most sensitive
techniques, e.g., *Escherichia coli* bactericidal test, bacteriophage
neutralization tests, passive hemagglutination, antigen-combining
globulin techniques, and even radioimmunoassay. By contrast, they
developed delayed and contact allergies very well. They usually
rejected skin allografts with vigor particularly in second set rejec-
tions (McKneally, 1970). Further, delayed allergic responses could
readily be transferred specifically to immunologically normal persons by injection of a sufficiently large inoculation of peripheral
blood leukocytes from such sensitized agammaglobulinemic patients
(Good *et al.*, 1959). Their lymph nodes (Fig. 1), showed very characteristic morphology. The far-cortical areas where germinal centers
usually appear were strikingly underpopulated, as were the medullary cords where plasma cells are usually found. Germinal centers
that I then called secondary lymphoid follicles, just like plasma
cells, did not appear in the nodes following secondary or tertiary
stimulation with potent antigens (Good, 1954a, b). The deep cortical
regions of the node showed proliferating cells, and the population
of cells in this region was regularly expanded by antigenic stimulation even though no demonstrable antibody or immunoglobulin was
produced. Later on, when studies were made of the thymus, this

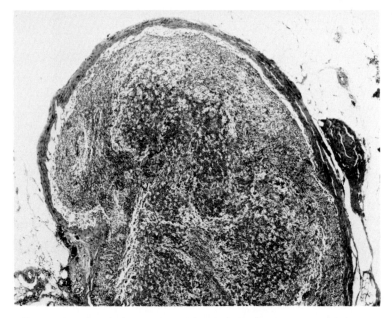

Fig. 1. Lymph node from patient with X-linked infantile agammaglobulinemia. Note deficiency of cells in far-cortical area, absence of germinal centers. By contrast, deep cortical areas show abundant cellularity.

organ was found to have no unusual features in children who had agammaglobulinemia associated with the extreme antibody deficiency syndrome (Peterson *et al.*, 1965). This rare disease was shown to be genetically X-linked. Figure 2 presents the characteristic appearance of the thymus and tonsil from such a case compared to the same lymphoid tissues from a similarly aged normal child who died accidentally. In the context of the observations on myeloma and other lymphomas, the spectrum of infections observed in the agammaglobulinemic children was most provocative. Life for these children we recognized to be a succession of threatening episodes of infection caused by pneumococci, *Hemophilus influenzae* bacillae, streptococci, meningococci, or *Pseudomonas aeruginosa*. To a much lesser extent, staphylococci and enteric pathogens caused trouble. Viral and fungal infections were not frequent, and clear evidence of immunity to such pathogens was observed.

On the basis of these clinical and early experimental studies it was possible for us as early as 1955 to begin to speak of two immunity systems, rather than one, and to contrast humoral immunity associated with plasma cells and cellular immunity focused in lymphocytes (Good, 1957).

These concepts were fortified by our detailed studies of the immunity mechanisms in patients with Hodgkin's disease (Kelly et al., 1959; Lamb et al., 1962; Kelly and Good, 1968). These patients not only were frequently anergic, as Schier et al. (1956) had found, but often rejected allografts poorly, failed to develop delayed allergy, and could not be readily stimulated to develop delayed allergic reaction or contact allergies by appropriate stimulation. This defect was progressive with progression of disease. Although a flurry of controversy was introduced into this field by a study carried out at the NIH (Brown et al., 1967), the essential elements of our original work have now been extensively confirmed (Aisenberg, 1965, 1966; Eltringham and Kaplan, 1972), and the immunologic defect in Hodgkin's disease can be described as an early and progressive deficit of cell-mediated immunities coupled with almost completely normal immunoglobulin synthesis and antibody response to many antigens. As mentioned above, associated with this immunologic defect, patients with Hodgkin's disease are susceptible to a spectrum of microorganisms quite different from that which plagues the patients with myeloma or X-linked infantile agammaglobulinemia.

This beginning new classification of the microbial world, in terms of a genetically based interaction in the evolution of the bodily defense of the eukaryotes and genetic adaptations of the microbial organisms, has been placed in bold relief by another extraordinary Experiment of Nature—the patients with fatal or so-called chronic granulomatous disease. This is an X-linked disorder that my students and I described in the late 1950's (Berendes et al., 1957; Bridges et al., 1959). I had first encountered such patients when I returned from New York to Minnesota and was deeply impressed by the lethality of the disease and its reality as a definable, genetically determined entity. In short, my graduate student Holmes and I, with Quie and Page (Holmes et al., 1966a, b, 1967; Quie et al., 1967), identified in these children a characteristic defect of phagocytic function. This defect seems to be based on a metabolic abnormality

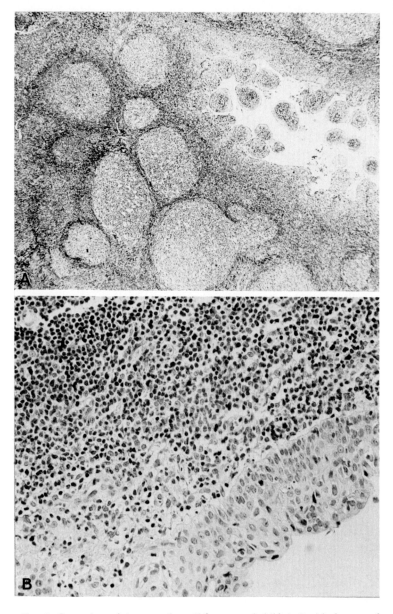

Fɪɢ. 2. Comparison of thymus and tonsil from normal child A, B with thymus and tonsil from child with Bruton-type agammaglobulinemia C, D. Note the abundant

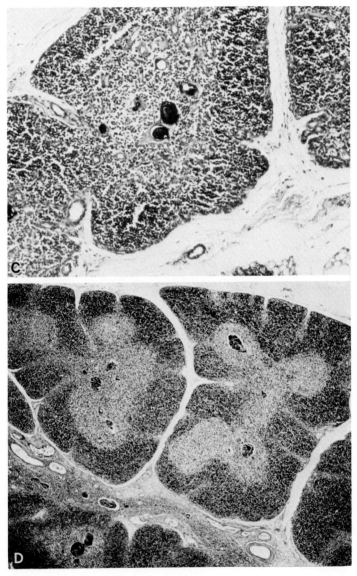

germinal centers in tonsil of normal child and the presence of only a small number of lymphocytes in the tonsil of child with Bruton-type agammaglobulinemia. Thymus from agammaglobulinemic child does not differ in any significant parameters from that of the immunologically normal child. Hassall's corpuscles, corticomedullary organization, characteristics of lymphocytes, are similar in the two.

that leads to failure to exhibit an increase in H_2O_2 synthesis during phagocytosis. Because of this metabolic defect the phagocytic cells cannot kill the catalase-positive bacteria and fungi which they ingest. By contrast they ingest and kill well catalase-negative pneumococci, streptococci, and hemophilus (Holmes-Gray and Good, 1971). Thus, the succession of granulomatous infections, often simulating tuberculous scrofula, cavitating and encapsulated pneumonias, granulomatous and purulent osteomyelitis, and granulomatous lesions of skin and other organs, can be attributed to failure to handle, and kill in normal fashion, staphylococci, Klebisella, aerobacteria, *Serratia marcescens*, salmonella, aspergillus, and other fungi. Once again a defect of the bodily defense as an Experiment of Nature can be used to gather together a strange group of microbial pathogens and reveal a basic defense mechanism in man for handling a significant component of the microbial world (Park *et al.*, 1972b) (Table II).

Directions for further revealing analyses of the lymphoid system and the bodily defense came from interpretation of another Experiment of Nature. A patient, first encountered by Richard Varco and me in 1952 (Good and Varco, 1955; MacLean *et al.*, 1957), had developed a severe immunodeficiency disease in temporal association

TABLE II

A CLASSIFICATION OF BACTERIA ACCORDING TO THE
BACTERICIDAL CAPACITY OF LEUKOCYTES FROM
PATIENTS WITH FATAL GRANULOMATOUS
DISEASE

Bacteria that are not killed (catalase positive)
1. Coagulase-positive staphylococci
2. *Escherichia coli*
3. *Aerobacter aerogenes*
4. *Paracolon hafnia* (Klebsiella)
5. *Serratia marcescens*

Bacteria that are killed (catalase negative)
1. *Lactobacillus acidophilus*
2. *Streptococcus viridans*
3. *Diplococcus pneumoniae*
4. *Streptococcus faecalis*

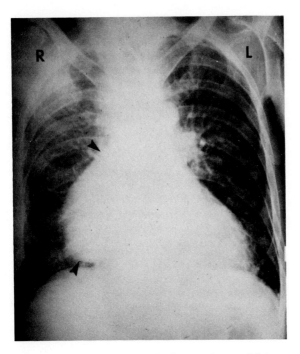

Fig. 3.   Chest X-ray from patient with thymoma-immunodeficiency syndrome.
Note mediastinal mass projecting to the right in the posterior–anterior roentgenogram.

with development of a huge mediastinal tumor. Extirpation of the
tumor showed it to be a 540-gm benign stromoepithelial thymoma.
Figures 3 and 4 depict the roentgenological and histopathological
characteristics of this lesion. This patient had defects of both cellular
and humoral immunity. He showed low levels of gamma globulin, a
deficiency of antibody responses as well as deficient allograft immunity, and deficient capacity to develop delayed allergic reactions.
Our reasoning that the conjunction of such a rare case of defective
immunity and an unusual pathologic entity, benign thymoma, were
unlikely to represent chance association has been amply supported
by subsequent experience (Gafni et al., 1960; Jeunet and Good, 1968;
Waldmann, 1968). We can now count more than 45 associations of
the two rare diseases. Such frequent conjunction establishes the

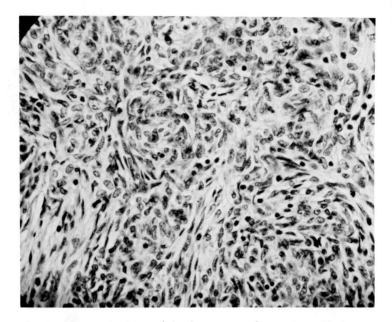

Fig. 4. Microscopic picture of the thymus tumor from patient with thymoma-immunodeficiency syndrome. Note that the tumor is comprised almost completely of spindle-shaped, stromal–epithelial cells.

relationship between benign thymoma and a severe broadly based immunodeficiency in such patients. The initial postulate that we derived from this encounter was that the normal thymus must play some critical role in maintaining the adequacy of the immune response. Tests of this postulate using thymic extirpation in small rabbits (as young as 4 weeks of age) revealed no detectable influence of the thymus on immunity by the techniques used in our study. Although we found this information to be somewhat discouraging, we stated clearly in the discussion of our most definitive presentation of the index case (MacLean *et al.*, 1957) that we trusted our Experiment of Nature more than we trusted our contrived laboratory studies and thus proposed to keep our minds open. Fortunately, we were then receptive to the events to be described below.

At the Federation Meetings in April, 1959, we learned that Harold Wolfe and his students had already begun to obtain evidence confirming an earlier discovery of Glick and associates (Glick *et al.*, 1956; Glick, 1964) that the bursa of Fabricius is essential for full immunological development in chickens. Papermaster, then a graduate student at Minnesota, visited Wisconsin where he was openly received, and he came roaring home with the conclusion that the bursa really is essential to the development of antibody production in chickens. He immediately went to work to elucidate the basis for this important influence. This new information struck us like a thunderbolt because my hematology professor, Hal Downey, had impressed on me that Jolly in 1911 and 1914 had considered the bursa to be the cloacal thymus. Jolly's view was based on morphologic and developmental similarity of the bursa to the thymus. Both are lymphoepithelial organs and both show striking development of mesenchymal lymphoid tissues in what is at first essentially an epithelial organ. Further, both begin an involution about the time of sexual maturation. The involution of the bursa is even more rapid and more complete than that of thymus. Figures 5 and 6 compare the developmental characteristics of the two organs. Immediately, I launched Olga Archer on the problem. Archer was a young Australian Master's degree student, and she worked directly with me on the problem. She was given the task of studying the influence of extirpation of the thymus very early in life on the immunologic development of rabbits. J. C. Pierce, a surgical fellow with Varco, helped Archer with the surgical aspects of our study. By fall, 1960 we could already offer clear evidence that the thymus of rabbits, like the bursa of chickens, is essential to the development of immune capacity (Archer and Pierce, 1961; Archer *et al.*, 1962). Kersey, then a freshman medical student working with Martinez and me (Martinez *et al.*, 1962; Good *et al.*, 1962a) was assigned to carry out studies on the influence of neonatal thymectomy in inbred mice and on the development of allograft immunity. Papermaster, Finstad, and I began to look for the thymus and bursa of Fabricius in primitive fishes following the lead of Salkind (1915) and Hammar (1908). We found that we could readily trace thymus development from epithelial anlagen in even the most primitive fishes including the elasmobranch (Fig. 7). But we are still searching for the bursal equivalent in all species save birds. Later we studied the effect of neonatal thymectomy in rats, hamsters, and dogs. Still later, with

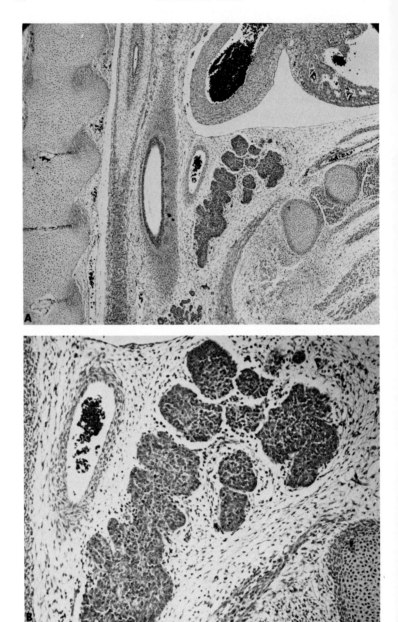

McKneally (McKneally and Good, 1971; McKneally *et al.*, 1971) and Mosser and Cooper (Mosser *et al.*, 1970), the influence of thymectomy coupled with total body irradiation on immune functions and responses of rabbits and mice was investigated. We presented at the American Association of Immunology meetings April 1961, both in written communication and in the discussions, our findings which we interpreted to indicate that the thymus is essential for full immunologic development in both rabbits and mice (Archer and Pierce, 1961). We had obtained, and so presented at that time, clear evidence that neonatal thymectomy in both rabbits and mice interferes with full immunologic development and influences many immune responses. In our first presentation we made it clear that both antibody production and cellular immune responses, such as

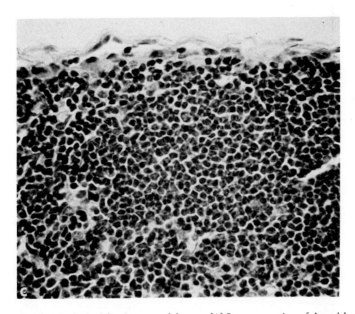

FIG. 5. Morphological development of thymus. (A) Low power view of the epithelial anlagen of the thymus of rabbit at 17 days of a 31-day embryonation period. (B) Higher power view showing epithelial anlagen without lymphocytes at 17 days. (C) High power view 5 days later showing abundance of lymphocytes. All these lymphocytes are derived from differentiating and proliferating mesenchymal stem cells that have entered the thymus.

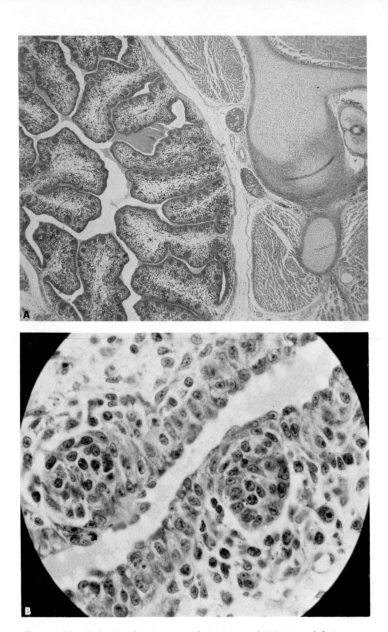

Fig. 6. Morphological development of the bursa of Fabricius. (A) Low power view of epithelial bursal anlage from chick embryo at 12 days of embryonation. Note the epithelial nature and beginning development of epithelial follicles. (B) High power view of bursal follicle at 14 days embryonation. Note the beginning development of lymphoblasts.

18

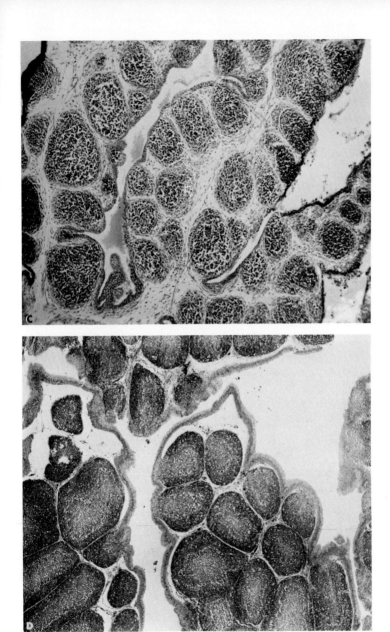

Fig. 6. (C) Eighteen-day embryonic bursa. The individual follicles are now predominantly lymphoid. (D) Mature bursa. Note follicular and cortical and medullary organization of a predominantly lymphoid organ. Each follicle relates intimately to the epithelium of the lower GI tract. (E) High power view of mature bursal follicles.

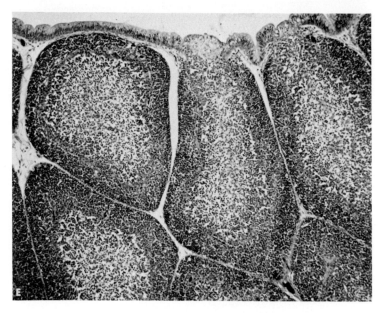

FIG. 6E. See legend to Fig. 6C and D.

allograft rejection and development of capacity to initiate graft-versus-host GVH reactions were inhibited by neonatal thymectomy. Coming at the question from a completely different perspective and apparently unaware of our work, Miller (1961) reported for the first time 3 months later in June of 1961 that the thymus is essential to development of certain immunities in mice. Extensive investigations in our own laboratories, by Miller and associates (Miller, 1961, 1964) and also by Jankovic *et al.* (1962) in Waksman's laboratory quickly established that immunodeficiency of both humoral and cellular immunity is produced in rats, mice, rabbits, and chickens when the thymus is extirpated very early in life. The competition of the three laboratories really energized the field, and useful new information poured quickly from all sides. Figure 8 compares neonatally thymectomized and normal mice and reveals the characteristic wasting and runting of the thymectomized animals. The wasting disease observed especially in some strains of mice, like the C3H and A, was less prominent in others, such as C57Bl. Indeed, resistance to wasting seemed to be directly proportional to the degree of development of the peripheral lymphoid tissue at the time of birth. Germ-free environments and specific pathogen-free environments (Jones *et al.*, 1971) seemed to mitigate against both the striking runting phenomenon and early death usually observed in neonatally thymectomized mice in conventional environments. In most colonies, neonatal thymectomy of mice produced high mortality, as revealed in Table III, which represents a single typical experiment carried out in our laboratory by Kalpaktsoglou. Thymectomy at 2 and 4 weeks of age appeared to be much less hazardous to the animals than was neonatal thymectomy.

Figure 9 presents data reflecting the strong influence of neonatal thymectomy on capacity of peripheral lymphoid cells to initiate a graft-versus-host reaction. It will be seen from these data that in several strains of mice development of ability to initiate a graft-versus-host reaction could be eliminated by neonatal thymectomy, but that grafting a new thymus from syngeneic or even from allogeneic donors reconstituted this function (Dalmasso *et al.*, 1964). In the reconstitution experiments, syngeneic thymus transplants always worked best (Dalmasso *et al.*, 1962, 1963; Stutman *et al.*, 1967). Thymus transplants across major histocompatibility barriers although sometimes effective often failed completely to restore the immunologic functions, resistance to runting and wasting and the capacity to survive in the ordinary laboratory environment. Transplants of thymus to genetically disparate mice matched at the H2 histocompatibility locus, although less effective than syngeneic

TABLE III

EFFECT OF THYMECTOMY ON SURVIVAL OF C3H MICE

	Newborn	2 Weeks	4 Weeks
Number of mice operated	109	75	72
Survival to 6 weeks	54	61	64
Dead by 6 weeks	55	14	8
Mortality (%)	51	18.7	11

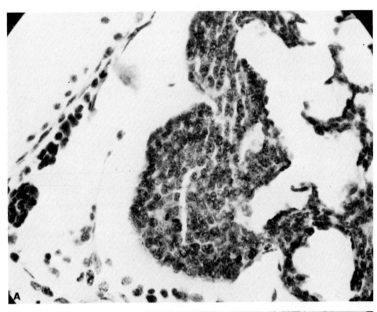

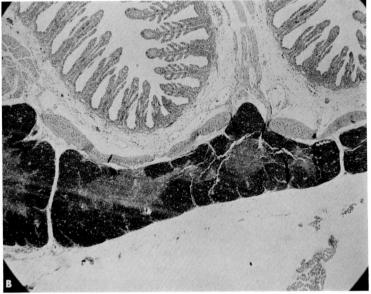

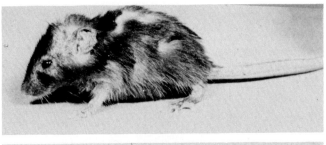

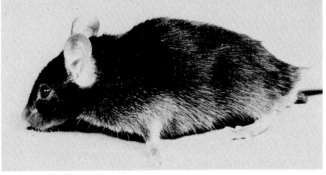

FIG. 8.   Comparison of neonatally thymectomized runted mouse and sham-operated control. Note severe wasting and runting and ruffled fur of the thymectomized mouse.

thymus, restored quite well the neonatally thymectomized recipients (Stutman *et al.*, 1969c). By contrast, transplants of thymus from donors mismatched at major barriers often but not always failed to reconstitute.

With G. Dalmasso, E. Yunis, and O. Stutman, we also studied the influence of peripheral lymphoid cells, e.g., spleen and lymph node cells, as reconstituting factors in neonatally thymectomized mice. Here again large numbers of syngeneic cells could be shown to restore such animals, prevent runting and wasting, and even reverse

FIG. 7.   Thymus development in a primitive fish. (A) Thymic epithelial anlage in an embryonic ray. (B) Mature thymus in a young ray. Note that the thymus shows all the morphological characteristics that feature the thymus of mammals and man. Cortex and medulla, lobular structure, and Hassall's corpuscles are apparent.

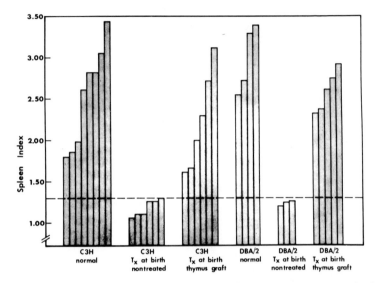

FIG. 9. Defect of capacity to initiate graft-versus-host reaction with lymphoid cells from neonatally thymectomized (T_x) mice. Note the deficiency in spleen index of A and DBA/2 mice when spleen cells used to initiate GVH reaction are taken from a neonatally thymectomized mouse. Reconstitution of this capacity occurs in neonatally thymectomized mouse transplanted with syngeneic thymus.

an already existing wasting syndrome. The neonatally thymectomized mice we found to be very susceptible to allogeneic disease induced by cells from donors differing from recipients by major (H2) histocompatibility determinants (Dalmasso et al., 1964). Even thymus grafts from donors mismatched with recipients at H2 determinants often induced lethal allogeneic diseases after restoring immunologic capacity in some combinations. The latter influence was not observed when thymuses were obtained from donors matched with recipients according to the major (H2) histocompatibility determinants (Stutman et al.,1969c).

One finding which we published with Yunis in 1965 seemed even then to have potential therapeutic importance. Peripheral lymphocytes from partially matched donors, matched at the H_2 locus, given in very large numbers to neonatally thymectomized recipients produced a long-term reconstitution of health and immunologic capacity and did not result in fatal graft-versus-host disease (Yunis *et al.*, 1965). By contrast, peripheral lymphoid cells from donors differing from neonatally thymectomized recipients at major histocompatibility determinants regularly produced early death from graft-versus-host disease. In the discussion of this paper, we pointed out clearly that these relationships might be therapeutically significant in attempting to correct immunodeficiency with transplants of hematopoietic or lymphoid cells.

After considerable study and some confusion, it was possible to conclude that a major influence of thymectomy early in life in mice, rats, hamsters, and chickens regards the cellular immunities. Allograft rejection, ability to initiate graft-versus-host reactions, and ability of lymphocytes to respond to phytohemagglutinin in culture (Rodey and Good, 1969) (Fig. 10) are all deficient in neonatally thymectomized mice. Always, however, we, along with all others who were studying the influences of thymectomy, showed that antibody responses to certain antigens, for example, sheep red blood cells, simple soluble protein antigens, certain bacteriophage antigens, and *Salmonella* H antigens, were defective in neonatally thymectomized mice. The latter finding seemed to be paradoxical because antibody responses to other antigens, for example, *Brucella* organisms, *Salmonella* organisms, pneumococcal polysaccharide as well as levels of all immunoglobulins studied seemed to develop

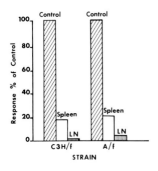

FIG. 10.   Deficiency of phytohemagglutinin (PHA) responding cells in neonatally thymectomized mice. Note that both lymph node (LN) and spleen cells from neonatally thymectomized mice respond poorly with DNA synthesis following stimulation with PHA.

normally in neonatally thymectomized mice (Jankovic *et al.*, 1962; Fahey *et al.*, 1965; Mosser *et al.*, 1970). This paradox was not clarified until Claman *et al.* (1966) discovered that the T-cell immunity system in mice often acts in cooperation with cells derived from bone marrow to achieve full antibody production. This discovery, extensively amplified by the work of Miller and associates (Mitchell and Miller, 1968; Nossal *et al.*, 1968; Miller and Mitchell, 1969, 1970), has been thought by many to represent a primary raison d'être of the thymus-dependent immunologic system. To us, several arguments stand against the view that, in the body economy, T-cell function regularly is essential for vigorous B-cell function (Good and Finstad, 1971).

Failure of normal development of the cellularity of lymphoid tissue is one feature of neonatally thymectomized animals (Metcalf, 1966). Focusing first on lymph nodes in mice, Parrott, deSoussa, and East (1966) showed that certain regions of the lymphoid tissues, for example, the deep cortical regions of the node, were most profoundly influenced by neonatal thymectomy. By contrast, medullary cords, plasma cells, far cortical areas, and germinal centers were not deficient. Further, antigenic stimulation effective in producing antibody responses in thymectomized mice induces plasma cell and germinal center responses. Our early contention that plasma cells and plasma cell responses (Good *et al.*, 1962a) are depressed in neonatally thymectomized mice was attributable to the fact that we were comparing plasma cells in lymphoid tissues of thymectomized and normal mice that had been repeatedly stimulated with thymic-dependent antigens, for example, soluble protein antigens and sheep red blood cells. Even though the B-cell system is not deficient in such animals, B-cell responses may be diminished when the antigenic stimulus cannot be vigorous because of the lack of T-cells, and this leads to the observed differences in number of plasma cells. Here again when full understanding emerged, everyone was right in what seemed at first to be irresolvable controversy.

Usually, however, when mice made grossly deficient in thymus-dependent lymphoid cell populations were kept long enough in a conventional environment, excessive proliferation of plasma cells and increase in all the thymus-independent regions was apparent. Figure 11 contrasts normal lymph node and lymph node of the

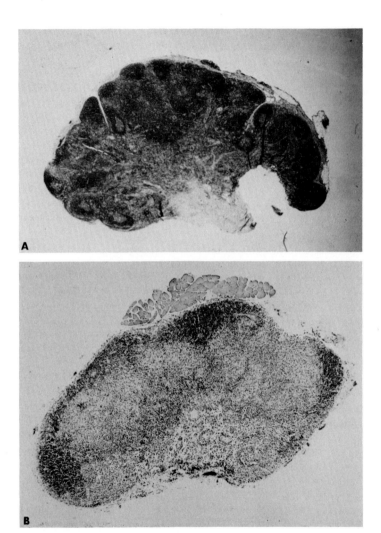

FIG. 11. Comparison of lymph node from normal mouse (A) and neonatally thymectomized mouse (B). Note abundance of cells in the deep cortical areas of the normal mouse. Note also the marked cellular deficiency in the deep cortical areas in the neonatally thymectomized mouse and the preservation of both medullary cords and far cortical concentrations.

neonatally thymectomized mouse illustrating the thymus-dependent regions of the node.

By the time the thymus conference was held in Minneapolis in 1962, much was already known but much confusion still reigned as to the nature of the influence that the thymus exerts on the development and maintenance of immunity. It is to the credit of this conference that the working interaction, in spite of its side show struggles for priority and dominance, focused many of the remaining questions and stated a number of useful hypotheses which guided the development of the field for nearly a decade (Good and Gabrielsen, 1964a). An important suggestion was made at this conference by Warner and Szenberg (1964) from studies of hormonally manipulated chickens. These workers had concluded that the thymus controls development of allograft immunity, while the bursa functions for development of antibody production. Their important insight was confounded by their contention that development of delayed allergies relates to the bursa and that capacity to initiate graft-versus-host reactions did not seem to be under developmental control of either bursa or thymus. Since this division of labor in the lymphoid system did not agree with the sorting of immune responses we had already carried out (Good, 1957; Good et al., 1957), largely from interpretation of the experiments of nature represented by Hodgkin's disease, myeloma and the X-linked agammaglobulinemic children the proposal generated some negative reaction especially from me even though it clearly reported a refreshing new view. Because there was so much confusion, we were determined to carry out clarifying studies. R. D. A. Peterson and later Max D. Cooper in my laboratories went to work to design experiments to clarify the relation of bursa and thymus to immunological development. Peterson developed collaborative relations with B. Burmester at East Lansing that permitted study of quarantined chickens. Cooper and Peterson also began to work with chickens on our own campus at the University of Minnesota. Both investigations produced important results and clearly established the separate roles of bursa and thymus in controlling immunologic development in the chicken. Cooper's studies employed complete bursal and thymic extirpation in newly hatched chickens and with these he coupled giving near lethal total body irradiation. In irradiated thymectomized newly hatched chickens one of two clearly separable populations of lymphocytes was prevented from developing as were all forms of cell-mediated immunity. Plasma cells, germinal centers, immuno-globulin concentrations and circulating antibody responses all developed normally. By contrast, bursectomy plus near lethal total body irradiation in newly hatched chickens regularly produced agammaglobulinemia and severe antibody deficiency syndrome. In addition, these manipulations prevented development of certain lymphocytes, all germinal centers and plasma cells. From these studies (Cooper *et al.*, 1965, 1966), it became clear that these two central lymphoepithelial organs, the thymus and the bursa exercised entirely different functions. Each guides differentiation and develop-ment of a separate system of cells responsible for immunity. The thymus was shown to be essential to development of a large popula-tion of relatively small lymphocytes essential to expression of the cell-mediated immunities. The bursa subserves development of a system of lymphoid cells responsible for humoral immunity. Thus, each of the central lymphoid organs in chickens appeared to subserve differentiation and development of a different population of lymph-oid cells. Table IV summarizes the influence of thymus and bursa on development of lymphoid tissue and immunologic functions. These findings were coupled with studies of the traffic of cells and develop-ment of immune functions in irradiated mice by C. E. Ford (1966)

TABLE IV

Role of Thymus and Bursa in Immunologic and Lymphoid Development

Bursa essential for	Thymus essential for
1. Humoral immunity	1. Cell-mediated immunities
2. Immunoglobulins	2. Deep cortical areas of node
3. Germinal centers	3. Perivascular areas of spleen
4. Plasma cells	4. $\theta+$ T-cells, small lymphocytes
5. B lymphocytes	5. Defense against facultative intra-cellular bacterial pathogens, fungi, and many viruses
6. Defense against encapsulated bacterial pathogens	

and with studies by Moore and Owen (1965, 1966) tracing origin of cells in the chicken bursa. When this information was viewed in light of knowledge of genetically determined perturbations of development of the immunity systems in man, we could formulate the two-component scheme of immunological development (Cooper et al., 1968c, d). This concept is illustrated in Fig. 12.

With this new clarification at hand, we promptly attempted to relate the known disturbances of development of the immunity systems in man to this scheme and found we could readily realize real success in this venture (Peterson et al., 1965; Good et al., 1968). DiGeorge (1968) recognized that the abnormalities of the lymphoid tissues and the peculiar deficiencies of lymphoid function in athymic children made sense in our new perspective of the lymphoid system. This insight acted as a catalyst to provoke us to bring this new look at the immunodeficiency diseases of man to formal conference, so we organized one on Immunologic Deficiency Diseases of Man to be held on Sanibel Island off the coast of Florida in 1967. At the conference, it was obvious that we were already on the way to useful new understanding of the immunologic apparatus. Projections for new approaches to treatment of immunodeficiency popped up frequently at that gathering (Good and Bergsma, 1968). In

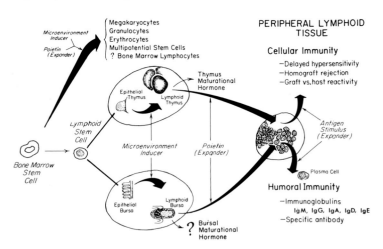

FIG. 12. Scheme of two-component concept of immunological development.

TABLE V

1. Chromosomal markers—CBA T₆ system
2. Surface differentiation isoantigens—TL
   and θ in mouse
3. Functional markers—response to
   PHA
   Concanavalin A
   Allogeneic cells *in vitro*
4. Formation of rosettes with SCBC at
   37°C

careful subsequent studies, Stutman *et al.* (1970a, b; Stutman and
Good, 1971) in our laboratories, Kincade *et al.* (1970; Kincade and
Cooper, 1970) in Alabama, Moore and Owen (1965, 1966), Warner
(1965), and Thorbecke *et al.* (1968) have brought forward much
new evidence that we believe establishes the reality of the two-
component model of lymphoid system development and function
that we originally proposed (Peterson *et al.*, 1965). In the most
telling of these studies, surface isoantigens (differentiation isoantigens), functional responses of cells, and chromosome markers
have been the critical parameters used to trace traffic and differentiation of lymphoid cells. The markers found most useful to us in
working out the development of the T-cell system have been those
listed in Table V. These include chromosome markers, especially the
T₆T₆ and T₆ markers used extensively in CBA mice by C. E. Ford
(1966), functional markers like capacity to respond by blast transformation *in vitro* to PHA, concanavalin A, or allogeneic cells, and
the surface differentiation isoantigens TL and θ so extensively
studied by Boyse *et al.* (1966, 1968). We have used these parameters
to trace the development and differentiation of both T- and B-cells.
In doing such studies, particular care must be taken in preparation
and absorption of anti-θ isoantisera to avoid the misleading conclusions derived from polyvalent and nonspecific anti-θ antiserum
used by many investigators (Raff, 1971; Raff and Cantor, 1971;
Stutman, 1970). Stutman and Good (1971) have shown that θ
negative prethymic cells of the yolk sac, fetal liver, or bone marrow
can enter the thymus, divide, and differentiate to θ+ cells which

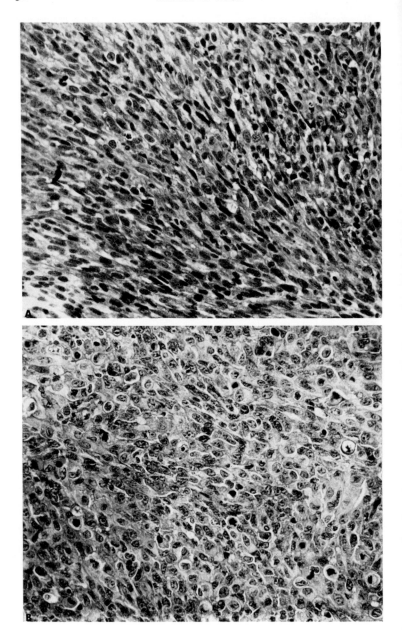

leave the thymus and can remain as recirculating cells in the peripheral lymphoid tissues. These postthymic cells may be long-lived or short-lived (Stutman, 1973) and are not necessarily fully competent at first, but become so after a period of dependence on an indirect long-range influence of the thymus. Raff and Cantor (1971) have shown that T_1 cells can be driven to T_2 cells by antigenic stimulation. The latter influence can be exercised by thymus grafts in cell-impenetrable chambers (Osoba and Miller, 1963) and by stromal epithelial tumors of the thymus (Stutman *et al.*, 1968, 1969a), which have the capacity to maintain and expand but not fully to differentiate a thymus-dependent population of lymphoid cells. Figure 13 shows such a functional thymoma. These tumors occasionally develop after injections of 7,12-dimethylbenzanthracene directly into the thymus. They represent few among many thymic tumors produced in this way that more frequently are lymphosarcomas, sometimes "Hassall's corpuscleomas," and occasionally rhabdomyosarcomas. Prethymic stem cells are present in yolk sac, fetal blood, fetal liver, and bone marrow and peripheral blood. Immediate postthymic T_1 cells are present in late fetal liver, spleen, bone marrow, and blood. Fully differentiated postthymic T_2 cells represent a recirculating sometimes long-lived population of T-cells which upon encounter with antigen can undergo blast transformation, proliferate to expand their number, and produce lymphokines. They seem to be the cells which act to achieve the biologic amplification influence involved in T-cell immunity by production of lymphokines. The differentiation of T-cells is associated with appearance of θ isoantigens at the surface of T-cells. This isoantigenic marker remains with these cells as an identifying marker throughout the life of these cells as the latter percolate and recirculate in the peripheral lymphoid system (Raff, 1971; Stutman *et al.*, 1970a, b; Raff and Cantor, 1971).

Similarly, it is clear from our own studies (Cooper *et al.*, 1966) and from the studies of Warner (1965) that the thymus of birds

---

Fig. 13. Morphological characteristics of the slowly growing stromal epithelial thymoma which can expand but cannot differentiate the T-cells system. Note the spindle-shaped nature of the cells. These tumors represented few among many induced by direct injection of the 7,12-dimethylbenzanthracene into the thymus.

TABLE VI

T-Cell System

Cell	Location	Characteristics
Prethymic	Yolk sac, fetal liver, bone marrow	θ neg., not immunologically competent; radiosensitive; traffic to thymus and bone marrow
Postthymic T_1	Fetal liver, spleen of neonatal mouse; peripheral lymphoid tissue; bone marrow	Not immunocompetent; sensitive to humoral inductive influence of thymus, $\theta+$, receptor not yet defined
Postthymic T_2	Blood, thoracic duct lymph, peripheral lymphoid tissues, thymus dependent areas; recirculating in blood and lymph	$\theta+$, immunocompetent long-lived recirculating cell; receptor not yet defined
Postthymic T_3	Peripheral lymphoid system, blood inflammatory exudates	Not recirculating, $\theta+$, produces lymphokines, selectively traffics to inflammatory site
Postthymic T_4	Spleen, lymph node, bone marrow	Radioresistant, $\theta+$, memory cell capable of engaging radiosensitive, nonspecific marrow cells to achieve delayed allergic reaction and cellular immunity
Postthymic T_5	Spleen, lymph node, thymus-dependent areas of peripheral lymphoid tissue, blood, and thymus cortex	Radiosensitive, corticosteroid sensitive; short-lived T-cells, short-lived memory cells; function unknown, may have helper function; separate population like this may produce lymphokines

exercises the same function, as does the thymus of mammals (Thorbecke et al., 1968). This function is to differentiate and expand a T-cell population that subserves the cell-mediated immunities. The bursa of Fabricius, on the other hand, is essential for differentiation of all the cells capable of synthesizing and secreting the known immunoglobulins and antibodies. Yolk sac, fetal liver and marrow cells can travel through the bursa, where they differentiate first to committed B_1 stem cells, then to B_2 cells capable of producing surface immunoglobulins. These are differentiated first to B_{2p} cells that can produce but not secrete immunoglobulins. They are distinguished by having fine irregular deposits of immunoglobulins at their surface. They in turn can be differentiated to B_{2s} immunoglobulin-secreting cells, apparently an end stage differentiation, by contact with specific antigen. Tables VI and VII define the T- and B-cell populations, and Table VIII records marker systems thus far used to trace differentiation of B-cells. It should be pointed out here that, even for the chickens, the data on the traffic and sojourns of the B-cell population are less well defined than are those for the T-cell population. On the other hand, the receptor immunoglobulins

TABLE VII

B-Cell System

Cell	Location	Characteristics
Prebursal	Blood islets of yolk sac, fetal liver, bone marrow	Not immunologically competent, capable of traffic to differentiative site in bursa or equivalent
Postbursal B_1	Bursal medulla; bone marrow and spleen late	Multipotential lymphocytes capable of providing long-term reconstitution of agammaglobulinemic bursaless animals
Postbursal B_{2p}	Medulla of bursa, far-cortical areas of lymph node—germinal centers, periarteriolar accumulations in Malpighian corpuscles of spleen; efferent lymph following antigenic stimulation; thoracic duct lymph, circulating blood	Capable of synthesis of antibody, but not specialized for secretion of large amounts of ab; C3 receptor of Nussenzweig present; probably specific antibody at all such cell surfaces
Postbursal B_{2s}	Bone marrow, medullary cords of lymph nodes, red pulp of spleen, lamina propria of GI tract and secretory glands, interstitial tissue of bone marrow, occasionally peripheral blood or lymph	Secretory lymphocyte, plasma cells; negative for Nussenzweig marker; specialized for both production and secretion of the several immunoglobulin classes; PC_1 antigenic marker in mouse; probably specific identifying antigens in other animals

TABLE VIII

Markers Useful for Tracing Development of
B-Cells

---

1. Chromosomal markers
2. Surface receptors and surface immunoglobulins
3. Functional markers—immunoglobulin and antibody production and secretion
4. Jerne plaque-forming units
5. Plasma cells

---

at the surface of B-cells serve to identify even the individual lymphocytes of this population. Telling experiments establishing the reality of this model of differentiation of B-cells have now been done by Moore and Owen (1965, 1966), Linna (1967), Kincade *et al.* (1970; Kincade and Cooper, 1970), Cooper *et al.* (1971), Toivanen *et al.* (1972a, b), and Toivanen and Linna (1971).

Our experiments with bursectomy performed *in ovo* have been most useful (Cain *et al.*, 1968; Van Alten *et al.*, 1968; Cooper *et al.*, 1969; Choi and Good, 1972). Differentiation of B-cells seems to occur from yolk sac, fetal liver, or bone marrow stem cells, which can enter the bursa and differentiate first to IgM producing cells, then in succession to IgG- and possibly IgA-producing cells (Kincade, 1970; Kincade *et al.*, 1970). Capacity for immunoglobulin or antibody secretion appears to represent a terminal differentiative step that requires stimulation of the cell by antigen. Thus, secretory B-cells or plasma cells seem not to develop without antigenic stimulation. IgM-producing cells appear in the bursa at 13–15 days of embryonation. They begin to move to the periphery between 17 and 19 days. If complete extirpation of the bursa is accomplished between day 15 and day 17, this procedure alone can yield agammaglobulinemic chickens lacking not only all immunoglobulins and ability for antibody response, but also plasma cells, germinal centers, and B-cells which have identifying surface immunoglobulins. Bursectomy *in ovo* on day 18–19, coupled with near lethal total body irradiation at hatching, regularly produces agammaglobulinemic chickens which have a perfectly normal T-cell population. Such animals have no germinal centers, plasma cells, or circulating B-cells with immunoglobulins in receptor pattern or irregular distribution at their surface. Complete bursectomy at 18 or 19 days of embryonation without irradiation often yields chickens capable of synthesis and secretion of IgM but not capable of producing or secreting IgG immunoglobulins. Such chickens may live quite well under conditions of conventional husbandry, but they fail ever to develop an IgG-producing population of cells. This is true even if such animals are extensively stimulated with a variety of antigens.

Recently Kincade *et al.* (1970) presented evidence that seems convincingly to show that in the chickens the differentiation of IgG-producing cells involves a step where the cells must first have been IgM producers. The switch from IgM to IgG production occurs only in the bursa of Fabricius. Using a model of agammaglobulinemia developed by Lerman and Weidanz (1970) and modified in our laboratories by Linna *et al.* (1972), Toivanen *et al.* (1972a, b) have studied extensively the development and differentiation of the chicken B-cells. They have been able to show that at the proper stage of development yolk sac or marrow cells can enter the bursa and develop into stem cells for the B-cell system that can be found in the bursa for several months. Such stem cells are capable of fully reconstituting, both in short and long term, the immunoglobulin- and antibody-producing system of agammaglobulinemic chickens. At a later stage of development of the bird, yolk sac and fetal liver cells cannot be differentiated by the bursa. Beginning about the time of earliest involution of the bursa, cells capable of fully reconstituting, for many months, immunoglobulin- and antibody-producing capacities seem to leave the bursa and take up residence in both bone marrow and spleen. The essential features of these several analyses are included in the consideration underlying the construction of Figs. 14–16 which represent our most recent attempt to illustrate schematically the definitions of the development of the two lymphoid systems.

II. THE QUEST FOR A BURSAL EQUIVALENT

Studies especially from human pathology and from comparative experiments in mice, rats, and chickens leave no question but that there are two separate immunity systems, one subserving cellular

immunity, and one subserving humoral immunity in all phylogeneti-
cally recent forms. The thymus in all species where studies have
been adequate can be shown to be essential for differentiation of the
system of cells responsible for the cellular immunities. This organ
seems not to play an essential role in the development of most of the
immunoglobulin-producing system of cells. Thus, it is essential to
view the development of the B-cell population as one requiring an
influence equivalent to that exercised in birds by the bursa of
Fabricius. Many investigators have concluded that in mammals and
man the bursal influence is exercised by the bone marrow. Indeed,
Stutman in our laboratories (1973) has recently obtained evidence
that B-cells, defined as immunoglobulin-producing cells, can
differentiate in the spleen of irradiated recipients from yolk sac or
fetal liver precursors. The evidence presented by the work of
Toivanen and Toivanen argues, however, that it may be possible for
the essential influence of even a crucial central lymphoid organ to
change with the state of development. Thus, more definitive experiments with both chickens and mammals are essential before we can
decide whether or not the bursal equivalent function is exercised in
mammals and man by the bone marrow and by other hematopoietic
sites such as spleen or by some more precise bursal equivalent organ,

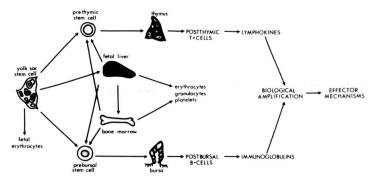

FIG. 14. Scheme of development of the two-cell system. Using chromosome
markers and functional and surface marker characteristics of the cells, the traffic
patterns indicated have been worked out. Each solid line represents an established
pathway of traffic and development.

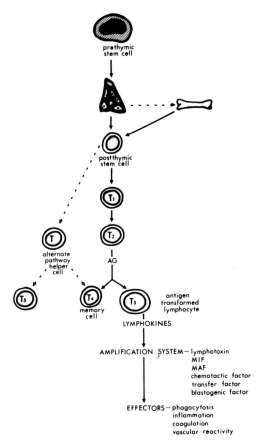

Fig. 15. Scheme of differentiation of T-cells. Prethymic cells are cells that lack θ isoantigen and are capable of traffic to the thymus. Postthymic T_1-cells possess the thymic differentiation isoantigens, but do not necessarily possess full immunocompetence. They depend on the indirect influence of thymus for their maintenance and further differentiation. Fully immunocompetent T_2-cells possess θ isoantigen. T_1-cells can be driven to be T_2-cells by antigenic stimulation. T_3-cells are θ+ cells that have been induced to transformation and to proliferation by contact with specific antigen. T_4 is a radioresistant thymus-dependent memory cell. Alternate pathway of short-lived and long-lived helper cells are suggested by studies already available, but the exact nature of these elements has not been clarified. Short-lived T_5 memory cells have been described.

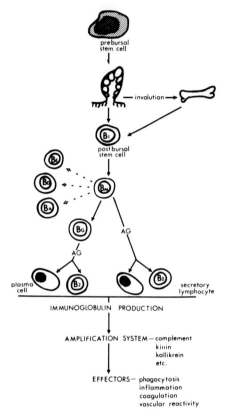

FIG. 16. Scheme for development of B-cells. In the chicken a B_1-cell exists in the immature chicken bursa which can leave the bursa at the early stages of involution and then reside in marrow or spleen. It acts as stem cell to replace the entire bursal dependent lymphoid system. In birds and probably also in mammals, all immunoglobulin-producing B_{2p}-cells seem to need to go through an IgM-producing stage. Immunoglobulin-secreting B_{2s}-cells are derived by terminal differentiation of B_{2p}-cells after contact with antigen.

perhaps associated with the distal gut and only transiently present. Characteristics by which we should be able to identify the bursal equivalent are present in Table IX.

On Table X are listed the basic functions of T-cells, and on Table XI the basic functions of B-cells. Tests for the adequacy of these

TABLE IX

Bursa and Bursal Equivalent Site

1. Most likely a lymphoepithelial site
2. First site in "B" lymphoid system to possess immunoglobulin-forming cells
3. First site to have lymphoid cells forming readily demonstrable μ chains
4. Later, also, the first site to have cells forming γ chains
5. Only site to have appreciable number of cells forming both μ and γ chains in large amounts at the same time. Thus, cytoplasm stains specifically for both IgG and IgM
6. A site where antigenic stimulation does not alter either the number or time of appearance of μ- or γ-containing cells and the follicles producing these cells
7. Site which involutes early in life
8. A site where many cells produce heavy chains lacking galactose residues

TABLE X

Major Functions of T-Cells

1. Initiate delayed allergic reactions and Jones-Mote reactions
2. Initiate graft-verus-host reactions
3. Respond with blast transformation to PHA or to mitomycin-treated or irradiated allogeneic cells *in vitro*
4. Participate in killer function against tumor cells
5. Participate in solid tissue allograft rejection
6. Contribute a major specific component in one of the bulwarks of bodily defense against certain viruses, fungi, and facultative intracellular bacterial pathogens
7. Participate in immunosurveillance against cancer

TABLE XI

Major Functions of B-Cells

1. Produce immunoglobulin receptors made up of specific antibodies in receptor distribution
2. Secrete immunoglobulins and antibodies
3. Provide primary defense against high grade encapsulated bacterial pathogens
4. Detoxify proteins, polypeptides, and other toxins
5. Prevent recurrences of virus and certain bacterial infections

TABLE XII

Tests for Adequacy of T-Cell Function

1. Quantitative response of cells in whole blood to phytohemagglutinin (PHA), *in vitro* transformation
2. Dose-response analysis of PHA responsiveness *in vitro*
3. *In vitro* response of lymphocytes to allogeneic, irradiated, or mitomycin-treated, lymphocytes
4. Development of delayed allergy to ubiquitous antigens, SK-SD, mumps, *Candida*, trichophyton, PPD
5. Development of contact allergy to 2,4-dinitrochlorobenzene
6. Small lymphocyte count
7. Capacity to reject allograft of skin
8. Presence of an abundant cell population in deep cortical areas of lymph node following antigenic stimulation
9. Vigorous defense against fungi, virus, and facultative intracellular bacterial pathogens
10. In mice, number of $\theta+$ cells.

TABLE XIII

Tests for Adequacy of B-Cell Function

1. Quantitation of levels of all major immunoglobulin classes by radial immunodiffusion or radioimmunoassay
2. Evaluation of fractional catabolic rate and/or synthesis rates for individual immunoglobulins
3. Antibody concentration to antigens widely distributed in nature, e.g., isohemagglutinins, ASO, Schick test, antiviral antibodies
4. Quantitation of antibody response to killed poliovirus vaccine—Pasteur Institute
5. Quantitation of antibody response to diphtheria and tetanus toxoids
6. Antibody responses to polysaccharide antigens from pneumococcal, meningococcal, and hemophilic polysaccharides
7. Concentration of IgA and analysis of form of IgA in saliva
8. Quantitation of immunoglobulin subclasses
9. Specific identification of bacteria causing frequent pneumonia, sepsis, conjunctivitis, and meningitis. The organisms that particularly plague patients with B-cell defects include pneumococci, streptococci, hemophilic influenza, meningococci, and *Pseudomonas aeruginosa*
10. Specific immunofluorescence against γ, μ, α, δ, ϵ, κ, and λ determinants after staining in the cold

cell systems are recorded in Tables XII and XIII. With these approaches, it is now possible to look critically and often to quantify perturbations of immunologic function in human disease. The most recent studies permitting quantitation of numbers and percentages of each of the separate classes of B-cells using the receptor immunoglobulin technique should prove most useful as a clinical tool (Pernis and Kunkel, 1971). Figure 17 illustrates immunoglobulin-producing and immunoglobulin-secreting cells. For example, quantitation of the numbers of each class of B-cells can be made by counting the total population of lymphocytes and then establishing the percentage of circulating lymphocytes that are IgM, IgG, or IgA producers (Fig. 17C). These immunoglobulin-producing cells with immunoglobulins at their surface in presumed receptor distribution are not the immunoglobulin-secreting cells. The latter must derive from these lymphocytes by stimulation with an antigen that in turn initiates proliferation and terminal differentiation (Fig. 17A and B). Secreting cells can also be quantified by applying the specific immunohistochemical techniques to evaluate the numbers of cells containing immunoglobulins within their cytoplasms. Such cells can be demonstrated in smears or imprints of bone marrow, lymphoid organs, or blood.

Similarly, new methods have been forthcoming to permit approximate quantitative evaluation of the number of T-cells in the circulation in man as well as in experimental animals (Park and Good, 1972). A technique we currently favor is one that involves quantitation of the uptake of tritiated thymidine during short-term cultures of whole blood in the presence of phytohemagglutinin. Since the only cells in the circulating blood that respond by nucleic acid synthesis to stimulation by PHA in solution are the T-cells, the amount of tritiated thymidine incorporated in such short-term direct cultures of blood seems a good measure of the number of circulating T-cells. Unfortunately as yet for man, specific surface antigens with which to identify T-cells have not yet been defined. Individual T-cells can now be identified in blood and peripheral lymphoid tissues. It is clear that they usually represent some 50–75% of peripheral blood lymphocytes. Among the peripheral blood lymphocytes we now include T-cells, B-cells, M-cells (monocyte precursors), multipotent stem cells, and various kinds of committed

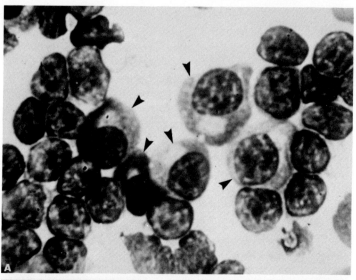

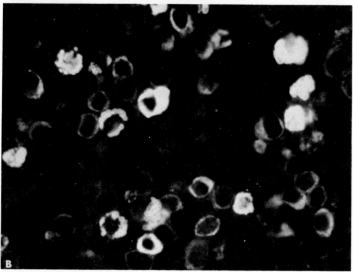

Fig. 17. (A) Plasma cells stained with Giemsa. Note excentric nucleus, perinuclear Hof region of the Golgi, and intense basophilia of cytoplasm. (B) Immunoglobulin producing and secreting cells are identified as the cells containing IgM, IgG, IgA, IgD, and IgE. Immunofluorescence staining with antibodies specific for the individual heavy chain, μ, γ, α, δ, ϵ, or with anti-κ and anti-λ antiserum can be used to demonstrate these cells. These are B_{2s}- or secretor B-cells stained with anti-μ.

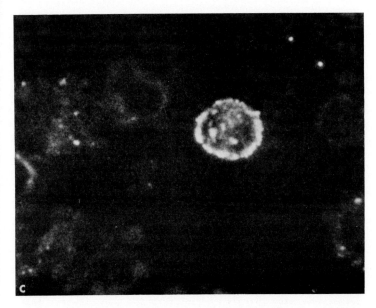

Fig. 17. (C) Surface immunoglobulin staining specific for IgM, IgG, or IgA can be used to quantify these B$_{2p}$-cells in circulation or lymphoid tissues. These are the immunoglobulin-producing but not immunoglobulin-secreting B-cells.

stem cells—at least 5 identifiable categories of cells, each with a different function. New methods for enumerating T-cells have recently been developed (Wybran *et al.*, 1972) and our results confirm the clinical usefulness of this technique.

III.   Correction of DiGeorge Syndrome

With all the new information about lymphoid system development and differentiation, it seemed likely at the Sanibel conference (Good and Bergsma, eds., 1968) that certain human immuno-deficiencies should be correctable. Some patients having DiGeorge syndrome are born without parathyroid or thymus. They often present clinically as cases of neonatal tetany which are readily correctable by appropriate treatment with vitamin D and dehydrotachysterol. In such patients when the thymus fails to develop at all, the lack of T-cells is revealed by failure to develop delayed or contact allergic reactions and failure to reject skin allografts. By contrast with normal persons, PHA responses of peripheral blood cells do not occur, and the patient's lymphocytes do not respond by proliferation to stimulation by irradiated or mitomycin-treated allogeneic cells. Immunoglobulin levels, on the other hand, develop normally, and antibody responses to some antigens also occur quite normally in these patients. We have recently studied the number of circulating lymphocytes in a child with apparently complete DiGeorge syndrome. We found that in normal persons 20–30% of lymphocytes in circulating blood possess immunoglobulin markers at their surface. In the blood of the child with DiGeorge's syndrome, more than 85% of circulating mononuclear cells are identifiable as B-cells (Gajl-Peczalska *et al.*, 1972). Table XIV and Fig. 18 illustrate the blood of such a patient showing the very large percentage of lymphocytes identifiable as B-cells by virtue of their finely spotted or rim staining with fluorescent antiserum specific for each of the separate immunoglobulin heavy chains. These patients may have no response whatever to PHA stimulation, and they may lack T-cells according to other markers.. Thus, patients with DiGeorge syndrome may have normal or near normal lymphocyte counts, but the lymphocytes are almost all identifiable as B-cells, and are not T-cells. Max Cooper (1972) has also encountered this

TABLE XIV

LYMPHOCYTES BEARING MEMBRANE-BOUND IMMUNOGLOBULINS

Source (No. of patients)	% IgG	% IgM mean (range)	% IgA	% Total mean
Control blood adults (7)	15.6 (14–19)	6.5 (4.4–9.5)	5.4 (3.6–9.4)	27.5
DiGeorge syndrome blood	32.9	26.6	23.7	83.2
Control lymph node infants (2)	9.9 (5.3–14.4)	5.8 (5.6–6.0)	4.4 (3.6–5.2)	21.1
DiGeorge syndrome lymph node	24.3	17.8	10.6	53.0

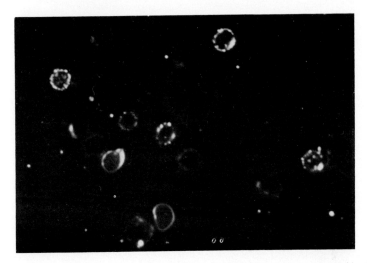

Fig. 18. Peripheral smear from patient with DiGeorge syndrome; 85–95% of circulating lymphocytes in this disease have been shown to be B_{2p}-cells with surface immunoglobulins in presumed receptor distribution. Fluorescent staining is anti-γ.

striking predominance of B-cells in other patients with DiGeorge syndrome as part of his extensive study of B-cells in patients with primary and secondary immunodeficiency. In one of our patients correction of the immunological deficiency by thymus transplantation resulted in a progressive decline in percentage of morphologically identifiable B-cells as the T-cell population increased.

Lymph nodes from patients with the complete athymic state and the DiGeorge's syndrome show very characteristic morphology of their lymph nodes. The far cortical areas of the nodes are well developed and germinal centers may be prominent. In the medullary cords, plasma cells are abundant. By contrast, the deep cortical areas are almost devoid of lymphoid cells. Having defined the DiGeorge syndrome immunologically as selective deficiency of T-cell development due to failure of differentiation of the thymus, it seemed likely that this abnormality should be correctable by thymus transplant. This approach has now apparently been successful using fetal thymus transplants on several occasions (Cleveland et al., 1968; August et al., 1968; Gatti et al., 1972; Biggar et al., 1972c).

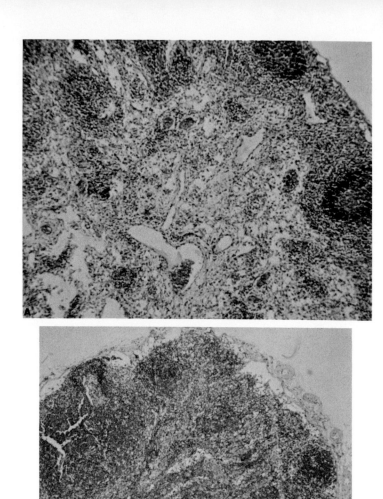

Fig. 19. (A) Lymph node of patient with DiGeorge syndrome before treatment with thymic transplant. Note the absence of cells in the deep cortical regions. By contrast, well developed far-cortical areas and germinal centers are present, and plasma cells are present in abundance in the medullary cords. (B) Lymph node of patient with DiGeorge syndrome taken 12 months after successful treatment by thymus transplant. Note the well developed deep-cortical or thymus-dependent regions.

Figures 19A and B show the lymph node of a patient with DiGeorge syndrome taken before and approximately 1 year after apparently successful immunologic reconstitution accomplished by thymus transplantation.

Fortunately, an experimental model of thymic deficiency like the DiGeorge syndrome has become available in the form of the nude athymic mice. Here an autosomal recessive trait leading to failure of thymic development and poor hair growth results in the lethal nude mouse syndrome. Such mice, sometimes completely lacking in T-cells, can be reconstituted immunologically by thymus transplant, but not by treatment with marrow cells (Wortis, 1971; Reed, referred to in Good and Wortis, 1971).

After the apparent reconstitution of the DiGeorge syndrome by thymic transplant, Dempster (1969) raised what appeared to be a valid criticism of the observations. Uncertainties were obvious when it became clear that the thymic deficiency in patients with DiGeorge syndrome either may not be present or may be incomplete (Lischner and DiGeorge, 1969). Dempster challenged us to show in any model of well established thymus deficiency that simple implantation of embryonic thymus could correct a T-cell defect. Douglas Biggar working with Stutman and me has now carried out the critical experiments in the mouse system. Working with epithelial membranes taken from the thymic anlagen of mouse embryos on day 11, 12, or 13 of embryonation, before the embryos have developed lymphoid tissues, we have been able fully to reconstitute immunologically the neonatally thymectomized mice which lack T-cells. We can implant these tiny epithelial membranes under the renal capsule, where we can follow their development and show that within 21 days beautiful little thymuses are present at the implantation site (Fig. 20). When such small moist epithelial membranes representing thymic anlagen are introduced intraperitoneally into neonatally thymectomized mice, they prevent development of immunodeficiency and reconstitute the T-cell population (Biggar et al., 1972b). Further, in more recent studies, Biggar (1972) has shown that these thymic anlagen can even reverse the runting and wasting syndrome in thymectomized mice at a stage where thymus system expanding but not differentiating, functional thymus tumors or thymus grafts in Millipore chambers are ineffective.

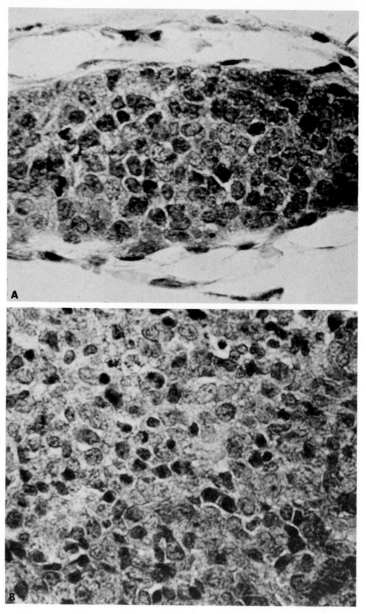

Fɪɢ. 20.   Transplant of thymus under the renal capsule in a mouse lacking a thymus.
(A) The epithelial anlage that was transplanted. (B) Beginning development of
lymphocytes 4 days posttransplant.

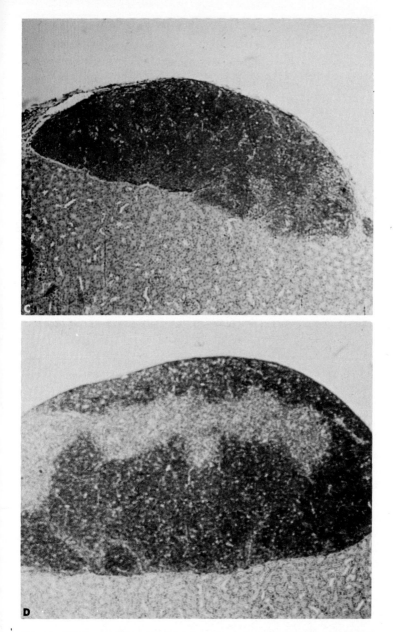

Fig. 20. (C) Lymphoid nature of the transplant 7 days after transplant. (D) Fully developed thymus structure 21 days after transplant. Note the cortical-medullary organization of the lymphoid tissue. Hassall's corpuscles are present.

If one transplants such thymic anlagen across strong or even weak (non-H2) histocompatibility barriers into thymectomized mice, immunologic reconstitution is accomplished without inducing graft-versus-host reactions. After immunologic reconstitution the transplant is rejected by the recipient, who now can recognize the implant as being foreign and eliminate it. How long the immunologic correction lasts in animals which have been reconstituted but have then rejected the thymus is an important point that needs further study. The parallelism of these new experimental findings with the reconstitution experiments in patients with DiGeorge syndrome is clear.

One puzzling aspect of each of the clinical situations in which DiGeorge syndrome has been corrected has been the amazing rapidity of the appearance of first signs of reconstruction of the T-cell functions. Only a few days need elapse after the embryonic thymus has been implanted before improvement of PHA responsiveness is seen. Like the others (August *et al.*, 1968), we too have (Biggar *et al.*, 1972a) recently observed this confusingly rapid response and now from our own experiences are convinced that it is real. Because it fits poorly with current dogma, we are determined to study it more completely. Ammann and Hong (1971) have observed a similar rapid improvement of T-cell immunity following thymus transplantation in patients with other syndromes that include defects of the T-cell population. The most likely explanation for these findings is that the embryonic thymus provides an expander, poietin, for an already partially differentiated population or provides a factor that finishes an almost completed differentiation. These and other possibilities should provoke exciting new experiments.

For the purposes of this lecture, it seems sufficient to emphasize that the correction of the DiGeorge syndrome by embryonic thymic transplantation serves at once as a most relevant analysis of DiGeorge syndrome and also a critical Experiment of Nature testing our developing concepts concerning the organization, development and function of the lymphoid systems. This observation we believe illustrates the ultimate usefulness of an Experiment of Nature like the DiGeorge syndrome which can provide a crucial testing ground for our new views of the lymphoid development. It is a final challenge to the new understanding that had been derived from continued and extensive laboratory studies. These studies in turn had been generated by another Experiment of Nature which years before, had sent us to the laboratory in search of understanding of the role of the thymus in immunobiology.

IV. DUAL-SYSTEM IMMUNODEFICIENCY

Another of the immunodeficiency diseases of man that has served to test our new understanding of lymphoid development and function is the combined immunodeficiency syndrome, or dual system immunodeficiency. It was our proposal in 1965 that in this so-called Swiss-type agammaglobulinemia the defect should be located at a point where the two immunologic systems are still one. In this disease both T-cells and B-cells of all kinds are grossly deficient. Figure 21 illustrates the typical lymphoid system histology of this disease. Plasma cells, germinal centers and far cortical accumulations as well as deep cortical accumulations of lymphocytes representing the T-cell population are lacking. Stimulation with antigen produces no plasma cell or lymphoid cell response. In the extreme cases, the lamina propria of the gastrointestinal tract is devoid of lymphoid cells and no Peyer's patches or lymphoid accumulations are to be seen in the tonsils. Few or no small lymphocytes are present in the circulation. In less extreme cases, gross deficiencies of all lymphoid populations are recognizable, but a few small lymphocytes may be seen and a few plasma cells can be encountered in the usual locations. Hoyer et al. (1968) felt that the X-linked form of the disease is distinguishable from the autosomal recessive form by a characteristic thymic morphology and less complete depletion of lymphoid elements. Our position has been challenged and considerable phenotypic variation has been encountered in both autosomal and X-linked recessive forms of the combined immunodeficiency syndrome (Hitzig, 1968; Hitzig et al., 1971). As, evidence concerning development of the peripheral lymphoid tissues by a continuing differentiative contribution of the central lymphoid organ on stem cells of marrow origin accumulated, it became reasonable to postulate that severe combined immunodeficiency might be correctable by marrow or fetal liver transplantation. This therapy was tried on several occasions including once with fetal liver and a thymus transplant in our clinic.

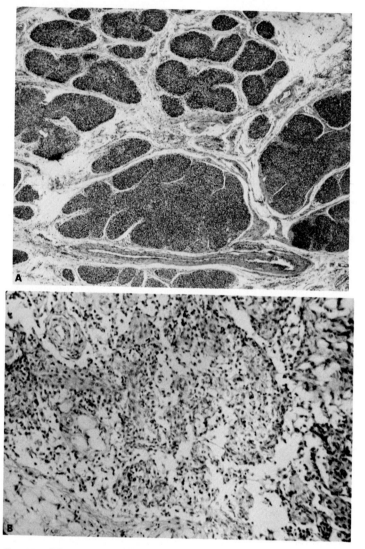

FIG. 21. (A) Thymus; (B) lymph node; (C) appendix; and (D) tonsil of patient with severe dual-system immunodeficiency. Note failure of development of essentially all lymphoid tissues.

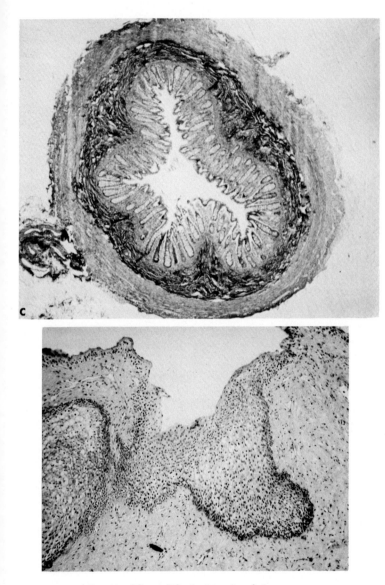

F1G. 21. (C) and (D). See legend on facing page.

The fetal liver cell transplant apparently corrected both B- and T-cell function leading to prompt rejection of a skin allograft that had been in place for 2 months prior to transplantation (Hong *et al.*, 1968b). Further, production of immunoglobulins and responsive production of antibodies all were observed. The triumph of the biological reconstitution was short-lived, however, when the child developed fatal graft-versus-host reaction probably attributable to the successful transplant and/or a small transfusion of fresh blood. A number of efforts at reconstruction of the immunologic system, which have several times corrected, at least in part, the immuno-deficiency only to lead to lethal graft-versus-host reaction, have been recorded.

V. The Minnesota System for Studying Transplant Immunity

This disconcerting clinical impasse was resolved by another set of laboratory analyses. When we at Minnesota first tried to confirm the work of the British investigators (Billingham *et al.*, 1953) on immunological tolerance in the mid 1950's, we were unable to do so. The reason, in part, was that we had first chosen too great a histo-compatibility barrier and bridging that barrier A strain (H_2A) to $C57Bl_6$ (H_2B) by tolerance induction proved to be too much for the methodology of the moment. Thus, we began to try other strain combinations and weaker histocompatibility barriers. We finally succeeded (Mariani *et al.*, 1958) in producing tolerance in the male–female syngeneic system of Eichwald and Silmser (1955). In this system we could readily produce tolerance not only in newborn, but also even in adult, mice (Mariani *et al.*, 1959). Further, mice matched according to the H2 allogeneic system Ce to C3H, C3H to Ce (both Ce and C3H are H2K) and BALB/c to DBA/2 and DBA/2 to BALB/c (BALB/c and DBA/2 are both H2D) (Shapiro *et al.*, 1961) were also easy to manipulate and the so-called tolerance could be readily produced.

Once we were able to produce tolerance in these situations char-acterized by H2 matching, we did many rather fantastic experiments. We could establish orthotopical pituitary allotransplants in hypo-physectomized tolerant recipients, and these grafts would exercise all known functions of the pituitary (Martinez *et al.*, 1956). We achieved successful ovarian allotransplants that functioned normally (Martinez *et al.*, 1956, 1958). J. B. Aust and his students even produced pure Ce offspring from C3H mice using C3H castrated females that had been orthotopically transplanted with Ce ovaries and were then bred to Ce males. These were exciting experiments. Among the studies using these H2 matched, weak histocompatibility situations were those that showed that fatal graft-versus-host reactions of infant F_1 mice required that the alloantigens in the F_1 recipient must differ from those of parent strain lymphoid cells being used to induce the GVH by major histocompatibility barriers, e.g., H_2 (Table XV) (Good, 1970).

In mice the H2 system represents the dominant genetic influence of a region on a somatic chromosome which controls major histocompatibility determinants. A similar inheritance of major histocompatibility differences has been found in rats in relation to the *AgB* locus, chickens at the *B* locus, dogs at the *DL-A*, monkeys at the *ML-A*, pigs at the *PL-A* and man at the *HL-A* region. Basically in this form of inheritance, there is a single chromosome region for each species at which multiple genetic determinants or alleles can

TABLE XV

GRAFT-VERSUS-HOST REACTIONS IN DIFFERENT MOUSE STRAIN
COMBINATIONS—NEONATAL F_1 MODEL

Strain	No. dead[a]/No. tested
H_2 Differences	
A (A × C57BL)F_1	20/20
A (A × C3H)F_1	10/10
A (A × CBA)F_1	9/10
C3H (C3H × C57BL/1)F_1	12/12
C57BL (C3H × C57BL)F_1	14/15
Non-H_2 Differences	
Ce (Ce × C3H)F_1	0/20
C3H (C3H × Ce)F_1	2/15
BALB/c (BALB/c × DBA/2)F_1	1/10
DBA/2 (DBA/2 × BALB/c)F_1	2/17

[a] Death before 30 days.

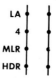

FIG. 22. Simplified scheme of relations in the somatic chromosome region controlling histocompatibility relationships. It now seems clear that a separate locus controls LA and 4 series of alleles in the HL-A system, and that both the LA and 4 series are under separate control from the determinants that are responsible for most mixed leukocyte culture reactions and probably also from many cellular immunity reactions.

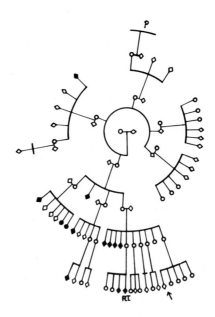

C FAMILY

FIG. 23. Family tree of patient with apparent X-linked recessive severe dual system immunodeficiency. The uniformly lethal disease present in this propositus was completely corrected by marrow transplantation. The solid figures represent the children who died in infancy. R. T. was extensively studied in Boston and found to have severe combined immunodeficiency.

operate. In man and mouse the system is polygenic and polyallelic and at least 3 separate and possibly 4 separate segregating systems have been found to be operative (Fig. 22). In general, however, the genetic region is transmitted as a single unit and contributions of one determinant from each parent establishes the major histocompatibility antigens of the offspring. This means that whereas the chance of obtaining a match in a nonfamily member of an outbred population may be very small, the chance of having a match in a sibling can be expected to occur approximately one time in four. Once we had figured out this relationship, we knew where to go in our efforts to correct a severe combined immunodeficiency (Hong *et al.*, 1968a). Fortunately, after our initial proposal we soon had such an opportunity when we encountered a child who was the propositus of the family tree shown in Fig. 23. This child had classical form of severe combined immunodeficiency and was grossly immunodeficient, severely symptomatic, and already desperately ill with recurrent pneumonias. He thus seemed to be an ideal candidate for attempted reconstitution of the immunologic apparatus by marrow transplant. Fortunately, he had four sisters, one of whom matched well but not perfectly at HL-A. This potential donor's lymphocytes were not stimulated by the child's lymphocytes in mixed leukocyte culture. The mismatch at HL-A has been analyzed genetically and found to be explained by a recombination involving the LA allelic series (Gatti *et al.*, 1971). The donor was of blood group O and the recipient child of blood group A. Marrow transplanted by the intraperitoneal route corrected completely the immunodeficiency (Table XVI) (Gatti *et al.*, 1968). The initial marrow from the female donor established a chimeric state and approximately 25% of the replicating cells of marrow became cells of female origin. After the successful transplant all the lymphocytes of the peripheral blood that responded to PHA by DNA replication were of female karyotype. As expected, although a GVH reaction occurred, the graft-versus-host disease was mild. The child was cured of his immunodeficiency disease. Both small lymphocytes and plasma cells that had been lacking appeared in the hematopoietic tissues. The child became capable of developing cellular immunities and delayed-type hypersensitivity. He developed immunoglobulins of all classes which climbed promptly up to normal levels. He be-

TABLE XVI

IMMUNOLOGIC DATA BEFORE AND AFTER MARROW
TRANSPLANT

Data	Before	After
Phytohemagglutinin response	—	+
Dinitrofluorobenzene skin test	—	+
Small lymphocytes	—	+
Anti-B isohemagglutinin	—	+
Immunoglobulins	Very low	Normal
Typhoid antibodies	—	+
Plasma cells		+
Secretory IgA (stools)		+
Thymus shadow	—	+

came able to respond to antigenic stimulation. Cells appeared in the peripheral blood that could respond to phytohemagglutinin and to allogeneic cells in mixed leukocyte culture. The sister's lymphoid cells which had been obtained from this O blood group donor then began to react to the A antigens on the hematopoietic and peripheral blood cells of the recipient child. This reaction produced first a hemolytic anemia, then aregenerative pancytopenia, which became life threatening 3 months after the initial successful marrow transplant.

The immunologically induced, aregenerative anemia and pancytopenia represented substitution of a potentially fatal, iatrogenically induced, immunologic disorder for the certainly fatal inherited disorder. To correct the new disease, iatrogenic aregenerative pancytopenia, we carried out a second marrow transplant (Good, 1969), which established virtually an entire new marrow of donor origin as was revealed by karyotype analysis of the squash preparation of the bone marrow cells. Further, we switched the blood type of the recipient child from A to O as is shown in Fig. 24. More than 4 years after the successful transplant, this child remains fully reconstituted immunologically. He responds well with both his humoral and cellular immune system and defends himself with vigor against organisms he encounters in his environment using the resources of both the cellular and humoral immunity. His blood

cells are all of blood group O. All the PHA responding and proliferating lymphocytes in blood are of female karyotype. There is
no evidence whatever of ongoing graft-versus-host reaction. He is,
indeed, a healthy normally growing child living in good health as
a consequence of our efforts at cellular engineering, which have
corrected in his case two separate fatal diseases (Good, 1970; Gatti
and Good, 1971b). The results of this new treatment surely represents a striking testimony to the understanding that derives from
fundamental analyses of an Experiment of Nature. This one case in
which both a genetic and an acquired disease have been cured by a
process of cellular engineering would by itself have been a very
stirring experience. But the case does not stand alone. Almost
simultaneously Bach *et al.* (1968) in Wisconsin corrected the
immunodeficiency of a child with Wiskott–Aldrich syndrome.
There have now been 21 successful corrections of severe combined
immunodeficiency around the world. We ourselves have achieved
full immunologic reconstitution in six such patients by marrow
transplantation and have corrected the T-cell deficiency of two
patients, with DiGeorge syndrome by thymus transplantation.

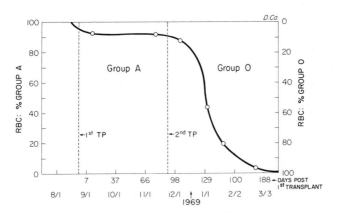

FIG. 24.   Complete switching of blood type by two marrow transplants in a patient
with the X-linked form of severe dual-system immunodeficiency. The first marrow
transplant corrected the genetically determined dual system immunodeficiency. The
second marrow transplant, leading to complete switching of blood type from A to O,
corrected an immunologically based aregenerative pancytopenia, an acquired disease.

Sir McFarlane Burnet (1971a) has criticized me publicly for having made these efforts to treat little children who were destined to die of inherited abnormality. His advice is to leave well enough alone and allow the children to die of their inherited deficiency. He believes they and we are all better off if they are out of their misery. To him I answer only that in conscience as a physician I would deem it immoral to learn from these patients and not to attempt to treat the disease from which they suffer. Further, already our matched sibling marrow approach which was first successful in treating not only this child's immunodeficiency but his immunologically induced acquired aregenerative anemia and pancytopenia promises to be effective in treating many patients with otherwise fatal idiopathic aregenerative anemia and pancytopenia. Patients like ours, with their rare, often genetically determined, diseases, represent crucial model systems in which our growing knowledge can be tested and our approaches to cellular engineering perfected and developed. They teach us, further, how the vigorous immunity system is developed and what machinery is necessary for each of us to survive as individuals in the ecological niche we have selected through eons of adaptation. Each as a person is precious to his family and each has many new lessons to teach us as physicians and students of biology. The genetic load that could be introduced by complete reconstitution of these children is of little consequence to equilibrium gene frequencies (Rendel, 1970). Rendel has addressed Burnet's general question which, as I interpret it, challenges all of modern medical philosophy and has refuted the logic behind at least one component of the argument, i.e., the increased genetic load. My philosophy derives from Hippocratic forebears in a Judeo-Christian ethic, and thus I must reject out of hand the remainder of the argument. On the bright side, it seems certain that these successes represent but the toddling steps in what will develop into an era in which medical therapy can be based on cellular, enzymatic, and genetic engineering.

Time will surely address further the pessimism that pervades all of Burnet's most recent writings (Burnet, 1971b), and the answers will exceed any verbal eloquence as heretofore has so often been the case. To argue that one must look to modern molecular biology only as a plaything, a game of cards, if you will, for intellectual satisfaction is surely a nonsense that fails to appreciate the creative potential of human behavior when applied to the problems of human disease.

VI. The Basis of the Chimerism

Presented in Tables XVII and XVIII are data from three cases in which full corrections of the immunologic system have been accomplished that may explain the self-limited nature of the mild graft-versus-host reactions these patients have experienced. It can be seen from the tables that although no overt evidence of immunologic

TABLE XVII

REACTION OF LYMPHOCYTES WITH TARGET-CELL FIBROBLASTS[a]

	Target cells	Lymphoid cells	Mean cpm ± SD[b]	Target cell loss (%)
Case 1				
	Recipient	Recipient	5158 ± 227	48
	Recipient	Donor	9342 ± 332	7
	Recipient	Control[d]	7785 ± 342	22
T/L[c] 1/1000	Control	Recipient[d]	8231 ± 415	18
	Control	Donor[d]	8044 ± 376	20
	Control	Control	9150 ± 398	9
Case 2				
	Recipient	Recipient	3924 ± 163	61
	Recipient	Control[d]	7112 ± 321	29
T/L[c] 1/1000	Control	Recipient[d]	7382 ± 311	26
	Control	Control	8721 ± 354	13
Case 3				
	Recipient	Recipient	4487 ± 186	55
	Recipient	Control[d]	8891 ± 371	11
T/L[c] 1/200	Control	Recipient[d]	8815 ± 384	12
	Control	Control	9486 ± 376	5

[a] Taken from Jose *et al.* (1971b).

[b] Mean counts per minute and standard deviation of six microcultures after adjustment of maximum activity per microculture in each experiment to 10,000 cpm.

[c] T/L, target-cell to lymphocyte ratio.

[d] HL-A nonidentical.

TABLE XVIII

INHIBITION OF CELLULAR IMMUNITY BY WHOLE SERUM, IMMUNOGLOBULIN-
FREE SERUM, AND PROTEIN ELUTED FROM SOLID IMMUNOGLOBULIN
ADSORBENT

	Serum in microcultures	Mean cpm ± SD	Target cell loss (%)
Case 1			
Recipient target cells with recipient lymphocytes	Donor: whole serum	5724 ± 263	43
	Donor: Ig-free serum	3193 ± 245	68
	Donor: eluted Ig	6630 ± 274	34
	Recipient: whole serum	9474 ± 215	5
	Recipient: Ig-free serum	5200 ± 386	48
	Recipient: eluted Ig	9865 ± 291	1
	Case 2: whole serum	7657 ± 293	23
	Case 3: whole serum	7891 ± 268	21
Control target cells with recipient lymphocytes[b]	Recipient: whole serum	8894 ± 256	11
	Recipient: Ig-free serum	6924 ± 215	31
	Recipient: eluted Ig	9408 ± 310	6
Recipient target cells with control lymphocytes[b]	Recipient: whole serum	9316 ± 234	7
	Recipient: Ig-free serum	7625 ± 365	24
	Recipient: eluted Ig	9641 ± 281	4
Case 2			
Recipient target cells with recipient lymphocytes	Control: whole serum	4431 ± 179	56
	Control: Ig-free serum	3241 ± 254	68
	Control: eluted Ig	5187 ± 231	48
	Recipient: whole serum	9216 ± 243	8
	Recipient: Ig-free serum	4594 ± 310	54
	Recipient: eluted serum	8631 ± 284	14
	Case 1: whole serum	6943 ± 215	31
	Case 3: whole serum	7587 ± 247	24
Case 3			
Recipient target cells with recipient lymphocytes	Control: whole serum	5126 ± 302	49
	Recipient: whole serum	9687 ± 359	3

[a] Taken from Jose *et al.* (1971b).
[b] HL-A nonidentical.

assault of donor cells on the host remains, the chimeric children each possess lymphocytes that will selectively destroy their own fibroblasts in tissue culture. Standing against such destruction seems to be a circulating IgG "blocking" antibody that can protect the host cells from such injury (Jose *et al.*, 1971b). Thus, in this model it is not tolerance of the new immunologic system or of the host by the new immunologic system but a form of immunodeviation that accounts for the harmonious chimeric state. This finding is consonant with prior observations by Hellström *et al.* (1970) which showed that chimeric dogs created by fatal total body irradiation coupled with marrow transplantation likewise seem to exist with a foreign hematopoietic system by virtue of this form of immunodeviation. Recent analysis with modern immunobiologic tools of many systems once thought to represent the tolerant state reveal not a complete tolerance, as we were first taught to conceive of it, but a form of apparent immunodeviation. Thus, central tolerance of viral infection cannot be established. Chimeric dogs salvaged from fatal irradiation by successful marrow transplants are immune in a special way and are not tolerant. Toleration of many malignancies surely foreign to the host seems to represent a form of immunodeviation (Hellström and Hellström, 1970). Even the classical models of tolerance studied in the early British work often show some evidence of immunity and may represent not a complete negative adaptation when carefully studied by more modern methods. Of special interest are the tetraparental mice where the two immunity systems seem not to be tolerant of one another but mutually reactive bodies. These findings represent information damaging to present concepts of tolerance. Since a positive immunological adaptation may be easier to work with pragmatically than are negative ones, this evidence encourages us to seek means of specific immunization that may favor activation of the B-cell system over activation of the T-cell system and thus the achievement of the desired immunodeviation. Further studies to define the nature of true self-tolerance are sorely needed.

VII.   Peripheral versus Central Correction

Although it seems likely that in our first successful case and one case corrected by DeKoning *et al.* (1969) with marrow stem cells represent stem cell reconstitution, the Stiehm case (Stiehm *et al.*, 1972), in which the marrow does not possess donor cells, and several cases with immunologic correction that we have studied at postmortem suggest that *peripheral* lymphoid reconstitution may be a second way of correcting severe combined immunodeficiency by marrow transplantation. In the cases we have observed, reconstruction of vigorous cellular and humoral immunity has occurred without evidence that the thymus has been morphologically reconstructed or that marrow has become chimeric. These are important observations since they recall the experiments of Yunis *et al.* (1965) which showed that long-lived reconstitution of the thymus system can be achieved by giving large numbers of peripheral lymphoid cells from donors matched with recipients at the major histocompatibility determinants. In recent studies with the Toivanens, evaluating reconstitution of the B-cell system in chickens, we have found that the entire B-cell immunity system can be reconstituted from B system stem cells that have shifted from the bursa to the bone marrow. Perhaps it is the high frequency with which peripheral reconstitution is accomplished by marrow transplantation that accounts for the repeated failure of transplants of fetal liver cells to reconstitute the immunodeficiency patient or to produce any influence on immunodeficiency as has been stressed in the studies of Githens *et al.* (1969).

VIII. Approaches to Crossing the Major Histocompatibility Barrier or of Using Donors from the General Population in Immunologic Reconstitution

The major obstacle to general application of marrow transplants to the treatment of many diseases is absence of availability of matched sibling donors. Over and over again attempts to correct immunodeficiency with marrow or other lymphoid tissues from nonmatched donors have proved disastrous. Even when donors perfectly matched with recipients at the HL-A genetic determinants have been located in the general population fatal graft-versus-host reactions have occurred when marrow transplantation has been attempted. These experiments have pressed for better understanding of the contributions of the independently segregating influences of the somatic chromosomal region that controls the major histocompatibility differences. It is already clear from studies by Yunis and Amos (1971), Gatti *et al.* (1971), Park *et al.* (1972b), Dausset *et al.* (1970), and Dupont *et al.* (1971) that our earlier simple view of the influence of the HL-A system is not complete and is probably incorrect. In every possible combination, we have been able genetically to separate the determinants of MLC reactivity, for example, from the determinants of HL-A characteristics. Further, we have obtained excellent evidence that HL-A determinants alone cannot account for the severity of GVH reactions. Indeed, the determinants of graft-versus-host reactions like those of the MLC may be completely dissociated from the HL-A system. In a recent study with Dupont *et al.* (1973) in Copenhagen, it has been possible partially to reconstitute immunologically a child with severe combined immunodeficiency by marrow transplantation by electing a maternal uncle who differed in all HL-A determinants from the recipient child but whose cells were not stimulated in MLC by the patient or the patient's mother. This observation reveals one direction for future progress in this field, namely to achieve matching according to the truly relevant determinants in the general population. The task might not be as difficult as it once seemed. It may be quite possible when improved micromethods for MLC matching are fully exploited, and if and when appropriate serological methods can be developed to achieve more meaningful matching according to determinants presently only recognizable by matching with the relatively awkward MLC techniques.

IX. REPEATED SMALL INOCULA OF MARROW CELLS

Biggar *et al.* (1972c) recognized that large inocula of marrow cells often lead to fatal GVH reactions when the donor differs from recipient across major histocompatibility determinants. To obviate this obstacle, we have attempted to reconstitute patients with severe combined immunodeficiency by giving extremely small numbers of marrow cells from the mismatched donor. Although complete success of crossing the major barrier by this technique has thus far eluded us, we have experienced what we consider to be several very near misses by using this methodology.

In one instance, where paternal donor and recipient represented a clear HL-A haplotype mismatch and mixed leukocyte cultures showed the cells of the donor to be responsive to cells of the recipient in MLC, we were able fully to reconstitute both T- and B-cell responses and to maintain this correction over a 4-month period by repeated small (1–10 million) marrow cell transplants. Unfortunately, this child died of a persistent, antibiotic-resistant and progressive infection with a microorganism that had been troublesome even before the first marrow transplant had been accomplished. Using the small inocula of foreign marrow cells described above, the GVH reaction, although identifiable after the first transplant, was never a severe or life-threatening disease.

X. GVH IN GERM-FREE OR ANTIBIOTIC-TREATED ANIMALS

Jones *et al.* (1971) at Notre Dame have described the course of GVH reactions in germ-free mice. Under the conditions prevailing in their laboratory these investigators have been successful in initiating GVH reactions across major histocompatibility barriers which have not been lethal. The implication of these findings is that a part of the lethal GVH disease involves contributions of the microbial flora.

Keast (1968) in Perth has contributed important information in this perspective. He showed that treatment of rats with broad spectrum antibiotics can lessen the mortality of the GVH reaction in this species. Although these important contributions do not agree with observations of others, they do suggest an avenue to be tested in efforts to transplant marrow to immunodeficient recipients across major histocompatibility determinants. Thus far, our clinical efforts in this direction using all means to sterilize the bowel and the essentially germ-free environment of laminar flow units have not revealed clear evidence of reduction in the severity of the GVH or of mortality from GVH in man. Although somewhat discouraging at this juncture, efforts in this direction should continue since the fatal issue in human GVH disease often is an overwhelming microbial infection.

XI. OTHER FORMS OF IMMUNODEFICIENCY

In addition to the above three polar forms of primary immunodeficiency in man, a congeries of other diseases have been described in which severe perturbations of the immune response represent a major portion of the disease from which the children suffer. In each of these instances genetic factors play a major determining role. Like the three primary immunodeficiencies described above, each of these forms of immunodeficiency has unique features which have already taught us much about the normal immune system and about the function of its components in the body economy. Of special significance in this context are the immunodeficiencies associated with ataxia–telangiectasia, Wiskott–Aldrich syndrome, common variable form of primary immunodeficiency disease, and the isolated absence of circulating IgA.

XII.   ATAXIA-TELANGIECTASIA

The syndrome described by Louis-Bar (1941) and extensively collected and reported by Boder and Sedgwick (1972, 1963)* and Lambrechts and Snoijink (1971) is featured by progressive cerebellar ataxia, strange telangiectasis noticeable on ocular sclerae, on the eyelids, and on the skin of the antecubital and popliteal spaces. The appearance of the telangiectasis in a child with this syndrome is presented on Fig. 25. This is an uncommon, but not extremely rare, disease and some 440+ cases have been described around the world. Although ataxia–telangiectasia has been accepted as a genetically determined disease with autosomal inheritance, Lambrechts and Snoijink (1971) have questioned this and proposed that it may represent the consequences of an isoimmunization. The reason for this extrapolation is that in the most complete analysis of cases from the literature and from their own experience they have found consanguinity not to be of sufficiently great frequency. Within certain families too many cases are to be found. Further, these investigators have observed a progressive increase in severity of the neurological disease with successive cases in some families. The latter relationship was especially noticeable in a family having 4 involved children which Lambrechts and Snoijink (1971) have studied carefully in Antwerp and reported in great detail. If this be

* In all of our work with ataxia–telangiectasia, we have been fortunate to collaborate with Dr. Elena Boder who has been the major custodian of experiences with ataxia–telangiectasia patients. It is she who originally tabulated malignancies in these patients.

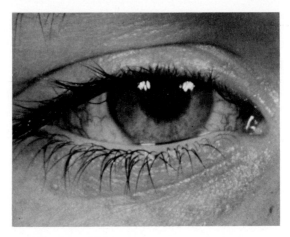

Fig. 25.   Telangiectasias of the sclerae in a patient with ataxia-telangiectasia.

the case, consideration should be given to the possibility that the isoantigen involved is the human equivalent of the θ isoantigen that is distributed on T lymphocytes and in both skin and brain (J. Finstad, cited by Good, 1970).

The immunodeficiency of ataxia–telangiectasia was defined by my colleagues and me (Peterson *et al.*, 1964b). We found that these patients regularly show readily demonstrable deficiencies of cell-mediated immunities. In addition, as was first noted by Thieffry *et al.* (1961), they frequently, 60–70%, lack IgA in their circulation. They also lack IgA in their saliva (Peterson *et al.*, 1964b). In even higher percentage they have a low level or lack of IgE (Biggar *et al.*, 1970). First-degree members of their families frequently show similar deficiency of IgE. Taken together, all these abnormalities account for the increased susceptibility to sinopulmonary infection that plagues these children. Those cases having the most severe immunologic deficiency seem to have the greatest trouble from infection. However, from study of the families of these children it is clear that isolated absence of IgE does not predispose to increased numbers of respiratory infections.

Biopsy studies of the lymph nodes of patients with ataxia-telangiectasia revealed a regular deficiency of cells in the deep cortical areas. Often, germinal centers are lacking in the cortex, and the tonsils may be poorly developed. Regularly, however, an abnormality of the thymus is encountered (Peterson *et al.*, 1964b; Peterson and Good, 1968). The thymus of children with ataxia–telangiectasia consistently shows absence of certain features of the normal thymus. Instead of being comprised of the usual cortical and medullary organization of lymphoid cells and having abundant Hassall's corpuscles, the thymus in ataxia–telangiectasia was found to be very deficient in lymphoid cells, to lack cortical and medullary differentiation and to lack Hassall's corpuscles completely (Fig. 26). Thus the thymus of these children being about one-fourth to one-fifth the normal size regularly has an appearance reminiscent of the embryonic thymus. Microscopically, the thymus is similar to the thymus of a 17–18-day-old rabbit embryo or a 12–13-day-old mouse embryo. In these species full gestation requires 31–32 days and 20–21

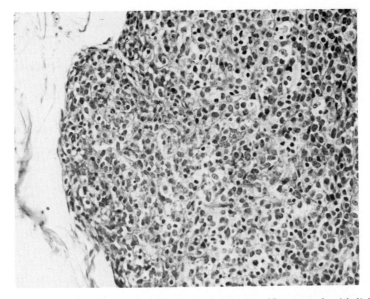

Fig. 26.   Thymus from patient with ataxia–telangiectasia. Note stromal–epithelial composition of the thymus, absence of Hassall's corpuscles, and absence of cortico-medullary lymphoid organization. The thymus is generally quite small—about one-fourth to one-third the size of a normal thymus.

days, respectively. These patients as an Experiment of Nature raise many questions. Important among them is the question concerning how the frequent lack of IgA and IgE relate to the defective development of the thymus.

Recent studies of the immunologically deficient nude mice which are born with incompletely developed thymi reveal that, like the patients with ataxia–telangiectasia, these mice regularly lack or are deficient in IgA (Wortis, 1971). They also show a deficiency of circulating levels of IgG_{2a}, one of the immunoglobulin G subclasses (Wortis, 1971; Good and Wortis, 1971). Just how these interesting perturbations of immunoglobulin development relate to the defects of thymic development remains a most provocative question. Fortunately, models for analysis of this question with the potential of thymic transplantation and cellular engineering promise to provide important answers in the near future. Especially to be focused in this regard is the fact that patients with DiGeorge's 3rd and 4th pharyngeal pouch syndrome accompanied by absence of the thymus often seem to show a normal pattern of development of immunoglobulins, even of IgA. This is the sort of conflict which when resolved can bring improved understanding of the entire immunity system and the relations of structure to function within it.

XIII. Wiskott–Aldrich Syndrome

Another of the primary immunodeficiencies that has been extensively investigated in our laboratories at the University of Minnesota is the immunodeficiency accompanying the Wiskott–Aldrich syndrome (Krivit and Good, 1959; St. Geme *et al.*, 1965; Cooper *et al.*, 1968a, b). Patients having this X-linked recessive disorder show the constellation of low and abnormal platelets leading to frequent life-threatening bleeding, eczema with distribution suggesting that of so-called atopic eczema, marked increased susceptibility to all manner of infections, especially infections with viral, fungal, enteric bacterial pathogens, *Pseudomonas aeruginosa*, and pneumococci. The propensity to bleed is often made worse by a drop of platelets to very low levels during or following an infection. The nature of the immunodeficiency in patients with the Wiskott–Aldrich syndrome has been extensively studied by Cooper *et al.* (1968a, b) in our laboratories and by my former student Blaese with Waldmann (Blaese *et al.*, 1968) at the NIH. These two sets of investigations complement one another and define a most interesting immuno-deficiency disease. Regularly there is a defect of cellular immunity which appears to progress with the duration of the disease in some patients. This defect is associated with inability normally to reject allografts of skin and to develop delayed allergic response. These patients also have a deficiency of the number of responding T-cells in the circulation. Krivit and I (1959) discovered that these patients regularly have absent or low levels of isohemagglutinins in their circulation. The latter abnormality seems intimately associated with both their failure to produce IgM normally and to the more rapid than normal degradation of the IgM that has been described (Blaese *et al.*, 1971). By contrast, serum concentrations of IgA and IgE may be extremely high and IgG levels tend to be normal or only slightly increased over those found in normal persons. This strange "dysimmunoglobulinemia" then is associated with a peculiar pat-tern of antibody deficiency syndrome. We discovered that these patients do not produce antibodies at all to certain polysaccharide antigens a finding that has been extensively studied, confirmed, and extended by Blaese *et al.* (1971). Thus, heterolysins fail to develop, as do antibodies to the red cell isohemagglutinins. The patients do not form antibodies to pneumococcal polysaccharide, Vi antigen or any of several other polysaccharide antigens studied. Yet both IgM and IgG antibodies are formed quite vigorously to appropriate protein antigens such as *Salmonella* H, diphtheria toxoid, and tetanus toxoid. Blaese *et al.* (1971) have modified the possible conclusions from our original study in which we postulated a defect on the afferent limb of the immune response. They found that the *in vitro* responses of lymphocytes to both polysaccharide and small molecular protein antigens are defective in such cases (Blaese *et al.*, 1972). Here again, much study is still needed ultimately to unravel the interrelationships of the components of this fascinating immuno-deficiency. It is certain, however, that important questions focusing on as yet unresolved problems of antigenic handling, antigenic stimulation, antibody response and the association of cell-mediated immunodeficiency with control of antibody and immunoglobulin production are being asked by these patients as an Experiment of

Nature. Morphologically the thymus of these children regularly has a normal appearance (Fig. 27), yet the defect of their cellular immunity system and deficiency of function of their T-cell population is progressive and may become as profound as that observed in children with the ataxis–telangiectasia syndrome who have such a distinct morphologic abnormality of the thymus. Excitement has been created by the claims of Fudenberg and his associates (Levin *et al.*, 1970) that much improvement in this disease can be induced by treatment of patients with the Wiskott–Aldrich syndrome using the so-called dialyzable transfer factor prepared from normal lymphocytes after the method of Lawrence (1969). The impressive anecdotal experience with treatment of this awful disease reported by these investigators demands controlled studies because the disease is one in which clinical expression sometimes varies without explanation.

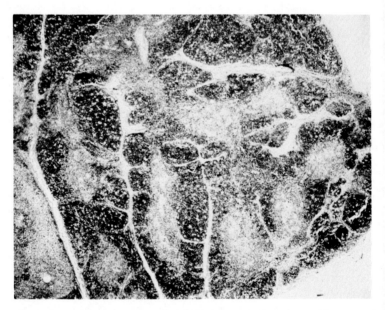

Fɪɢ. 27.   Thymus from a patient with Wiskott–Aldrich syndrome. Note normal lymphoid structure, normal corticomedullary organization, and Hassall's corpuscles. Although T-cell deficiency in these patients may be severe, the thymus itself seems to be morphologically normal.

Perhaps of even greater importance these findings demand that a molecular definition of transfer factor and its powerful influence on immune reactions be achieved (Good, 1972a).

XIV.   COMMON VARIABLE IMMUNODEFICIENCY

Much has been written about immunodeficiencies associated with dysgammaglobulinemia (Rosen et al., 1968), sporadic hypogamma-globulinemia, acquired hypogammaglobulinemia and various hered-itary patterns of immunodeficiency of dominant and recessive nature (Wolf et al., 1963; Seligmann et al., 1968; Fudenberg et al., 1971). Although it is quite certain that a number of separate diseases are included in this category, we have found it impossible to use pre-vious classifications, for example, of different forms of dysgamma-globulinemia, to work with or understand these patients. Many forms seem to be variable from time to time in the same patient and from patient to patient in the same family. Thus, some as yet obscure control mechanism, appears to be perturbed in many of these patients and members of their families. Certain families have been encoun-tered (Fudenberg et al., 1962; Wolf et al., 1963), in which extra-ordinary constellations of autoimmune disorders, malignancy, and immunodeficiency have presented along with examples of immuno-globulin deficiency. Figure 28 illustrates one such family. In this family the propositus suffered from hypogammaglobulinemia, rheumatoid arthritis, intestinal malabsorption syndrome, and an immunodeficiency involving readily demonstrable defects of both T- and B-cell function. The patient's mother suffered for many years from hyperglobulinemia and thrombopenic purpura and ultimately died of lupus. A half-brother of the patient has hyper-globulinemia and thrombopenia and a half-sister frank and typical deforming rheumatoid arthritis. The mother's brother died of lupus erythematosus, and his young daughter of what was thought to be Hodgkin's disease after apparently expressing clinical lupus for several years. A maternal uncle and a maternal aunt had lupus erythematosus, the grandmother rheumatoid arthritis. A maternal cousin suffered from regional enteritis and acquired valvular heart disease. In addition to finding that many members of the family had antinuclear antibody in their circulation, the family studies revealed

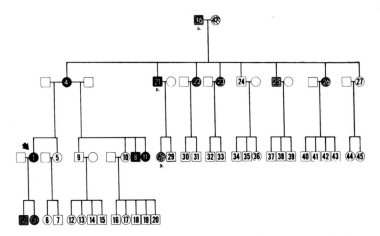

FIG. 28. Family tree of patient with common variable form of immunodeficiency.
Note the frequent "autoimmune" diseases and definite immunodeficiencies in this
patient's family. Key to cases of agammaglobinemia and mesenchymal diseases:
1 (propositus), acquired agammaglobinemia and rheumatoid arthritis; 46, difficulty
in healing; 47, rheumatoid arthritis; 21, lupus erythematosus; 28, Hodgkin's disease;
23, nose bleeds and eczema; 22, possible lupus erythematosus with skin rash and joint
pains; 2, neonatal lymphadenopathy; 25, possible lupus erythematosus, hyperpro-
teinemia; 26, bleeding, breast cancer; 40, rheumatic fever; 11, hypergammaglobinemia
and joint pains; 24, low γ-globulin, deficiency β_2A and β_2M; 33, low γ-globulin,
deficiency β_2M; 7, low γ-globulin, absence of β_2A and β_2M; 4, idiopathic thrombocytopenia purpura (ITP); 8, ITP.

three members representing three generations who had clearly
abnormal immunoelectrophoretic patterns. Quantitation of immunoglobulins confirmed these abnormalities. Each of the anomalies
would have to be classified as a different form of dysgammaglobulinemia. Thus, in this family some hereditary perturbation of the
immune system has occurred that is transmitted as an apparent
dominant trait which has been variously expressed as increased
susceptibility to a variety of mesenchymal diseases, autoimmunity
dysgammaglobulinemia of each of several types and possibly increased susceptibility to malignancy. To date the nature of a control
mechanism that must be perturbed in this form of inherited immunodeficiency remains obscure. This and many other families we and
others have studied have made it impossible to accept the concepts

of dysgammaglobulinemia that have previously been proposed. These families and their individual members stand forth as additional provocative Experiments of Nature which when fully analyzed should yield much new understanding of the controls operating on the lymphoid system that are perturbed in autoimmunity. Still other family studies suggest that autosomal recessive mechanisms may control a variant or variants of the common variable form of immunodeficiency. In our experience, patients with these forms of immunodeficiency quite regularly have defects of T-cell as well as defects of B-cell function. It seems without question that further analysis will ultimately separate several or even many different forms of immunodeficiency from this group. As the several forms become sufficiently well defined, they can be removed from this wastebasket and given their own definition, hopefully in genetic and enzymatic terms (Fudenberg *et al.*, 1971).

XV. Immunodeficiency and Cancer

No less commanding as Experiments of Nature have been the occurrence of malignancy in patients with immunodeficiency (Gatti and Good, 1971a; Good, 1972b). In 1958 when Thomas first stated his immunosurveillance postulate he predicted that the patients with immunodeficiency should not only suffer from increased suscepti- bility to overt microbial infections, but should be expected to be far too susceptible to the development of malignant diseases as well (Thomas, 1959). Surely Thomas expected, from the context of his remarks, that the increased susceptibility to malignancy would be expressed primarily in those immunodeficiencies in which allograft rejection and the delayed allergic responses are deficient. To him, it seemed unthinkable that the cellular immunity system had meaning only to stand as an obstacle to the surgeon wishing to transplant tissues or as the tool of the physician for skin testing to facilitate the diagnosis of ongoing or prior microbial infections. Seeking a deeper meaning for a system so sensitive to differences in cellular antigenicity, he postulated that the cellular immune system stands as a bulwark against malignant differentiation. At this point in time, there can be no question that Thomas' postulate has been useful, for it has generated a veritable mountain of data supporting

the view that immunosurveillance does stand against the potentiality of malignant differentiation. From the point of view of the
patients with immunodeficiency likewise, there can be no question
but that a corollary of his major postulate has also been borne out.
Patients with many different forms of primary immunodeficiency
have developed cancer in frequency far in excess of that occurring at
comparable age in the general population. Table XIX summarizes
relevant data collected from the cases of malignancy and immunodeficiencies reported from around the world. It will be seen from the
table that the incidence of malignancy in patients with Bruton's
sex-linked infantile agammaglobulinemia, the common variable
immunodeficiency, ataxia–telangiectasia, (Boder and Sedgwick,
1972; Sedgwick and Boder, 1972), Wiskott–Aldrich syndrome and
even in the patients with the lethal, short-lived combined immunodeficiency have experienced malignancy far too frequently to be
explained by chance association. In the Bruton X-linked infantile
agammaglobulinemia, cancer has occurred in nearly 10% of all
reported cases. In ataxia–telangiectasia malignancy has appeared in
10–15% of cases, in Wiskott–Aldrich syndrome in approximately
10%, and in the common variable immunodeficiency in the neigh-
borhood of 5% of instances. These are extraordinary figures which
say clearly that to have an immunodeficiency is to have the door

TABLE XIX

MALIGNANCIES IN PATIENTS WITH PRIMARY IMMUNODEFICIENCY

Primary disease	Approximate number of malignancies collected	% Cancer
Bruton-type agamma-globulinemia	5 Cases, all leukemia	5–10
Ataxia–telangiectasia	42 Cases, many forms of cancer	10–15
Wiskott–Aldrich syndrome	13 Cases, mostly but not exclusively lymphoreticular malignancies	>10
Common variable immunodeficiency	More than 30 cases, many forms of cancer	5–10
Severe dual-system immunodeficiency	3 Cases	1–10

opened wide to the development of cancer. In children of the general population by contrast, the frequency of cancer at a comparable age to that in which cancer is turning up so frequently in the immunodeficiency children is only 6–10 per 100,000. Thus, having certain forms of immunodeficiency increases the likelihood of developing cancer by a factor of 100–1000. It is not yet known why this door to cancer is ajar in immunodeficiency patients, but a reasonable possibility is that they cannot defend themselves against malignancy when it first appears. Other possibilities include deficiency in defense against an oncogenic or helper infectious agent. Whatever its basis, the patients with immunodeficiency tell us that our immunologic systems stand in some important way between us and many malignancies. The kinds of malignancy developing in patients with different kinds of immunodeficiency are of interest because here, as with the microbial world, study of the occurrence of different forms of cancer in patients with different kinds of immunodeficiency may offer insights leading to a meaningful new classification of cancers. For example, in patients with X-linked infantile immunodeficiency, leukemias have been the only kind of malignancy yet encountered. The increased incidence of leukemia, often beginning in the thymus and occurring in patients who have vigorous cell-mediated immunity but who form antibodies very poorly, surely suggests that antibody formation plays a special role in resistance to certain forms of leukemia. By contrast, the malignancies occurring in patients with the common variable form of immunodeficiency often are carcinomas (nearly 50%) and frequently involve the stomach and the small and large bowel. The latter immunodeficient patients also develop much lymphosarcoma, fibrosarcoma, reticulum cell sarcoma, other solid tissue neoplasms as well as leukemias. That these patients frequently show deficits of cell-mediated immunities and of T-cells as well as deficiencies of B-cells argues that T-cell immunity, perhaps together with humoral immunities plays an important role in defense against such cancers. In both the Wiskott–Aldrich syndrome and the ataxia–telangiectasia syndromes the kind of malignancy that develops is lymphoreticular in very high frequency. Other malignancies have been reported in both groups, but reticulum cell sarcomas, lymphomas, and lymphosarcomas are predominant. It seems certain that the deficiencies of resistance in both groups of patients include mechanisms of resistance against these cancers. Both in a general sense and in the highly specific sense these patients represent extraordinary Experiments of Nature which can lead to increased understanding of cancer. In a family reported by Haerer *et al.* (1969), for example, two members with ataxia–telangiectasia, aged 19 and 21, developed carcinoma of the stomach and died of this malignancy. Such a malignancy is almost unheard of at that age in the general population, and here two young people in one family with ataxia–telangiectasia developed this neoplasm. Such an association tells us a great deal about both carcinoma of the stomach and ataxia–telangiectasia and asks crucial questions that must be answered by further clinical and experimental investigation.

XVI. PREVENTION OF MALIGNANCY BY CENTRAL LYMPHOIDECTOMY

In 1944 Jacob Furth and associates (McEndy *et al.*, 1944) discovered that leukemia in AKR mice is prevented by removal of thymus early in life. Similarly thymectomy in young mice interferred with development of viral and irradiation-induced leukemia. The best analysis of this influence derives from studies by Kaplan (1950), Rappaport and Baroni (1962), and Siegler and Rich (1963), who showed that in different forms of leukemia preventable by neonatal thymectomy the malignancy is thymus-dependent because it begins as a malignant differentiation in the thymus itself. One might, however, encounter thymus-dependent malignancies that start as foci in the thymus or by transformation of cells anywhere within the thymus-dependent system. The alternative possibility of a B-cell malignancy based on similar mechanisms is clearly focused by experiments carried out under the leadership of R. D. A. Peterson of our laboratories in collaboration with the East Lansing group (Peterson *et al.*, 1964a, 1966). We showed that the bursa of Fabricius in chickens is essential to the development of a form of visceral lymphomatosus caused by the RPL_{12} viruses. If the bursa of Fabricius had been removed at hatching or shortly thereafter, visceral lymphomatosus did not develop in birds infected with the etiological agent that causes this form of cancer. This influence of bursectomy was found to parallel the influence of thymectomy when Dent *et al.* (1967) showed that the transformation to visceral lymphomatosus develops in few of many, perhaps 1 of 200 to 1 of 400, bursal follicles. If the bursa is absent, this form of malignancy cannot develop. It seems reasonable to extrapolate from these findings that thymus-dependent and bursal-dependent T and B forms of malignancy can be expected. An agent that acts preferentially to induce malignant differentiation in any subline of the T-cell population should be expected to be reduced or eliminated by neonatal thymectomy. Similarly any malignancy which develops in B-cells at any stage of their maturation should be preventable by early bursectomy. If these findings can be extrapolated from the experimental animal to man, we can expect to find lymphoreticular malignancies that originate in T-cells, those that originate in B-cells and those that originate in M-cells (monocyte precursors) or those that originate in various kinds of stem cells and partially differentiated committed stem cells. Looking back to our earlier studies of the Experiments of Nature represented by Hodgkin's disease and myeloma, it seems reasonable to conclude that in Hodgkin's disease the malignancy involves T cells or in some way depresses the function of these cells (Dent *et al.*, 1969). Myeloma obviously involves the secretory B-cells or plasma cells and depresses in a general way the functions of this entire system. During the past year it has been possible to define many cases of chronic lymphatic leukemia as malignancies of the B-cell line (Preud-homme *et al.*, 1971). Studies by several investigators using the analysis of surface immunoglobulins by specific immunofluorescent staining in the cold shows that in chronic lymphatic leukemia the disease almost certainly represents a malignant monoclonal expansion of B_{2p} cells. These cells usually possess immunoglobulins in the surface or so-called receptor distribution. Usually the monoclonal expansion of malignant B-cells represents cells possessing one kind of light chain, kappa or lambda, and one kind of heavy chain, most frequently mu. However, cases of chronic lymphatic leukemia where the malignant monoclonal lymphocytes are featured by the presence in surface distribution of immunoglobulins which contain gamma or alpha heavy chains have occasionally been encountered. Similarly in myeloma one sees a malignant monoclonal expansion of plasma cells, this time located at the stage of secretory B-cells or B_{2s}. Definition of the kinds of cells being expanded monoclonally in chronic myeloid leukemia, seems obvious, but further analysis will be required to define the kind of cells being deviated and expanded monoclonally in acute lymphatic leukemia, so-called acute myeloid leukemia, and in the many different forms of lymphosarcoma and lymphoma. From analyses of normal cellular development I would predict, for example, that when adequate studies are made the so-called benign follicular lymphoma of Brill-Symmers will be found to represent a monoclonal expansion of B-cells in which the malignant deviation has occurred at a stage of differentiation proximal to that which is deviated in chronic lymphatic leukemia, perhaps even at the stage where the cells are present in the bursa equivalent itself.

XVII. Iatrogenic Immunodeficiency and Malignancy

With the demonstration in 1958 that 6-mercaptopurine can act as an immunosuppressive agent (Schwartz and Dameshek, 1960), the potentiality for clinically successful organ transplantation was at hand (Meeker et al., 1959; Pierce et al., 1961; LaPlante et al., 1962; Gabrielsen and Good, 1967). During the past 10 years some 7000 renal transplants have been attempted. In the best centers throughout the world improving immunosuppression permits long-term survival and function of transplanted kidneys from live donors between 75 and 85% of the time. With matched sibling donors long-term successes of renal transplants have been much higher—more than 95%. Thus, with effective immunosuppression based primarily on adrenal corticosteroids, antimetabolites, cytotoxic drugs, and antilymphocyte serum, the era of successful organ transplantation, especially vis-à-vis kidneys, is at hand. In the context of our present discussion it is of interest that malignancies are occurring too frequently in such immunosuppressed transplant recipients. At least 9 instances of "successful" transplantation of cancer occurred inadvertently, and in 4 of these the cancer became widely disseminated throughout the body as metastases (reviewed by Gatti and Good, 1971a). In several of these the only treatment needed to eliminate the widely disseminated cancer was cessation of immunosuppressive treatment. This manipulation led to the complete elimination of the disseminated cancer. Since immunosuppression for renal transplantation has become widely used, *de novo* malignancies have been recorded from many different clinics and laboratories where renal transplantation has been used to treat end-stage kidney disease. Approximately 75 malignancies have been encountered. Even though it is frequently stated that the malignancies occurring in these patients are predominantly malignancies of the lymphoreticular system, it is clear from study of the cases presented in the literature and those encountered in Minneapolis that this is not quite the case. These *de novo* cancers occurring in immunosuppressed patients have been of epithelial origin in approximately 50% of instances. Nonetheless, the basis for the high frequency of lymphoreticular malignancies and the other malignancies in such patients requires explanation. By contrast with the transplanted malignancies, those developing *de novo* under immunosuppression have not regressed after cessation of immunosuppressive regimens. In the transplantation experience at Minneapolis, 5 malignancies have been observed. None of these have been of lymphoreticular nature, but rather each has been a carcinoma. In experimental animals several studies have linked immunosuppression to increased incidence of malignancies. Here enhanced occurrence and earlier than usual appearance of virus-induced cancer have been most closely linked to immunosuppression, but so-called spontaneous cancers and some chemical carcinogen-induced malignancies have also apparently been favored by immunosuppressive therapy.

XVIII. Susceptibility to Transformation by SV40 Virus in Immunodeficient Patients

Studies by Todaro and co-workers have linked susceptibility to malignancy in patients with Fanconi's anemia, Down's and Kleinfelter's syndromes (Todaro, 1968) to susceptibility of the fibroblast population of such patients to transformation to a cancer-like state using the SV40 virus of monkey origin. The patients with each of these syndromes possess fibroblastic cells that in culture will be transformed approximately 10 times more readily than are similar cultures of fibroblasts from members of the general population. This correlation of increased susceptibility of fibroblasts from such patients to transformation induced by a possible oncogenic virus is most provocative. Particularly since certain patients with primary immunodeficiency disease, e.g., patients with ataxia–telangiectasia may have chromosomal abnormalities, it was deemed important to study the susceptibility of fibroblast cell lines from these patients to the transforming influences of the SV40 virus (Kersey *et al.*, 1972) Evaluations to define transformation have included measurements to detect the two different kinds of cytoplasmic and surface antigens that Rapp (1971) and others have linked to SV40 virus-induced cell transformation.

In short, our data, summarized in Table XX have shown that fibroblast cell strains established from patients with X-linked infantile agammaglobulinemia, common variable immunodeficiency, immunodeficiencies with ataxia–telangiectasia, and Wiskott–Aldrich syndrome and dual-system immunodeficiency have not shown increased transformability with the SV40 virus. Thus, a real difference in this regard exists between fibroblasts from these immunodeficient groups of patients who are susceptible to malignant adaptation and patients with Down's syndrome, Fanconi's syndrome, and Kleinfelter's syndrome who also are susceptible to malignancy. The latter high incidence may be explained, at least in part, by the greater than normal impulse to malignant differentiation under influence of viral (and perhaps other) oncogenic agents. This finding is compatible with, but of course does not establish the concept that the increased incidence of malignancy in patients with primary immunodeficiencies is consequent to a deficiency in immunosurveillance.

XIX. IMMUNODEFICIENCY AND AUTOIMMUNITY

As patients with immunodeficiency are described and studied in increasing numbers, it becomes apparent that in several different forms of primary immunodeficiency disease, autoimmunities, such as Coombs positive hemolytic anemia, thrombocytopenia, rheumatoid joint disease, pernicious anemia, and even amyloidosis, have been occurring far more frequently than should be explained by chance alone. This association seems also to be true of gastric atrophy, nontropical sprue or malabsorption syndrome, dermatomyositis, and other apparent autoimmune disorders. In some series of patients, this constellation of diseases of presumed autoimmune

TABLE XX

Susceptibility of Fibroblasts from Patients with Immunodeficiency Diseases to Transformation by SV40[a]

Patient	Age	Sex	Early T antigen (% of cells positive for T antigen)[b]	Late T antigen (number of colonies per coverslip)[b]
Normal				
RD	49	M	1.3 (1.3, 1.7, 0.8)	1.7 (0, 0, 5.0)
Highly susceptible				
SH	27	F	4.8 (4.4, 4.0, 6.1)	13.3 (8.0, 12.0, 20.0)
Sex-linked agammaglobulinemia				
DH	10	M	0.6 (0.7, 0.5)	0 (0)
IgA deficiency				
CW	6	F	0.85 (0.7, 1.0)	0 (0)
Variable (late onset) immunodeficiency				
VJ	40	F	0.5 (0.5)	1.0 (1.0)
LL	38	M	0.8 (0.8)	1.0 (1.0)
CL	33	M	2.9 (2.9)	6.0 (6.0)
AR	7	M	1.4 (1.3, 1.5)	0 (0)
GR	5	M	1.0 (1.0)	3.0 (3.0)
SE	24	M	1.1 (1.1)	1.0 (1.0)
Ataxia–telangiectasia				
VC	17	F	1.3 (1.3)	2.0 (2.0)
LD	4	F	0.7 (0.4, 1.0)	1.0 (1.0)
Wiskott–Aldrich syndrome				
RM	4	M	0.3 (0.3)	2.0 (2.0)
SG	8	M	0.3 (0.3)	1.0 (1.0)
Severe combined system immunodeficiency				
DC	3	M	0.3 (0.3)	1.0 (1.0)
EF	3	F	0.3 (0.3)	1.0 (1.0)
CM	2	M	0.2 (0.2)	2.0 (2.0)

[a] Kersey et al. (1972).
[b] Expressed as mean of individual experiments. Results of individual experiments are given in parentheses.

nature was occurring as often as 30 times more frequently than in the general population (Good, 1962; Good et al., 1957, 1961, 1962b; Good and Gabrielsen, 1964b; Twomey et al., 1970). The association of the presumed autoimmune diseases with demonstrable autoantibodies, too, has been variable in these disorders. In patients with primary immunodeficiency who themselves retained some antibody-forming capacity, autoantibodies such as rheumatoid factor, anti-thyroid and antinuclear antibodies have been found in serum in high frequency. In others, the so-called autoimmune diseases seem to have occurred without demonstrable autoantibodies in the serum. As was mentioned earlier in regard to many patients with the common variable form of immunodeficiency, members of the family showed a high frequency of autoimmune phenomena and apparent auto-immune disease (Fudenberg, 1971). Rheumatoid arthritis and tenosynovitis occurring in patients with agammaglobulinemia can often be treated with good results by regular administration of normal gamma globulin in large amounts. This paradoxical occur-rence of far too much autoimmunity and far too much autoantibody production in patients with primary immunodeficiency may be most dramatically seen in certain populations of patients who have an isolated absence of IgA and lack an effective local IgA immunity system. As first observed by Cassidy *et al.* (1966) and also reported by Huntley *et al.* (1967), patients with rheumatoid arthritis and lupus erythematosus lack circulating IgA more frequently than do members of the general population. Further, patients lacking circulating IgA have in very high frequency not only autoantibodies such as those represented by rheumatoid factor but too high an incidence of rheumatoid arthritis, other autoantibodies, and even of precipitating antibodies directed toward bovine serum proteins present in milk, e.g., bovine serum albumin (Buckley and Dees, 1969; Ammann and Hong, 1971). This has been a puzzling set of observa-tions which may be better understood when it is realized that barriers to absorption of intact protein may include both the local and systemic antibody system. We all eat proteins immunologically closely related to those of our own cells, tissues, and circulating proteins. Lack of the normal immunological barrier to absorption of these molecules may be an important opening to an exposure that results in stimulation of the remaining immunological systems when one system like the IgA system is lacking. Such stimulation could be a means of developing autoantibodies or autoimmune disease (Good and Rodey, 1970). Recently, Walker *et al.* (1972a, b) have brought forward evidence testing these relationships and have shown by

careful quantitative analysis that immunization via the oral route
leading to local immunity in turn leads to significantly decreased
absorption of proteins from the bowel. Similarly systemic immunization also decreases absorption of protein from the bowel. A nice
relationship of this same general nature may have been brought
forward by Polmar *et al.* (1972) working at the NIH. In the latter
studies it was found that respiratory manifestations were frequent if
IgA were lacking in the body but the IgE immunoglobulin system
present. When both IgA and IgE are absent, this form of respiratory
disease was not so frequent or prominent. It is this relationship that
led Hobbs to remark, "When you can't say A you may say E,"
which sums up graphically what may be a most important generalization. Perturbations basic to this analysis may represent a most
important source of disease in immunodeficient patients. If the
immune system is partly defective as, for example, if a defect of the
cellular immunity system exists while ability to form some antibodies remains intact, the persisting immunological system may be
excessively stimulated. This relationship could account for the
extremely high levels of IgA and the markedly elevated concentrations of IgE frequently seen in patients with the Wiskott–Aldrich
syndrome. It seems likely to me that a kind of immunological
imbalance resulting from stimulation of a remaining system or
systems when one or several systems are deficient may underly many
of the autoimmune phenomena, dysgammaglobulinemias, and
perhaps even the high frequency of amyloidosis that have been
associated with immunodeficiency. Further, such perturbations may
account for the frequent autoimmune diseases occurring in patients
with immunodeficiency and even in members of their families.

Both Burnet (1959) and Fudenberg (1971) have attempted to
explain these autoimmune disturbances occurring in the immunodeficient patients in terms of permission of persistence of forbidden
or aberrant clones of cells that produce the autoantibodies. However,
little or no molecular evidence has been brought forward to support
the view that forbidden clones exist in such patients. These findings
make me much more receptive to the view that it is antigens gaining
access to the body abnormally or persisting in the body abnormally
that account for the many autoimmunities in immunodeficient
patients. Thus, persisting or recurrent infections, uninhibited

antigenic absorption, more frequent, more variable, and quantitatively greater antigenic stimulation represent the source of the otherwise forbidden antigens that seem the more likely basis of the immunologic diseases and autoimmunities that occur in immunodeficient patients with far too great a frequency.

XX. IMMUNODEFICIENCY AND AGING

Recent studies by Walford (1969) and Makinodan (1972) and the extensive investigations by Yunis *et al.* (1972) and Teague *et al.* (1973) on the immunologic perturbations occurring with aging reveal that immunodeficiency is a common concomitant of aging in experimental animals and man. In our own studies we found that in different strains of mice deficiencies of T-cell immunities occur at different times and progress at different rates with aging. In NZB mice for example, deficiencies of T-cell functions are already far advanced when the animals are 10 months of age. Similarly the T-cells as revealed by analyses with anti-θ antiserum and by T-cell functions have been lost in large part at this juncture (Stutman, 1972). Beginning at this time, the autoimmunities advance rapidly, resulting in progressive hemolytic anemia and kidney destruction. The latter is probably based on an indirect immune assault by antigen–antibody complexes as occurs in human lupus. The antigen–antibody complexes accumulate in the capillaries on the epithelial side of the renal basement membranes and yield a characteristic morphological lesion. In addition to its occurrence in NZB mice susceptibility to autoimmunity is present also in mice of other genetic lines. The strains we have found to be susceptible to autoimmune disease include NZB, NZW, C57Ks, A/J, and A/UMC, in which the thymus and T-cell immunities involute relatively early in life. By contrast, autoimmune-resistant strains are those in which T-cell immunities do not involute until much later in life, the CBA strain for example. Thus NZB and A/J strain mice are immunologically old mice relatively early in life while CBA mice that resist autoimmunities retain their full immunological vigor and their T-cells much longer. In several of these strains we have been able to shift the curve of development of autoimmunity and that of decline of cellular immunity to the left by removal of the thymus early in life. Shifting of the curve of development of autoimmunity and cellular immunodeficiency to the right has been much more difficult to accomplish. Nonetheless, reversal of certain autoimmune processes in A strain mice has been accomplished by giving the recipients lymphoid cells from young immunocompetent syngeneic donors (Teague *et al.*, 1970, 1972; Teague and Friou, 1969). Not only in mice, but in rabbits (Sutherland *et al.*, 1965; Kellum *et al.*, 1965) and man certain autoimmunities and autoimmune phenomena and amyloidosis seem to be reciprocally related to deficiencies of T-cell or both T- and B-cell immunity systems. It is this relationship that may be present in extreme form in patients with certain primary or secondary immunodeficiency diseases.

XXI. Manipulations of Separate Systems Separately

If there are not one but two separate immunologic systems, as so many data now indicate, it would be desirable to be able separately to manipulate each system independently. Already progress toward this goal has been forthcoming. In our own laboratories using appropriate doses of pure inhibitors of DNA synthesis, e.g., hydroxyurea, we have been able selectively to depress cell-mediated immunity while permitting humoral immunity to be expressed with little apparent depression (McKneally *et al.*, 1966). Similarly cytosine arabinoside has been reported (Griswold *et al.*, 1972) to prevent antibody synthesis while leaving cell-mediated immunity intact, and L-asparaginase (Friedman, 1971) has been shown to depress cell-mediated immunity while to some extent sparing humoral immunity. The most impressive selective manipulations of cellular and humoral immunity systems accomplished to date, however, have been seen with use of specific antilymphocyte serums which selectively depresses the very mobile T-cell system while leaving relatively intact the more sessile B-cell immunity system. Also a single injection of cyclophosphamide will depress B-cell based humoral immunity and even result in increased cell-mediated immunities, e.g., in Jones Mote reactions (Turk and Poulter, 1972). By contrast, chronic restriction of protein intake has been shown by Jose *et al.* (1971a; Jose and Good, 1971, 1972) and W. C. Cooper and Good (1971) to reduce B-cell dependent humoral immunity selectively while leaving cellular immunities (T-cell immunity) completely intact or even more vigorous than normal. Such separate manipulations of the two immunity systems are, of course, to be expected. As such manipulations are further developed they may bring powerful new tools for prevention of malignancy, prevention of development of autoimmunity and perhaps tools useful even for manipulating the rate of development of the immunologic involution and immunologic perturbations so frequently accompanying aging in man and experimental animals. If this is the case such manipulations may alter the development or propensity to develop autoimmune disease and autoimmune phenomena with aging.

XXII. B-Cells in Immunodeficiency Diseases of Man

In 1970 Pernis (Pernis *et al.*,1970) adapted a technique used earlier by Möller (1961) to study surface isoantigens to permit identification and quantitation of the number of circulating lymphocytes that produce receptor immunoglobulins. Several investigators, particularly Grey *et al.* (1971), Cooper *et al.* (1971), Pernis and Kunkel (1971), and Preud'homme *et al.* (1971) have used this method to quantify the numbers of B lymphocytes of different immunoglobulin classes in patients with primary immunodeficiency diseases. Dr. Gajl and I, too, have used this method to analyze the numbers of B-lymphocytes in the circulation of our patients with primary and secondary immunodeficiency diseases (Gajl-Peczalska and Good, 1972). The results of this analysis have been most interesting. Summarized on Table XXI are data recording some of our experiences with this method to date. It will be seen from the table that, as in Grey's experience, the patients we refer to as Bruton's X-linked infantile immunodeficiency show with this method also virtually no circulating B-cells. Both Pernis and Kunkel (1971) and Cooper *et al.* (1971), however, have found some patients with apparent X-linked infantile agammaglobulinemia who have an appreciable number of B-cells in the blood. Surface immunoglobulin possessing lymphocytes in circulating blood and lymph node have been almost completely lacking in our patients with X-linked infantile agammaglobulinemia. By contrast, in the DiGeorge syndrome B-cells may reach 85–95% at a time when quantitation of T-cell responses may show no evidence that any PHA-responding T-cells are present in

TABLE XXI

"B" Cells in Primary Immune Deficiency Disease

Type of deficiency	Blood surface Ig% (mean)			
	Total	G	A	M
Normal subjects (12)	30 (24–46)	16.7	5.8	7.8
Bruton (3)	<1	0.6	0.1	0.2
Common variable (11)	11 (2–23)	6.1	2.1	3.6
Selective IgA (3)	27	10.4	8.8	7.8
Wiskott–Aldrich (2)	36	21.5	5.5	9.0
Ataxia–telangiectasia (2)	31	9.2	11.8	10.2
DiGeorge syndrome (1)	84	32.9	23.7	26.6

the circulation. This finding represents a striking figure for circulating B-lymphocytes when it is compared to the normal numbers of 15–30%. Further, effective treatment by thymic transplantation of the DiGeorge syndrome in one of our patients led to a dramatic reduction of both absolute and relative numbers of B-cells in the blood as the T-cell responses increased.

Patients with the common variable form of immunodeficiency, although sometimes having immunoglobulin levels as low as those seen in our children with X-linked infantile agammaglobulinemia, quite regularly showed substantial numbers of B-cells of each immunoglobulin class in the circulating blood. As has been observed by others, patients having a selective absence of IgA in blood and in secretions possessed at least normal numbers of IgA producing B lymphocytes in the circulating. Special notice should be given to the high levels of IgA possessing B-lymphocytes in patients with ataxia–telangiectasia. This finding is particularly striking since these patients often are completely lacking IgA in their serum and secretions. In the Wiskott–Aldrich syndrome where IgM levels are low, normal numbers of cells with IgM surface immunoglobulins as well as normal numbers of cells with the IgA and IgG in surface distribution are to be found in the circulation. It is suggested from these findings that in some diseases of immunodeficiency a block exists at the level of secretion of the immunoglobulins and antibodies while in others a block exists at an earlier stage and both synthesis and secretion are defective.

XXIII. Studies of Immunodeficiency by Techniques of Molecular Biology

To date the several immunodeficiency diseases of man have been defined reasonably well in terms of the morphological abnormalities of their lymphoid tissues. The deficiencies in these patients have been studied effectively by immunohistochemical techniques and analyzed in terms of functional deficits. The abnormalities of these patients have even been critically investigated in genetic and developmental terms, but little has been done to elucidate and compare the abnormalities of the cells of these patients using the tools of modern molecular biology. Y. S. Choi, whose earlier studies with Lennox (Choi *et al.*, 1971a, b) together with those of Uhr and co-workers (Shapiro *et al.*, 1966; Sherr and Uhr, 1971) have contributed much to the understanding of the processes of synthesis and secretion of immunoglobulin molecules in the malignant cells obtained from patients with multiple myeloma, has begun comparative investigations in molecular terms of the lymphoid cells of patients suffering from the several forms of immunodeficiency. These investigations had their point of departure in studies of the lymphoid cells from the bursa of Fabricius in birds and in studies of synthesis and secretion of immunoglobulins in lymphoid tissue of agammaglobulinemic chickens produced by in ovo bursectomy. Studies by Choi (Choi and Good, 1972) and later by Kiszkiss and Choi (Kiszkiss *et al.*, 1972) in my laboratory had confirmed our investigations which earlier had established that birds bursectomized *in ovo* late in embryonic life (15–17 days of a 21-day embryonation) are often agammaglobulinemic and cannot produce immunoglobulins or antibodies of any type (Good and Finstad, 1971). Similarly birds bursectomized at 18–19 days of embryonation that have been given, in addition, near-lethal total body irradiation at hatching also regularly show agammaglobulinemia and do not produce antibodies to antigenic stimulation. Such chickens make vigorous cell-mediated immune responses that are dependent on T-cells. These birds can develop allograft rejection reactions of great vigor and can show normal delayed allergic reactions. They have cells that initiate GVH reactions just as effectively as do the cells of immunologically normal birds. In confirmation of earlier observations by Dent (Good and Finstad, 1971) in my laboratory we have recently reinvestigated rosette-forming cells in agammaglobulinemic birds. Using all the most sensitive modern methods, we have failed to find in such agammaglobulinemic chicks any sign of rosette-forming lymphocytes. The agammaglobulinemic chickens will not develop such rosette-forming lymphocytes even after extensive stimulation with sheep red blood cells. Thus, in our model system for study of agammaglobulinemia it was possible to show that T-cells without a B-cell contribution are not the lymphocytes that form rosettes with sheep red blood cells, even when the so-called delicate rosettes are sought. By contrast these T-cells have the capacity to initiate and execute all other known cell-mediated immune responses. These findings have convinced us that rosettes based on antibody and even so-called special "T-cell rosettes" of mice and chickens have nothing to do with the receptor mechanism that is the basis of specificity in cell-mediated immunities. T-cell rosettes not a function of antibody against sheep cells do, however, seem to be a marker for T-cells of man. Choi found further that cells from the bursa of Fabricius, may not produce and secrete immunoglobulins with characteristic light and heavy chains, but the cells contain but do not secrete an immunoglobulin having a heavy chain class that we have called H_o (Choi and Good, 1972). This immunoglobulin, although immunochemically possessing heavy chains with apparent μ determinants, has a heavy chain that lacks the galactose residues which normally are attached to the heavy chains in the process of secretion of the molecule. Thus, this heavy chain is smaller than the normal heavy chain (Choi and Good, 1972). Agammaglobulinemic, bursaless chickens, even after antigenic stimulation, cannot be shown either to synthesize or secrete any known immunoglobulins. These studies employ extremely sensitive methodologies for labeling the immunoglobulin molecules that are being synthesized and secreted. The observations thus establish, consonant with many other recent studies, that T-cell immunity either does not involve synthesis of any of the usual immunoglobulin molecules or that it involves production of extremely small amounts of such molecules. This amount, if any is produced at all, must be at least several orders of magnitude smaller than that produced by B-cells which have readily demonstrable immunoglobulins at their surface. This amount, is even still that much smaller than the amount involved in the usual synthesis and secretion of immunoglobulin molecules by plasma cells.

Turning to human immunodeficiency, we are now certain that patients with X-linked infantile agammaglobulinemia like the agammaglobulinemic chickens do not possess or produce immunoglobulin-based rosette-forming lymphocytes.* As reported above they may lack demonstrable immunoglobulin in so-called receptor distribution at their surface that can be revealed by immunohistochemical analysis (Gajl-Peczalska *et al.*, 1972). By contrast, they develop cellular immunities normally. Y. S. Choi's studies showed further that the peripheral lymphocytes and lymph node cells from such patients neither synthesize nor secrete immunoglobulins in detectable amounts. By contrast, clear evidence of immunoglobulin synthesis can be demonstrated when the same methodology is applied to the peripheral blood and lymph node cells of patients with the common variable immunodeficiency who do have in their circulation abundant lymphocytes possessing surface immunoglobulins. However, lymphoid cells from the latter patients show little or no evidence of immunoglobulin secretion. Further, the lymphoid cells of such patients can be shown to synthesize immunoglobulins with H chains that seem to be like those produced by the cells in the bursa of Fabricius (Choi *et al.*, 1972). The heavy chains of such cells are smaller than are the μ or γ heavy chains secreted by the lymphoid cells of normal humans, and they lack the galactose residues present on normally secreted H chains. The parallelism between chicken and man again is striking. These efforts represent, we believe, initial steps to employ modern methods of molecular biology to define more precisely the immunodeficiency diseases. They must be considered to be only a beginning. We are certain that this beginning can ultimately be extended until a full molecular definition of each of the several immunodeficiency diseases has been accomplished.

* These children with Bruton-type X-linked immunodeficiency have, however, many rosette-forming lymphocytes, where the rosettes are formed at 37°C. Such rosettes are not antibody-based but are due to receptors on the T-cell. They are found on T-cells of man and some primates but not on T-cells of many other animal species.

XXIV. Primary Deficiency of Complement Components

Silverstein (1960) discovered that the serum of a healthy immunologist lacked the C2 component of complement and thus could not hemolyze sensitized sheep blood cells in the usual way. This defect turned out to be the first genetically determined deficiency of the complement system. When subsequently other cases of C2 deficiency turned up in healthy immunologists and their family members, some concluded that perhaps the complex complement system might be a sport of nature placed on earth to confound immunologists. Because Gewurz, Finstad, Muschel, and I (1966a) had been studying the development of the complex complement system in phylogenetic perspective and had found an extraordinary consistency of this complicated system of interacting proteins and enzymes over great eons of vertebrate evolution, we knew that this conclusion was incorrect. It was our view that patients with genetically determined deficiencies of the complement system would be discovered and that as with patients having primary immunodeficiencies the inherited defects of the complement system would reveal the importance of each of the separate complement components in the body economy. Perhaps unpopular, we argued this position at several national and international meetings. We began studying selective complement component deficiencies by trying to understand the relative good health of persons lacking C2. From this first study we could convince ourselves that, in spite of the defect of C2, such patients exercise important complement-dependent functions. For example, they can achieve immune adherence and a fairly vigorous bactericidal activity with their undiluted serum (Gewurz et al., 1966b). More recently patients with several forms of severe disease and deficiency of the bodily defense have been discovered to have isolated defects of the complement system. Alper et al. (1970) described a defect of a stabilizer of C3 that leads to recurrent pneumonias, Miller et al., (1968) and Miller and Nillson (1970) described defects of C5 leading to Leiner's disease. This disease can be corrected completely by giving C5 or whole plasma containing C5. Pickering et al. (1970) discovered a patient lacking C2 who was not healthy but had severe progressive renal disease. One of our patients with C2 deficiency subsequently developed lupus erythematosus (Day et al., 1973). We found another patient who had deficiency of Clr (Pickering *et al.*, 1970), who had severe renal disease; and Pondman *et al.* (1968) had a patient with selective Cls deficiency who had lupus. Subsequently Moncada *et al.* (1972) and Day *et al.* (1972) studied in some detail serums from two children of a Chicago family where the significance of an inborn error of the earlier complement components has been revealed in bold relief. The children whose sera we studied lacked a single subcomponent, Clr, of the trimolecular first complement component. Three children of this family had died showing increased frequency of infection and one had an apparent vasculitis. Two children were alive; both showed far too frequent infections, and one had serious skin, vascular, and renal disease resembling lupus. Several children in the family were normal. Thus, with apparent autosomal recessive inheritance of an inborn defect of production of Clr, the vital importance of this complement component has been revealed. It is not different with other components. C2 deficiency has now been associated with lupus (Agnello *et al.*, 1973; Day *et al.*, 1973), dermatomyositis (J. P. Leddy, personal communication), chronic glomerulonephritis (Pickering *et al.*, 1970), skin purpura (P. Lachman, personal communication), and increased frequency of infection (Agnello *et al.*, 1973; Day *et al.*, 1973). Several different forms of genetically determined deficiency of C3 (Alper and Rosen, 1971) have been associated with extraordinary susceptibility to infections. Even in experimental animals where defects of isolated components such as C4, C5, and C6 had earlier been thought to be compatible with good health and normal vigor, extraordinary vulnerability to infection and to other diseases have turned up after more complete analysis. These associations can be taken as a mere beginning. They represent, however, clear indications through study of Experiments of Nature, that the complement system and each individual component plays crucial roles of major survival advantage in the body economy. The individual defects when thoroughly analyzed can be expected to contribute to our understanding of the complement system just as the inborn and acquired defects of the specific immunity systems have contributed to the analyses of immune mechanisms.

In finishing my dissertation, I wish only to restate the beginning and urge all to reflect on the extraordinary power of Experiments of Nature, especially of those representative of inborn errors of metabolism. As a source of questions they give focus and relevance to our scientific endeavor. As a testing ground for the significance of our advancing knowledge, they are unexcelled in revealing the adequacy or inadequacy of experimental analysis. They are only made more important by technological advances. They deserve even more attention that we have paid them heretofore, and I commend them to you once again. I must insist, however, that to listen to them in good conscience requires that we develop means to alleviate their suffering. We must become skillful at treating effectively the diseases which they exhibit. This is a difficult but not impossible task. It can be and already is being addressed by the developing sciences of cellular and enzymatic engineering. Hopefully it will be addressed in the future by true genetic engineering.

ACKNOWLEDGMENTS

I am deeply indebted to Connie Finstad and Betty Sokolosky for assistance in the preparation of this manuscript.

REFERENCES

Agnello, V., de Bracco, M. M. E., and Kunkel, H. G. (1973). *J. Immunol.* (in press).

Aisenberg, A. C. (1965). *J. Clin. Invest.* **44,** 555–564.

Aisenberg, A. C. (1966). *Cancer Res.* **26,** 1152.

Alper, C. A., and Rosen, F. S. (1971). *Advan. Immunol.* **14,** 252.

Alper, C. A., Abramson, N., Johnston, R. B., Jandl, J. H., and Rosen, F. S. (1970). *N. Engl. J. Med.* **282,** 349.

Ammann, A. J., and Good, R. A. (1971). *Medicine* **50,** 223–236.

Ammann, A. J., and Hong, R. (1971). *Lancet* **1,** 1264–1266.

Archer, O., and Pierce, J. C. (1961). *Fed. Proc., Fed. Amer. Soc. Exp. Biol.* **20,** 26.

Archer, O. K., Pierce, J. C., Papermaster, B. W., and Good, R. A. (1962). *Nature (London)* **195,** 191–192.

August, C. S., Rosen, F. S., Filler, R. M., Janeway, C. A., Markowski, B., and Kay, H. E. M. (1968). *Lancet* **2,** 1210–1211.

Bach, F. H., Albertini, R. J., Joo, P., Anderson, J. L. Y., and Bortin, M. M. (1968). *Lancet* **2,** 1364–1366.

Bearn, A. G., Kunkel, H. G., and Slater, R. (1956). *Amer. J. Med.* **21,** 3–15.

Berendes, H., Bridges, R. A., and Good, R. A. (1957). *Minn. Med.* **40,** 309–312.

Biggar, W. D. (1972). *Fed. Proc., Fed. Amer. Soc. Exp. Biol.* **31,** 650.

Biggar, W. D., Lapointe, N., Ishizaka, K., Meuwissen, H., Good, R. A., and Frommel, D. (1970). *Lancet* **2,** 1089.

Biggar, W. D., Park, B. H., and Good, R. A. (1972a). Unpublished observations.

Biggar, W. D., Stutman, O., and Good, R. A. (1972b). *J. Exp. Med.* **135,** 793–807.

Biggar, W. D., Good, R. A., and Park, B. H. (1972c). *J. Pediat.* **81,** 301–306.

Billingham, R. E., Brent, L., and Medawar, P. B. (1953). *Nature (London)* **172,** 603.

Bing, J., and Plum, P. (1937). *Acta Med. Scand.* **92,** 415.

Bjoerneboe, M., and Gormsen, H. (1943). *Acta Pathol. Microbial. Scand.* **20,** 649.

Blaese, R. M., Strober, W., Brown, R. S., and Waldmann, T. A. (1968). *Lancet* **1,** 1056–1061.

Blaese, R. M., Strober, W., Levy, A., and Waldmann, T. A. (1971). *J. Clin. Invest.* **50,** 2331–2338.

Blaese, R. M., Oppenheim, J. J., Seeger, R. C., and Waldmann, T. A. (1972). *Cell. Immunol.* **4,** 228–242.

Boder, E., and Sedgwick, R. P. (1963). *Little Club Clin. Develop. Med.* **8,** 110–118.

Boder, E., and Sedgwick, R. P. (1972). *In* "Cellular and Molecular Basis of Neurological Diseases" (E. Goldensohn and S. Appel, eds.). Lea & Febiger, Philadelphia, Pennsylvania.

Boyse, E. A., Old, L. J., and Stockert, E. (1966). Immunopathology, *Int. Symp. 4th, 1965* pp. 23–40.

Boyse, E. A., Old, L. J., Stockert, E., and Shigeno, N. (1968). *Cancer Res.* **28,** 1280–1287.

Bridges, R. A., and Good, R. A. (1960). *Ann. N. Y. Acad. Sci.* **86,** 1089–1097.

Bridges, R. A., Berendes, H., and Good, R. A. (1959). *AMA J. Dis. Child.* **97,** 387–408.

Brown, R. S., Haynes, H. A., Foley, H. T., Godwin, H. A., Berard, G. W., and Carbone, P. P. (1967). *Ann. Int. Med.* **67,** 291–302.

Bruton, O. C. (1952). *Pediatrics* **9,** 722–728.

Buckley, R. H., and Dees, S. C. (1969). *N. Engl. J. Med.* **281,** 465.

Burnet, F. M. (1959). "The Clonal Selection Theory of Acquired Immunity." Vanderbilt Univ. Press, Nashville, Tennessee.

Burnet, F. M. (1971a). Unpublished address presented at 1st International Congress of Immunology, Washington, D.C.

Burnet, F. M. (1971b). "Genes, Dreams and Realities." Basic Books, New York.

Cain, W. A., Cooper, M. D., and Good, R. A. (1968). *Nature (London)* **217,** 87–89.

Cassidy, J. T., Burt, A., Sullivan, D. B., and Dickenson, D. G. (1966). *Arthritis Rheum.* **9,** 850.

Choi, Y. S., and Good, R. A. (1971). Unpublished observations.

Choi, Y. S., and Good, R. A. (1972). *J. Exp. Med.* **135,** 1133–1150.

Choi, Y. S., Knopf, P. M., and Lennox, E. S. (1971a). *Biochemistry* **10,** 659–667.

Choi, Y. S., Knopf, P. M., and Lennox, E. S. (1971b). *Biochemistry* **10,** 668–679.

Choi, Y. S., Biggar, W. D., and Good, R. A. (1972). *Lancet* **1,** 1149–1151.

Claman, H. N., Chaperon, E. A., and Triplett, R. F. (1966). *Proc. Soc. Exp. Biol. Med.* **122,** 1167–1171.

Cleveland, W. W., Fogel, B. J., Brown, W. T., and Kay, H. E. M. (1968). *Lancet* **2,** 1211–1214.

Coons, A. H., Leduc, E. H., and Connolly, J. M. (1955). *J. Exp. Med.* **102,** 49.

Cooper, M. D. (1972). Unpublished observations.

Cooper, M. D., Peterson, R. D. A., and Good, R. A. (1965). *Nature (London)* **205,** 143–146.

Cooper, M. D., Peterson, R. D. A., South, M. A., and Good, R. A. (1966). *J. Exp. Med.* **123,** 75–102.

Cooper, M. D., Chase, H. P., Lowman, J. T., Krivit, W., and Good, R. A. (1968a). *Amer. J. Med.* **44,** 499–513.

Cooper, M. D., Chase, H. P., Lowman, J. T., Krivit, W., and Good, R. A. (1968b).

In "Immunologic Deficiency Diseases in Man" (D. Bergsma and R. A. Good, ed.), pp. 378–387. National Foundation Press, New York.

Cooper, M. D., Perey, D. Y., Gabrielsen, A. E., Sutherland, D. E. R., McKneally, M. F., and Good, R. A. (1968c). *Int. Arch. Allergy Appl. Immunol.* **33**, 65–88.

Cooper, M. D., Perey, D. Y., Peterson, R. D. A., Gabrielsen, A. E., and Good, R. A. (1968d). *In* "Immunologic Deficiency Diseases in Man" (D. Bergsma and R. A. Good, ed.), pp. 7–16. National Foundation Press, New York.

Cooper, M. D., Cain, W. A., Van Alten, P., and Good, R. A. (1969). *Int. Arch. Allergy Appl. Immunol.* **35**, 242–252.

Cooper, M. D., Lawton, A. R., and Bockman, D. E. (1971). *Lancet* **2**, 791–795.

Cooper, W. C. and Good, R. A. (1971). *Fed. Proc., Fed. Amer. Soc. Exp. Biol.* **30**, 351.

Dalmasso, A. P., Martinez, C., and Good, R. A. (1962). *Proc. Soc. Exp. Biol. Med.* **111**, 143–146.

Dalmasso, A. P., Martinez, C., Sjodin, K., and Good, R. A. (1963). *J. Exp. Med.* **118**, 1089–1109.

Dalmasso, A. P., Martinez, C., and Good, R. A. (1964). *In* "The Thymus in Immunobiology" (R. A. Good and A. E. Gabrielsen, eds.), pp. 478–489. Harper (Hoeber), New York.

Dausset, J., Colombani, J., Legrand, L., and Fellous, M. (1970). *In* "Histocompatibility Testing" (P. I. Terasaki, ed.), pp. 53–75. Munksgaard, Copenhagen.

Day, N. K., Geiger, H., Stroud, R., deBracco, M., Moncada, B., Windhorst, D., and Good, R. A. (1972). *J. Clin. Invest.* **51**, 1102–1108.

Day, N. K., Geiger, H., Michael, A., and Good, R. A. (1973). *J. Clin. Invest.* (in press).

DeKoning, J., Dooren, L. J., van Bekkum, D. W., van Rood, J. J., Dicke, K. A., and Radl, J. (1969). *Lancet* **1**, 1223–1227.

Dempster, W. J. (1969). *Lancet* **1**, 468.

Dent, P. B., Cooper, M. D., Payne, L. N., Good, R. A., and Burmester, B. R. (1967). *In* "Perspectives in Virology" (M. Pollard, ed.), pp. 251–265. Academic Press, New York.

Dent, P. B., Gabrielsen, A. E., Cooper, M. D., Peterson, R. D. A., and Good, R. A. (1969). *In* "Textbook of Immunopathology" (P. A. Miescher and H. J. Müller-Eberhard, eds.), pp. 385–405. Grune & Stratton, New York.

DiGeorge, A. M. (1968). *In* "Immunologic Deficiency Diseases in Man" (D. Bergsma and R. A. Good, eds.), pp. 116–121. National Foundation Press, New York.

Dupont, B., Nielsen, L. S., and Svejgaard, A. (1971). *Lancet* **2**, 1336–1340.

Dupont, B., Andersen, V., Faber, V., Good, R. A., Henriksen, K., Juhl, F., Koch, C., M-Berat, N., Park, B., Svejgaard, A., and Wiik, A. (1973). *Transplant. Proc.* (in press).

Edelman, G. M., and Gall, W. E. (1969). *Annu. Rev. Biochem.* **38**, 415–455.

Edelman, G. M., and Poulik, M. D. (1961). *J. Exp. Med.* **113**, 861–864.

Eichwald, E., and Silmser, C. R. (1955). *Transplant. Bull.* **2**, 148–149.

Eltringham, J. R. and Kaplan, H. S. (1972). Presented at Int. Symp. on Hodgkin's Disease. Stanford Univ., Stanford, California, March 20–24, 1972.

Fagraeus, A. (1948). *Acta Med. Scand.* Suppl. 204 (accompanies Vol. **130**, 1).

100 ROBERT A. GOOD

Fahey, J. L., Barth, W. F., and Law, L. W. (1965). *J. Nat. Cancer Inst.* **35,** 663.

Ford, C. E. (1966). *Thymus. Exp. Clin. Stud. Ciba Found. Symp. 1965* pp. 131–158.

Friedman, H. (1971). *Science* **174,** 139–141.

Fudenberg, H. H. (1971). *In* "Immunobiology" (R. A. Good and D. W. Fisher, eds.), pp. 175–183. Sinauer Ass., Stamford, Connecticut.

Fudenberg, H., German, J. L. III, and Kunkel, H. G. (1962). *Arthritis Rheum.* **5,** 565.

Fudenberg, H., Good, R. A., Goodman, H. C., Hitzig, W., Kunkel, H. G., Roitt, I. M., Rosen, F. S., Rowe, D. S., Seligmann, M., and Soothill, J. R. (1971). *Pediatrics* **47,** 927–946.

Gabrielsen, A. E., and Good, R. A. (1967). *Advan. Immunol.* **6,** 91–229.

Gafni, J., Michaeli, D., and Heller, H. (1960). *N. Engl. J. Med.* **263,** 536–540.

Gajl-Peczalska, K. J. and Good, R. A. (1972). Unpublished observations.

Gajl-Peczalska, K. J., Biggar, W. D., Park, B. H., and Good, R. A. (1972). *Lancet* **1,** 1344–1345.

Garrod, A. E. (1924). *Brit. Med. J.* **2,** 747–752.

Gatti, R. A., and Good, R. A. (1971a). *Cancer* **28,** 89–98.

Gatti, R. A., and Good, R. A. (1971b). *J. Pediat.* **79,** 475–479.

Gatti, R. A., Meuwissen, H. J., Allen, H. D., Hong, R., and Good, R. A. (1968). *Lancet* **2,** 1366–1369.

Gatti, R. A., Meuwissen, H. J., Terasaki, P. I., and Good, R. A. (1971). *Tissue Antigens* **1,** 239–241.

Gatti, R. A., Gershanik, J., Levkoff, A. H., Wertelecki, W., and Good, R. A. (1972). *J. Pediat.* **81,** 920–926.

Gewurz, H., Finstad, J., Muschel, L. H., and Good, R. A. (1966a). *In* "Phylogeny of Immunology" (R. T. Smith, P. A. Miescher, and R. A. Good, eds.), pp. 105–116. Univ. of Florida Press, Gainesville.

Gewurz, H., Pickering, R. J., Muschel, L. H., Mergenhagen, S. E., and Good, R. A. (1966b). *Lancet* **2,** 356–360.

Githens, J. H., Muschenhein, F., Fulginiti, V. A., Robinson, A., and Kay, H. E. M. (1969). *J. Pediat.* **75,** 87–94.

Gitlin, D., Hitzig, W. H., and Janeway, C. A. (1956). *J. Clin. Invest.* **35,** 1199.

Gitlin, D., Janeway, C. A., Apt, L., and Craig, J. M. (1959). *In* "Cellular and Humoral Aspects of the Hypersensitive States" (H. S. Lawrence, ed.), p. 375. Harper (Hoeber), New York.

Glick, B. (1964). *In* "The Thymus in Immunobiology" (R. A. Good and A. E. Gabrielsen, eds.), pp. 343–358. Harper, New York.

Glick, B., Chang, T. S., and Jaap, R. G. (1956). *Poultry Sci.* **35,** 224–225.

Good, R. A. (1948). *Proc. Soc. Exp. Biol. Med.* **67,** 203–205.

Good, R. A. (1954a). *J. Lab. Clin. Med.* **44,** 803.

Good, R. A. (1954b). *Rev. Hematol.* **9,** 502.

Good, R. A. (1957). *In* "Host Parasite Relationships in Living Cells" (H. Felton *et al.*, eds.), pp. 68–161. Thomas, Springfield, Illinois.

Good, R. A. (1962). *In* "Conference on Host Response Mechanisms in Rheumatoid Arthritis," pp. 30–35. Arthritis and Rheumatism Found., New York.

Good, R. A. (1969). *Hosp. Practice* **4,** 41–47.

Good, R. A. (1970). *J. Amer. Med. Ass.* **214,** 1289–1300.

Good, R. A. (1972a). *Cell. Immunol.* **3,** i-iv.

Good, R. A. (1972b). *Proc. Nat. Acad. Sci. U.S.* **69,** 1026–1032.

Good, R. A., and Bergsma, D. (eds.) (1968). "Immunologic Deficiency Diseases in Man." National Foundation Press, New York.

Good, R. A., and Campbell, B. (1950). *Amer. J. Med.* **9,** 330–342.

Good, R. A., and Finstad, J. (1971). *In* "Cell Interactions and Receptor Antibodies in Immune Responses" (O. Makela, A. Cross, and T. U. Kosunen, eds.), pp. 27–40. Academic Press, New York.

Good, R. A., and Gabrielsen, A. E. (eds.) (1964a). "The Thymus in Immunobiology." Harper (Hoeber), New York.

Good, R. A., and Gabrielsen, A. E. (1964b). *In* "Streptococcus, Rheumatic Fever and Glomerulonephritis" (J. W. Uhr, ed.), pp. 368–403. Williams & Wilkins, Baltimore, Maryland.

Good, R. A., and Rodey, G. E. (1970). *Cell. Immunol.* **1,** 147–149.

Good, R. A., and Varco, R. L. (1955). *J. Lancet* **75,** 245.

Good, R. A., and Wortis, H. H. (1971). *In* "Progress in Immunology" (B. Amos, ed.), pp. 1271–1278. Academic Press, New York.

Good, R. A., and Zak, S. J. (1956). *Pediatrics* **18,** 109–149.

Good, R. A., Rotstein, J., and Mazzitello, W. F. (1957). *J. Lab. Clin. Med.* **49,** 343–357.

Good, R. A., Bridges, R. A., Zak, S. J., and Pappenheimer, A. M. (1959). *In* "Cellular and Humoral Aspects of the Hypersensitivity States" (H. S. Lawrence, ed.), pp. 437–441. Harper (Hoeber), New York.

Good, R. A., Venters, H., Page, A. R., and Good, T. A. (1961). *J. Lancet* **81,** 192–204.

Good, R. A., Dalmasso, A. P., Martinez, C., Archer, O. K., Pierce, J. C., and Papermaster, B. W. (1962a). *J. Exp. Med.* **116,** 773–796.

Good, R. A., Kelly, W. D., Rotstein, J., and Varco, R. L. (1962b). *Progr. Allergy* **6,** 187–319.

Good, R. A., Peterson, R. D. A., Perey, D. Y., Finstad, J., and Cooper, M. D. (1968). *In* "Immunologic Deficiency Diseases in Man" (D. Bergsma and R. A. Good, eds.), pp. 17–39. National Foundation Press, New York.

Grey, H. M., Rabelino, E., and Pirofsky, B. (1971). *J. Clin. Invest.* **50,** 2368–2375.

Griswold, D. E., Heppner, G. H., and Calabresi, P. (1972). *Cancer Res.* **32,** 298–301.

Haerer, F., Jackson, J. F., and Evers, C. G. (1969). *J. Amer. Med. Ass.* **210,** 1884–1887.

Hammar, J. A. (1908). *Arch. Mikrosk. Anat.* **73,** 1.

Hellström, I., Hellström, K. E., Storb, R., and Thomas, E. D. (1970). *Proc. Nat. Acad. Sci. U.S.* **66,** 65–71.

Hellström, K. E., and Hellström, I. (1970). *Hosp. Practice* **5,** 45.

Hitzig, W. H. (1968). *In* "Immunologic Deficiency Diseases in Man" (D. Bergsma and R. A. Good, eds.), pp. 82–87. National Foundation Press, New York.

Hitzig, W. H., Landolt, R., Müller, G., and Bodmer, P. (1971). *J. Pediat.* **78,** 968–980.

Holmes, B., Quie, P. G., Windhorst, D. B., and Good, R. A. (1966a). *Lancet* **1,** 1225–1228.

Holmes, B., Quie, P. G., Windhorst, D. B., Pollara, B., and Good, R. A. (1966b). *Nature (London)* **210,** 1131–1132.

Holmes, B., Page, A. R., and Good, R. A. (1967). *J. Clin. Invest.* **46,** 1422–1432.

Holmes-Gray, B., and Good, R. A. (1971). *In* "Immunobiology" (R. A. Good and D. W. Fisher, eds.), pp. 55–61. Sinauer Ass., Stamford, Connecticut.

Hong, R., Gatti, R. A., and Good, R. A. (1968a). *Lancet* **2,** 388–389.

Hong, R., Kay, H. E. M., Cooper, M. D., Meuwissen, H., Allan, M. J. G., and Good, R. A. (1968b). *Lancet* **1,** 503–506.

Hoyer, J. R., Cooper, M. D., Gabrielsen, A. E., and Good, R. A. (1968). *Medicine* **47,** 201–226.

Huntley, C. C., Thorpe, D. P., Lyerly, A. D., and Kelsey, W. M. (1967). *Amer. J. Dis. Child.* **113,** 411–418.

Janeway, C. A., Apt, L., and Gitlin, D. (1953). *Trans. Ass. Amer. Phys.* **66,** 200.

Jankovic, B. D., Waksman, B. H., and Arnason, B. G. (1962). *J. Exp. Med.* **116,** 159–176.

Jeunet, F., and Good, R. A. (1968). *In* "Immunologic Deficiency Diseases in Man" (D. Bergsma and R. A. Good, eds.), pp. 192–206. National Foundation Press, New York.

Jolly, J. (1911). *C. R. Soc. Biol.* **70,** 498.

Jolly, J. (1914). *Arch. Anat. Microsc.* **16,** 363–547.

Jones, J. M., Wilson, R., and Bealmear, M. M. (1971). *Radiat. Res.* **45,** 477.

Jose, D. G., and Good, R. A. (1971). *Fed. Proc., Fed. Amer. Soc. Exp. Biol.* **30,** 246.

Jose, D. G., and Good, R. A. (1972). *Lancet* **1,** 314.

Jose, D. G., Cooper, W. C., and Good, R. A. (1971a). *J. Amer. Med. Ass.* **218,** 1428–1429.

Jose, D. G., Kersey, J. H., Choi, Y. S., Biggar, W. D., Gatti, R. A., and Good, R. A. (1971b). *Lancet* **2,** 841–844.

Kaplan, H. S. (1950). *J. Nat. Cancer Inst.* **11,** 83.

Keast, D. (1968). *Immunology* **15,** 273.

Kellum, M. J., Sutherland, D. E. R., Eckert, E., Peterson, R. D. A., and Good, R. A. (1965). *Int. Arch. Allergy Appl. Immunol.* **27,** 6–26.

Kelly, W. D., and Good, R. A. (1968). *In* "Immunologic Deficiency Diseases in Man" (D. Bergsma and R. A. Good, eds.), pp. 349–356. National Foundation Press, New York.

Kelly, W. D., Good, R. A., Varco, R. L., and Levitt, M. (1959). *Surg. Forum* **9,** 785–789.

Kelly, W. D., Lamb, D. L., Varco, R. L., and Good, R. A. (1960). *Ann. N.Y. Acad. Sci.* **87,** 187–202.

Kersey, J. H., Gatti, R. A., Good, R. A., Aaronson, S. A., and Todaro, G. J. (1972). *Proc. Nat. Acad. Sci. US.* **69,** 980–982.

Kincade, P. W., and Cooper, M. D. (1970). *Fed. Proc., Fed. Amer. Soc. Exp. Biol.* **29,** 503.

Kincade, P. W., Lawton, A. R., Bochman, D. E., and Cooper, M. D. (1970). *Proc. Nat. Acad. Sci. U.S.* **67,** 1918–1925.

Kiszkiss, D., Choi, Y. S., and Good, R. A. (1972). *J. Immunol.* **109,** 1405–1407.

Koller, P. C., Davies, A. J. S., Leuchars, E., and Wallis, V. (1967). *In* "Germinal Centers in Immune Responses" (H. Cottier, N. Odartchenko, R. Schindler, and C. C. Congdon, eds.), pp. 157–160. Springer-Verlag, Berlin and New York.

Kolouch, F. (1938). *Proc. Soc. Exp. Biol. Med.* **39,** 147.

Kolouch, F., Good, R. A., and Campbell, B. (1947). *J. Lab. Clin. Med.* **32,** 749–755.

Krivit, W., and Good, R. A. (1959). *AMA J. Dis. Child.* **97,** 137–153.

Kunkel, H. G., Ahrens, E. H., Jr., Eisenmenger, W. Y., Bongiovanni, A. M., and Slater, R. J. (1951a). *J. Clin. Invest.* **30,** 654.

Kunkel, H. G., Slater, R. S., and Good, R. A. (1951b). *Proc. Soc. Exp. Biol. Med.* **76,** 190–193.

Lamb, D., Pilney, F., Kelly, W. D., and Good, R. A. (1962). *J. Immunol.* **89,** 555–558.

Lambrechts, A. F., and Snoijink, J. J. (1971). *In* "Ataxia-Telangiectasia. Morbus lympholyticus Congenitalis." Bushmann, Antwerp.

LaPlante, E. S., Condie, R. M., and Good, R. A. (1962). *J. Lab. Clin. Med.* **59,** 542.

Lawrence, H. S. (1969). *Advan. Immunol.* **2,** 195–266.

Leduc, E. H., Coons, A. H., and Connolly, J. M. (1955). *J. Exp. Med.* **102,** 61.

Lerman, S. P., and Weidanz, W. P. (1970). *J. Immunol.* **105,** 614–619.

Levin, A. S., Spitler, L. E., Stites, D. P., and Fudenberg, H. H. (1970). *Proc. Nat. Acad. Sci. U.S.* **67,** 821–828.

Linna, T. J. (1967). *Int. Arch. Allergy Appl. Immunol.* **31,** 313.

Linna, T. J., Frommel, D., and Good, R. A. (1972). *Int. Arch. Allergy Appl. Immunol.* **42,** 20–39.

Lischner, H. W., and DiGeorge, A. M. (1969). *Lancet* **2,** 1044.

Louis-Bar (1941). *Confin. Neurol.* **4,** 32–42.

McEndy, D. P., Boon, M. C., and Furth, J. (1944). *Cancer Res.* **4,** 377–384.

McKneally, M. F. (1970). Ph.D. Thesis, Univ. of Minnesota, Minneapolis.

McKneally, M. F., and Good, R. A. (1971). *Surgery* **69,** 166–174.

McKneally, M. F., Windhorst, D. B., Yarbro, J. W., and Good, R. A. (1966). *Surg. Forum* **17,** 258.

McKneally, M. F., Sutherland, D. E. R., and Good, R. A. (1971). *Surgery* **69,** 345–353.

MacLean, L. D., Zak, S. J., Varco, R. L., and Good, R. A. (1957). *Transplant. Bull.* **4,** 21–22.

McQuarrie, I. (1944). *In* "Experiments of Nature and Other Essays." Univ. of Kansas Press, Lawrence.

Makinodan, T. (1972). *In* "Tolerance, Autoimmunity and Aging" (M. M. Sigel and R. A. Good, eds.), pp. 3–17. Thomas, Springfield, Illinois.

Mariani, T., Martinez, C., Smith, J. M., and Good, R. A. (1958). *Proc. Soc. Exp. Biol. Med.* **99,** 287–289.

Mariani, T., Martinez, C., Smith, J. M., and Good, R. A. (1959). *Proc. Soc. Exp. Biol. Med.* **102,** 751–755.

Martinez, C., Aust, J. B., and Good, R. A. (1956). *Transplant. Bull.* **3,** 128–129.

Martinez, C., Smith, J. M., and Good, R. A. (1958). *Brit. J. Exp. Pathol.* **39,** 574–581.

Martinez, C., Kersey, J., Papermaster, B. W., and Good, R. A. (1962). *Proc. Soc. Exp. Biol. Med.* **109,** 193.

Meeker, W., Condie, R., Weiner, D., Varco, R. L., and Good, R. A. (1959). *Proc. Soc. Exp. Biol. Med.* **102,** 459–461.

Metcalf, D. (1966). *In Thymus, Exp. Clin. Stud.,* Ciba Found. Symp. p. 242.

Miller, J. F. A. P. (1961). *Lancet* **2,** 748–749.

Miller, J. F. A. P. (1964). *In* "The Thymus in Immunobiology" (R. A. Good and A. E. Gabrielsen, eds.), pp. 436–460. Harper, New York.

Miller, J. F. A. P., and Mitchell, G. F. (1969). *Transplant. Rev.* **1,** 3.

Miller, J. F. A. P., and Mitchell, G. F. (1970). *J. Exp. Med.* **131,** 675.

Miller, M. E., and Nilsson, U. R. (1970). *N. Engl. J. Med.* **282,** 354–358.

Miller, M. E., Seals, J., Kaye, R., and Levitsky, L. C. (1968). *Lancet* **2,** 60.

Mitchell, G. F., and Miller, J. F. A. P. (1968). *J. Exp. Med.* **128,** 821–837.

Möller, G. (1961). *J. Exp. Med.* **114,** 415–432.

Moncada, B., Day, N. K. B., Good, R. A., and Windhorst, D. B. (1972). *N. Engl. J. Med.* **286,** 689–693.

Moore, M. A. S., and Owen, J. J. T. (1965). *Nature (London)* **208,** 956.

Moore, M. A. S., and Owen, J. J. T. (1966). *Develop. Biol.* **14,** 40–51.

Mosser, G., Good, R. A., and Cooper, M. D. (1970). *Int. Arch. Allergy Appl. Immunol.* **39,** 62–81.

Nossal, G. J. V., Cunningham, A., Mitchell, G. F., and Miller, J. F. A. P. (1968). *J. Exp. Med.* **128,** 839–853.

Oppenheim, J. J., Blaese, R. M., and Waldmann, T. A. (1970). *J. Immunol.* **104,** 835.

Osoba, D., and Miller, J. F. A. P. (1963). *Nature (London)* **199,** 653.

Page, A. R., and Good, R. A. (1960). *AMA J. Dis. Child.* **99,** 288–314.

Park, B. H., and Good, R. A. (1972). *Proc. Nat. Acad. Sci. U.S.* **69,** 371–373.

Park, B. H., Biggar, W. D., and Good, R. A., (1972a). Unpublished observations.

Park, B. H., Holmes-Gray, B., and Good, R. A. (1972b). *In* "Pulmonary Disorders" (E. L. Kendig, Jr., ed.), Vol. 1, pp. 789–796. Saunders, Philadelphia, Pennsylvania.

Park, B. H., Yunis, E. J., and Good, R. A. (1972c). Unpublished observations.

Park, B. H., Biggar, W. D., and Good, R. A. (1973). *Proc. 4th Transplant. Soc.*, in press.

Parrott, D. M., deSoussa, M. A. B., and East, J. (1966). *J. Exp. Med.* **123,** 191–203.

Pernis, B., and Kunkel, H. (1971). *In* "Progress in Immunology" (B. Amos, ed.), p. 723. Academic Press, New York.

Pernis, B., Forni, L., and Amante, L. (1970). *J. Exp. Med.* **132,** 1001–1018.

Peterson, R. D. A., Burmester, B. R., Fredrickson, T. M., Purchase, H. G., and Good, R. A. (1964a). *J. Nat. Cancer Inst.* **32,** 1343–1354.

Peterson, R. D. A., Kelly, W. D., and Good, R. A. (1964b). *Lancet* **1,** 1189–1193.

Peterson, R. D. A., Cooper, M. D., and Good, R. A. (1965). *Amer. J. Med.* **38,** 579–604.

Peterson, R. D. A., Purchase, H. G., Burmester, B. R., Cooper, M. D., and Good, R. A. (1966). *J. Nat. Cancer Inst.* **36,** 585.

Peterson, R. D. A., and Good, R. A. (1968). *In* "Immunologic Deficiency Diseases in Man" (D. Bergsma and R. A. Good, eds.), pp. 370–377. National Foundation Press, New York.

Pickering, R. J., Naff, G. B., Stroud, R. M., Good, R. A., and Gewurz, H. (1970). *J. Pediat.* **78,** 30–43.

Pierce, J. C., Varco, R. L., and Good, R. A. (1961). *Surgery* **50,** 186–195.

Polmar, S. H., Waldmann, T. A., Balestra, S. T., Jost, M. C., and Terry, W. D. (1972). *J. Clin. Invest.* **51,** 326–330.

Pondman, K. W., Stoop, J. W., Cormane, R. H., and Hannama, A. J. (1968). *J. Immunol.* **101,** 811.

Preud'homme, J. L., Klein, M., Verroust, P., and Seligmann, M. (1971). *Rev. Eur. Etudes Clin. Biol.* **XVI,** 1025–1031.

Putnam, F. W., Shonda, T., Titani, K., and Wikler, M. (1967). *Science* **157,** 1050–1053.

Quie, P. G., White, J. G., Holmes, B., and Good, R. A. (1967). *J. Clin. Invest.* **46,** 668–679.

Raff, M. C. (1971). *In* "Cell Interactions and Receptor Antibodies in Immune Responses" (O. Makela, A. Cross, and T. U. Kosunen, eds.), pp. 83–90. Academic Press, New York.

Raff, M. C. and Cantor, H. (1971). *In* "Progress in Immunology" (B. Amos, ed.), pp. 83–93. Academic Press, New York.

Rapaport, H., and Baroni, C. (1962). *Cancer Res.* **22,** 1067.

Rapp, F. (1971). *Hosp. Practice* **5,** 49.

Rendel, J. M. (1970). *In* "The Impact of Civilisation on the Biology of Man" (S. V. Boyden, ed.), pp. 27–47. National University Press, Canberra, Australia.

Rodey, G. E., and Good, R. A. (1969). *Int. Arch. Allergy Appl. Immunol.* **36,** 399–407.

Rosen, F. S., Gotoff, S. P., Craig, J. M., Ritchie, J., and Janeway, C. A. (1966). *N. Engl. J. Med.* **272,** 18–21.

Rosen, F. S., Craig, J. M., Vawter, G., and Janeway, C. A. (1968). *In* "Immunologic Deficiency Diseases in Man" (D. Bergsma and R. A. Good, eds.), pp. 67–70. National Found. Press, New York.

Salkind, J. (1915). *Arch. Zool. Exp.* **55,** 81.

Schier, W. W., Roth, A., Ostroff, G., and Schrift, M. H. (1956). *Amer. J. Med.* **20,** 94–99.

Schwartz, R. S., and Dameshek, W. (1960). *J. Clin. Invest.* **39,** 952–958.

Sedgwick, R. P., and Boder, E. (1972). *In* "Handbook Clinical Neurology," Vol. 13. North-Holland Publ., Amsterdam.

Seligmann, M., Fudenberg, H., and Good, R. A. (1968). *Amer. J. Med.* **45,** 817–825.

Shapiro, A. L., Scharff, M. D., Maizel, J. V., and Uhr, J. W. (1966). *Proc. Nat. Acad. Sci. U.S.* **56,** 216.

Shapiro, F., Martinez, C., Smith, J. M., and Good, R. A. (1961). *Proc. Soc. Exp. Biol. Med.* **106,** 472–475.

Sherr, C. J., and Uhr, J. W. (1971). *J. Exp. Med.* **133,** 901.

Siegler, R., and Rich, M. A. (1963). *Cancer Res.* **23,** 1669.

Silverstein, A. M. (1960). *Blood* **16,** 1338.

Slater, R. J., Ward, S. M., and Kunkel, H. G. (1955). *J. Exp. Med.* **101,** 85.

Stiehm, E. R., Lawlor, G. J., Kaplan, M. S., Greenwald, H. L., Neerhout, R. C., Sengar, D. P. S., and Terasaki, P. I. (1972). *N. Engl. J. Med.* **286,** 797–803.

St. Geme, J. W., Jr., Prince, J. T., Burke, B. A., Good, R. A., and Krivit, W. (1965). *N. Engl. J. Med.* **273,** 229–234.

Stutman, O. (1970). *In* "Fifth Leukocyte Culture Conference" (J. Harris, ed.), pp. 671–681. Academic Press, New York.

Stutman, O. (1973). *Proc. 4th Transplant. Soc.* (in press).

Stutman, O., and Good, R. A. (1971). *Transplant. Proc.* **3,** 923–925.

Stutman, O., Yunis, E. J., Martinez, C., and Good, R. A. (1967). *J. Immunol.* **98**, 79–87.

Stutman, O., Yunis, E. J., and Good, R. A. (1968). *J. Nat. Cancer Inst.* **41**, 1431–1452.

Stutman, O., Yunis, E. J., and Good, R. A. (1969a). *J. Nat. Cancer Inst.* **43**, 499–508.

Stutman, O., Yunis, E. J., and Good, R. A. (1969b). *J. Immunol.* **103**, 92–99.

Stutman, O., Yunis, E. J., and Good, R. A. (1969c). *Transplantation* **7**, 420–423.

Stutman, O., Yunis, E. J., and Good, R. A. (1970a). *J. Exp. Med.* **132**, 583–600.

Stutman, O., Yunis, E. J., and Good, R. A. (1970b). *J. Exp. Med.* **132**, 601–612.

Sutherland, D. E. R., Archer, O. K., Peterson, R. D. A., Eckert, E., and Good, R. A. (1965). *Lancet* **1**, 130–133.

Szenberg, A., and Warner, N. L. (1962). *Nature (London)* **194**, 146–147.

Teague, P. O., and Friou, G. J. (1969). *Immunology* **17**, 663–673.

Teague, P. O., Yunis, E. J., Rodey, G., Fish, A. J., Stutman, O., and Good, R. A. (1970). *Lab. Invest.* **22**, 121–130.

Teague, P. O., Friou, G. J., Yunis, E. J., and Good, R. A. (1972). *In* "Tolerance, Auto-immunity and Aging" (M. M. Sigel and R. A. Good, eds.), pp. 33–61. Thomas, Springfield, Illinois.

Thieffry, St., Arthuis, M., Aicardi, J. and Lyon, G. (1961). *Rev. Neurol.* **105**, 390–405.

Thomas, L. (1959). *In* "Cellular and Humoral Aspects of the Hypersensitivity States." (H. S. Lawrence, ed.), p. 529. Hoeber-Harper, New York.

Thorbecke, G. J., Warner, N. L., Hochwald, G. M., and Ohanian, S. H. (1968). *J. Immunol.* **15**, 123.

Todaro, G. (1968). *Nat. Cancer Inst. Monogr.* **29**, 271–275.

Toivanen, P., and Linna, T. J. (1971). *Fed. Proc., Fed. Amer. Soc. Exp. Biol.* **30**, 529.

Toivanen, P., Toivanen, A., and Good, R. A. (1972a). *J. Immunol.* (in press).

Toivanen, P., Toivanen, A., and Good, R. A. (1972b). *J. Exp. Med.* (in press).

Turk, J. L., and Poulter, L. W. (1972). *Clin. Exp. Immunol.* **10**, 285–296.

Twomey, J. J., Jordan, P. H., Jr., Laughter, A. H., Meuwissen, H. J., and Good, R. A. (1970). *Ann. Int. Med.* **72**, 499–504.

Van Alten, P. J., Cain, W. A., Good, R. A., and Cooper, M. D. (1968). *Nature (London)* **217**, 358–360.

Waldmann, T. A. (1968). *In* "Immunologic Deficiency Diseases in Man" (D. Bergsma and R. A. Good, eds.), p. 394. National Found. Press, New York.

Walford, R. L. (ed.) (1969). "The Immunologic Theory of Aging." Williams & Wilkins, Baltimore, Maryland.

Walker, W. A., Cornell, R., Davenport, L. M., and Isselbacher, K. J. (1972a). *J. Cell Biol.* in press.

Walker, W. A., Isselbacher, K. J., and Bloch, K. J. (1972b). *Science* (in press).

Warner, N. L. (1965). *Aust. J. Exp. Biol. Med. Sci.* **43**, 439.

Warner, N. L., and Szenberg, A. (1964). *In* "The Thymus in Immunobiology" (R. A. Good and A. E. Gabrielsen, eds.), pp. 395–411. Harper (Hoeber), New York.

Warner, N. L., Szenberg, A., and Burnet, F. M. (1962). *Aust. J. Exp. Biol. Med. Sci.* **40**, 373.

White, R. G., Coons, A. H., and Connolly, J. M. (1955). *J. Exp. Med.* **102**, 83.

Wolf, J. K., Gokcen, M., and Good, R. A. (1963). *J. Lab. Clin. Med.* **61**, 230–248.

Wortis, H. H. (1971). *Clin. Exp. Immunol.* **8**, 305–317.

Wybran, J., Carr, M., and Fudenberg, H. H. (1972). *J. Clin. Invest.* **51,** 2537–2543.
Yunis, E. J., and Amos, B. (1971). *Proc. Nat. Acad. Sci. U.S.* **68,** 3031–3035.
Yunis, E. J., Hilgard, H. R., Martinez, C., and Good, R. A. (1965). *J. Exp. Med.* **121,** 607–632.
Yunis, E. J., Fernandes, G., Teague, P. O., Stutman, O., and Good, R. A. (1972). *In* "Tolerance, Autoimmunity and Aging" (M. M. Sigel and R. A. Good, eds.), pp. 62–119. Thomas, Springfield, Illinois.
Zinneman, H. H., and Hall, W. H. (1954). *Ann. Int. Med.* **41,** 1152–1163.

THE GENETIC CONTROL OF SPECIFIC
IMMUNE RESPONSES*

BARUJ BENACERRAF

Department of Pathology, Harvard Medical School,
Boston, Massachusetts

I. Introduction

THIS lecture will describe the identification and the properties of a new class of genes which control the ability to form specific immune responses. The products of these genes are endowed with a considerable degree of specificity in their ability to permit immune responses to be initiated to protein and polypeptide antigens and the determinants they carry.

In spite of the complexity of immune phenomena and of the numerous specificities against which immune responses can be formed, and therefore contrary to expectation, dominant Mendelian genetics have been shown to control specific immune responses (McDevitt and Benacerraf, 1969). Several autosomal dominant genes, each concerned with the ability to form specific immune responses to distinct antigens, have been identified in the past few years. An animal possessing such a gene can form a vigorous immune response against the corresponding antigen, a response characterized both by cellular immunity and sustained antibody synthesis. Animals lacking the gene never display cellular immunity and are either totally or partially deficient in their antibody response to the antigen (Benacerraf and McDevitt, 1972).

The discovery of specific immune response genes (*Ir* genes) has depended upon experiments wherein the immunological system is presented with a challenge of highly restricted heterogeneity and specificity. Three types of antigens have been used for this purpose: (1) synthetic polypeptides with limited numbers of different L-amino

---

* Lecture delivered October 21, 1971.

acids, and their hapten conjugates, to present the immunological mechanism with molecules of limited structural diversity; (2) *limiting* immunizing doses of complex multideterminant native protein antigens; that is, in a dose range which is immunogenic for only some individuals or certain inbred strains in a given species; (3) weak native isologous antigens.

These conditions limit considerably the possibilities of specific interaction between the antigens and immunocompetent cells.

These three methods have permitted the identification within a relatively short time of many specific immune response genes in the two species most intensively investigated, guinea pigs and mice. Most of the *Ir* genes detected with these antigens have been shown to be intimately linked with genes controlling major histocompatibility specificities and not with immunoglobulin structural genes, in several animal species. This class of *Ir* genes, characterized by their distinctive properties as the "histocompatibility linked *Ir* genes," control in each case highly heterogeneous antibody responses. A large number of these genes have been discovered in the last few years and are listed in Table I.

We must recognize, however, that another class of *Ir* genes is being presently identified in several laboratories; this second class of genes, in contrast to the histocompatibility linked genes, appear to be linked to immunoglobulin allotypes and thus to the structural genes of the immunoglobulin chains (Cohn, 1972). The "allotype linked genes" are being recognized in experiments where the response to antigens which stimulate the formation of clonal antibody with limited heterogeneity, such as polysaccharides, is studied (Eichman *et al.*, 1971). The data on this second class of genes are still fragmentary and will not be discussed this evening. We will concern ourselves with the identification and properties of the histocompatibility linked specific *Ir* genes. We shall first describe the guinea pigs *Ir* genes with which our work has been primarily concerned. We will also discuss the mouse immune response genes which have been studied most intensively by McDevitt and associates. I cannot emphasize too strongly, however, that the histocompatibility linked *Ir* genes in both species behave in an identical fashion in every respect.

TABLE I

HISTOCOMPATIBILITY LINKED SPECIFIC IMMUNE RESPONSE GENES

Antigens	Species	Linkage	Reference
PLL ⎫	Guinea pig	Strain 2 H specificity	Ellman *et al.* (1970a)
PLA ⎪ probably		Strain 2 H specificity	Ellman *et al.* (1970a)
$G^{60}L^{40}$ ⎬ same		Strain 2 H specificity	Ellman *et al.* (1970a)
DNP-PLL ⎭ gene		Strain 2 H specificity	Ellman *et al.* (1970a)
$G^{60}A^{40}$		Strain 2 H specificity	Bluestein *et al.* (1971c)
BSA (low dose)		Strain 2 H specificity	Green *et al.* (1970)
DNP-BSA (low dose)		Strain 2 H specificity	Green *et al.* (1970)
HSA (low dose)		Strain 2 H specificity	Green and Benacerraf (1971)
GT		Strain 13 H specificity	Bluestein *et al.* (1971c)
DNP-GPA		Strain 13 H specificity	Green *et al.* (1972)
(T,G)-A–L	Mouse	$H\text{-}2^{b,i}$	McDevitt and Chinitz (1969)
(H,G)-A–L		$H\text{-}2^{a,k,h}$	McDevitt and Chinitz (1969)
(Phe,G)-A–L		$H\text{-}2^{a,b,d,i,k,q}$	McDevitt and Chinitz (1969)
$G^{60}A^{30}T^{10}$		$H\text{-}2^{a,b,d,k}$	Martin *et al.* (1971)
$G^{60}A^{30}L^{10}$		$H\text{-}2^{a,b,d,k,s}$	Merryman and Maurer (1971)
GL Phe		$H\text{-}2^{d,q}$	Merryman *et al.* (1972)
Ovomucoid (low dose)		$H\text{-}2^{a,k}$	Vaz and Levine (1970)
Ovalbumin (low dose)		$H\text{-}2^{b,d,q}$	Vaz and Levine (1970)
Bovine gamma globulin (low dose)		$H\text{-}2^{a,k}$	Vaz *et al.* (1970)
Male (Y) transplantation antigen		$H\text{-}2^{b,i}$	Gasser and Silver (1971)
Mouse IgA myeloma		$H\text{-}2$	Lieberman and Humphrey (1971)
Mouse IgG myeloma		$H\text{-}2$	Lieberman and Humphrey (1972)
Autoimmune thyroiditis		$H\text{-}2$	Vladutiu and Rose (1971)
Porcine LDH-A_4	Rat	$H\text{-}1$	Wurzburg (1971)

II.   GUINEA PIG *Ir* GENES

Two inbred guinea pig strains, 2 and 13 (developed by Dr. Sewall Wright from a small closed colony) as well as random-bred lines, have been used to study the genetic control of specific immune responsiveness.

Figure 1 illustrates the antibody response of these inbred strains and of $(2 \times 13)F_1$ animals to limiting doses of human serum albumin (HSA) as an example of genetic control of the response to a native antigen in the low dose range (Green and Benacerraf, 1971). Identical results have been obtained with bovine serum albumin. The differences observed are specific, as strain 2 and 13 animals respond equally well to limiting doses of other antigens, such as ovalbumin or bovine γ-globulin.

The synthetic polypeptide antigens used in our studies are described in Table II.

The gene which controls the response to poly-L-lysine (PLL) was the first specific immune response gene identified (Levine *et al.*, 1963a). It controls responsiveness to PLL, poly-L-arginine, to

TABLE II

POLYPEPTIDE ANTIGENS, THE RESPONSES TO WHICH ARE
CONTROLLED BY SPECIFIC GUINEA PIG *Ir* GENES

A. *Homopolymers*		
1. Poly-L-lysine	PLL	
2. Poly-L-arginine	PLA	
B. *Copolymers of*:		
1. 60% L-Glutamic acid	GL	
40% L-Lysine		
2. 60% L-Glutamic acid	GA	
40% L-Alanine		
3. 50% L-Glutamic acid	GT	
50% L-Tyrosine		
4. 60% L-Glutamic acid	GAT	
30% L-Alanine		
10% L-Tyrosine		
C. *Hapten polypeptide conjugates*		
1. 2,4-Dinitrophenyl-poly-L-lysine		DNP-PLL
2. 2,4-Dinitrophenyl-GL		DNP-GL

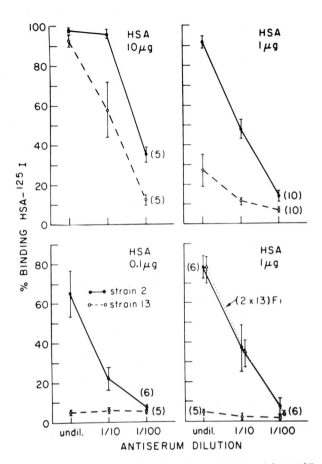

FIG. 1.   Anti-HSA antibody responses of strain 2, strain 13, and $(2 \times 13)F_1$ guinea pigs to 0.1, 1, or 10 µg HSA in complete Freund's adjuvant. Data are expressed as % binding of 0.7 µg HSA-^{125}I by globulin fraction of 0.1 ml of antiserum dilution. Mean values and standard errors are indicated. The number of animals per group is shown in parentheses. From Green and Benacerraf (1971), *J. Immunol.*, by permission of The Williams & Wilkins Co., Baltimore, Maryland.

copolymers of L-glutamic acid and L-lysine (GL) and to hapten conjugates of these polypeptides. The PLL gene is found in all strain 2 and some Hartley guinea pigs and is lacking in strain 13 animals.

As illustrated in Fig. 2, the immune response of guinea pigs to the

STRAIN 2
HARTLEY RESPONDERS

STRAIN 13
HARTLEY NONRESPONDERS

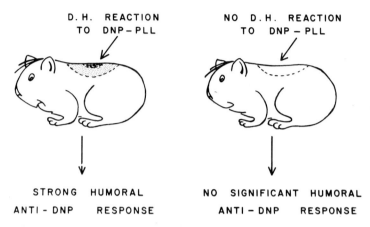

D.H. REACTION
TO DNP—PLL

NO D.H. REACTION
TO DNP—PLL

STRONG HUMORAL
ANTI—DNP RESPONSE

NO SIGNIFICANT HUMORAL
ANTI—DNP RESPONSE

FIG. 2.   Immune response of inbred strains and random-bred Hartley animals to 2,4-dinitrophenyl-poly-L-lysine (DNP-PLL).

antigens, the recognition of which is under the control of the PLL gene, is characterized by cellular immunity, and the synthesis of significant levels of specific antibody. Animals lacking the gene never develop delayed sensitivity and do not produce significant levels of antibodies under usual conditions of immunization. The activity of these immune response genes in guinea pigs is therefore responsible for clear-cut qualitative differences between responder and nonresponder animals. This is also illustrated in Fig. 3, where the antibody responses of strain 2 and strain 13 to the linear random copolymer of L-glutamic acid and L-alanine (GA), are presented (Bluestein *et al.*, 1971a).

As shown in Table III, the abilities of inbred guinea pigs to form immune responses to the synthetic polypeptide antigens, 2,4-dinitrophenyl (DNP)-PLL, GA, and L-glutamic acid and L-tyrosine copolymer (GT) and to limiting doses of native antigens and their hapten conjugates, bovine serum albumin (BSA), human serum albumin (HSA), DNP-BSA, DNP-guinea pig albumin (DNP-GPA) are inherited according to strict Mendelian genetics, indicating that the immune responses to these antigens are controlled by distinct dominant *Ir* genes. Thus, strain 2 but not strain 13 guinea pigs respond to DNP-PLL, GL, GA, and to low doses of BSA, HSA, and to limiting doses of DNP-GPA. All $(2 \times 13)F_1$ animals are responders to all these antigens, illustrating the dominant character of these responses.

Responsiveness to DNP-PLL, GA, and to low doses of BSA and DNP-BSA segregate together in 50% of $(2 \times 13)F_1 \times 13$ backcross guinea pigs. On the other hand, the abilities to respond to GT and to low doses of DNP-GPA are inherited together by 50% of $(2 \times 13)F_1 \times 2$ backcross offspring.

The genetic analysis can be pursued further taking advantage of the fact that in guinea pigs, contrary to mice, the *Ir* genes detected in inbred strains are also found in a significant proportion of random-

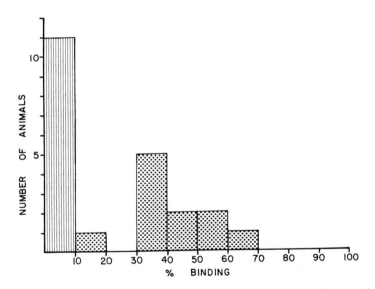

Fig. 3.   Antibody response to 0.5 mg of linear random copolymer of L-glutamic acid and L-alanine (GA) in complete Freund's adjuvant of individual inbred strain 2 (stippled bars) and strain 13 (vertical hatched bar) guinea pigs expressed as percent binding of GAT-^{125}I by 1–10 dilution of antiserum. From Bluestein *et al.* (1971a), by permission of The Rockefeller University Press, New York.

TABLE III

INHERITANCE OF SPECIFIC *Ir* GENES AND OF THE MAJOR HISTOCOMPATIBILITY LOCUS OF STRAIN 2 AND STRAIN 13 GUINEA PIGS BY (2 × 13)F₁ AND BACKCROSS ANIMALS

Antigens	Strain			(2 × 13)F₁ × 13		(2 × 13)F₁ × 2	
	2	13	(2 × 13)F₁	50%[a]	50%	50%	50%
DNP-PLL ⎫	+[b]	−[b]	+	+	−		
GL ⎭							
GA	+	−	+	+	−		
GT	−	+	+			+	−
BSA 0.1 μg	+	−	+	+	−		
HSA 1 μg	+	−	+				
DNP-BSA 1 μg	+	−	+	+	−	+	−
DNP-GPA 1 μg	−	+	+				
Major H Locus							
Strain 2	+[b]		+	+	−		
Strain 13		+	+			+	−

[a] Column identifies the same group of backcross animals.

[b] Plus indicates responsiveness and presence of major histocompatibility specificities; minus indicates nonresponsiveness and absence of major histocompatibility specificities of the inbred strains.

bred animals. The genes controlling immune responsiveness to GA, GT, and PLL are not inherited independently. As we have seen, the *GA* gene and the *PLL* gene are linked in strain 2 and (2 × 13)F₁ guinea pigs. Responsiveness to GA and PLL are also linked in most Hartley responder guinea pigs. However, there is a small proportion of Hartley guinea pigs which respond to GA and not to PLL or to PLL and not to GA, as illustrated in Fig. 4. The existence of random-bred animals which respond to GA and not to PLL which may result from crossover between the *PLL* gene and the *GA* gene may be considered evidence for the nonidentity of these two genes (Bluestein *et al.*, 1971b).

Similarly, the ability to respond to GT in random-bred Hartley animals is also not independent of the PLL or GA responder status. But in this case, responsiveness to GT tends to segregate away from

PLL and GA responsiveness, indicating allelism or pseudo-allelism between the *GT* gene on the one part and the *PLL* and *GA* genes on the other, in random bred animals (Fig. 5) (Bluestein *et al.*, 1971b).

In summary, distinct *Ir* genes have been identified in inbred strain 2 and 13 guinea pigs and in random-bred Hartley animals. In strain 2 guinea pigs, the genes controlling responsiveness, respectively, to PLL antigens, to GA, and to low doses of BSA are linked. Other genes have been identified in strain 13 guinea pigs which control, respectively, responsiveness to GT and to limiting doses of DNP-GPA. In random-bred animals, crossing over may have occurred between the *PLL* gene and the *GA* and *BSA-I* genes. Furthermore, the *GT* gene tends to behave as an allele or pseudo-allele to the *PLL* and *GA* genes.

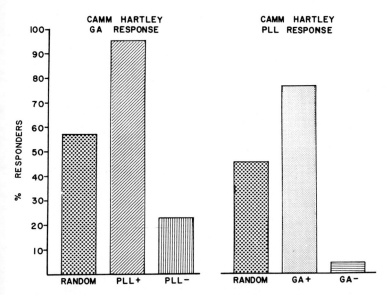

Fig. 4.   Frequency of responsiveness to GA as a function of PLL responsiveness, and frequency of PLL responsiveness as a function of GA responsiveness in random-bred Hartley guinea pigs simultaneously immunized with DNP-PLL and GA. Columns labeled "random" indicate the frequency of responders in the unselected population. PLL+ and GA+ indicate responders to these antigens. From Bluestein *et al.* (1971b), by permission of The Rockefeller University Press, New York.

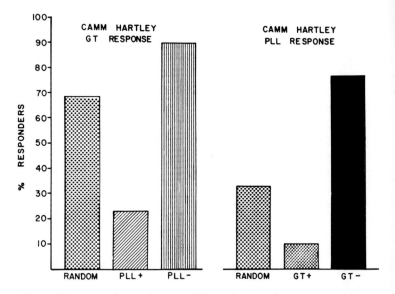

Fig. 5. Frequency of responsiveness to GT as a function of PLL responsiveness and frequency of PLL responsiveness as a function of GT responsiveness in random-bred Hartley guinea pigs immunized with DNP-PLL and GT. Columns labeled "random" indicate the frequency of responders in the unselected population. PLL+ and GT+ indicate responders to these antigens. From Bluestein *et al.* (1971b), by permission of The Rockefeller University Press, New York.

These relationships between individual guinea pig *Ir* genes will be better understood when the linkage between specific immune response genes and histocompatibility specificities detected originally in inbred strains is shown to be largely preserved in random-bred guinea pigs.

III. Mouse *Ir* Genes

Similar to what was found in guinea pigs, specific immune response genes controlling responsiveness to synthetic polypeptides and to limiting doses of protein antigens have been identified in mice. However, homopolymers and linear copolymers of 2 L-amino acids which are antigenic in guinea pigs are not immunogenic for mice (Pinchuck and Maurer, 1968). Immunogenicity for mice begins with copolymers of 3 L-amino acids. McDevitt and Sela (1965) have studied most thoroughly a set of branched multichain synthetic copolymers with a restricted range of amino acids; L-glutamic acid with L-tyrosine or with either L-histidine or L-phenylalanine, on a backbone of L-lysine and DL-alanine side chains, (T,G)-A–L, (H,G)-A–L and (Phe,G)-A–L. The ability of inbred mice to make antibodies, in response to each of these antigens, is a quantitative genetic trait controlled by autosomal dominant genes at a locus designated *Ir-1*. These polypeptides are not immunogenic in random-bred Swiss mice. It is not known whether the *Ir-1* locus is a single gene with multiple alleles, or three closely linked genes, although the evidence is most compatible with the latter interpretation. The immunogenicity of several linear terpolymers has similarly been found to be under dominant unigenic control and linked to *H-2* genotype in our and Maurer's laboratories. We should specially mention the response to one of these, a terpolymer of L-glutamic acid, L-alanine, and L-lysine (GAT), which is of particular interest because, in contrast with the branched polypeptides of McDevitt and Sela, the antibody response to GAT, as shown in Fig. 6, is completely dependent on the presence of the specific *Ir* gene (Martin *et al.*, 1971; Merryman and Maurer, 1971).

It is also very important to recognize that in mice the cellular or humoral immune response to several weak allogeneic antigens has been shown to be under *H-2* linked dominant unigenic control. We will mention only two of the most striking examples: (1) the capacity to form antibodies against allotypic determinants on IgA and IgG myelomas discovered by Lieberman and Humphrey (1971), and (2) the ability of female recipients to reject male syngeneic skin grafts and therefore to recognize a histocompatibility antigen controlled by the Y chromosome which was discovered by Gasser and Silvers (1971) (Table I).

IV. The Linkage of Specific *Ir* Genes with the Major Histocompatibility Locus of the Species in Inbred Mice and Guinea Pigs

From the genetic point of view, a remarkable feature of the immune response genes which we are discussing this evening is their intimate linkage in several species (Table I) with genes controlling

BARUJ BENACERRAF

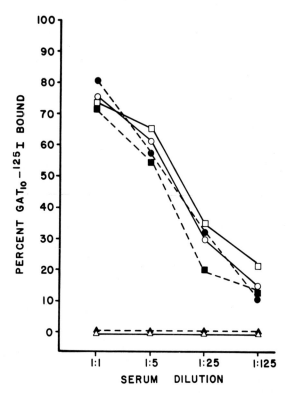

FIG. 6. Antibody response to GAT of several congenic mouse strains differing at the *H-2* locus. Antibody is expressed as % GAT-^{125}I bound by dilutions of pooled sera obtained 3 weeks after immunization. No significant binding was detected with sera from B10.P (△——△) or B10.S (▲ - - - ▲) mice. ○——○, B10; ● - - - ●, B10.A; □——□, B10.Br; ■ - - - ■, B10.D$_2$. From Martin *et al.* (1971), *J. Immunol.*, by permission of The Williams & Wilkins Co., Baltimore, Maryland.

histocompatibility specificities, as was shown in Fig. 6 with GAT in mice congenic at the *H-2* locus. The first evidence of such a linkage was provided in mice by the observations of McDevitt and Chinitz (1969) on *Ir-1* and *H-2*: that the responsiveness of inbred mice to (T,G)-A–L, (H,G)-A–L, and (Phe,G)-A–L could be predicted on the basis of their *H-2* genotype.

During the past 3 years extensive studies have been made by

McDevitt *et al.* (1972) to localize *Ir-1* in the *H-2* locus with mice bearing known recombinant *H-2* alleles. The result of these studies has established that *Ir-1* genes map in the middle of the H-2 chromosome region, lying just to the right of the *Ss* (serum substance) locus, and just to the left of the K region major specificities, in the right-hand part of the *H-2* locus (Fig. 7). It is important to stress, however, that these data did not establish nor rule out that *Ir-1* may code for distinct histocompatibility specificities.

In contrast to the linkage of *Ir-1* to *H-2*, this locus was shown *not* to be linked to the genes controlling allotypes of the H chains of mouse immunoglobulins (McDevitt and Benacerraf, 1969).

Similarly, the antibody response of mice to limiting doses of protein antigens was found by Vaz and Levine (1970) to be also

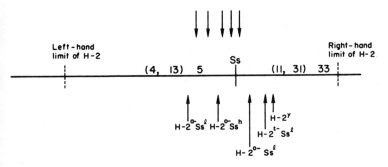

Fig. 7. Diagram of the organization of the *H-2* locus, with arrows indicating the approximate position of crossovers resulting in recombinant *H-2* alleles. The top arrows indicate a set of five reciprocal crossovers between *H-2ᵃ* and *H-2ᵇ* to give rise to *H-2ʰ* and *H-2¹* recombinant alleles. All five of these recombinant alleles localize *Ir-1* to the right of the crossover event. The three bottom arrows indicate a set of three reciprocal crossovers between *H-2ᵈ* and *H-2ᵏ*, giving rise to *H-2ᵃ⁻Ss¹*, *H-2⁰⁻Ss¹*, and *H-2⁰⁻Ssʰ*. Once again, *Ir-1* is located to the right of these crossovers. *H-2ᵗ⁻Ss¹* was derived from a crossover between *H-2ᵃ⁻Ss¹* and *H-2ˢ*, and *Ir-1* is located to the left of this crossover. *H-2ʸ* is derived from a crossover between *H-2ᵃ* and *H-2ᵠ*, and in this crossover event there was an outide marker (brachyury, T) which established that the crossover was a single crossover event. *Ir-1* was also localized to the left of this crossover. Since *Ir-1* is to the left of the last two crossovers, and the crossovers are known to be to the right of the serum substance (*Ss*) locus, these results definitely localize *Ir-1* between the *Ss* locus and the *K* region *H-2* antigenic specificities. From B. Benacerraf and H. O. McDevitt (1972). Reprinted from *Science* **175,** 273–279. Copyright 1972 by the American Association for the Advancement of Science.

TABLE IV

Analysis of Inheritance of Specific *Ir* Genes and Major
Histocompatibility Specificities in Inbred Guinea Pigs

---

1. $(2 \times 13)F_1$ animals are backcrossed with parental strains.
2. The response of the backcross offspring to the relevant antigens is studied.
3. The lymph node cells of individual animals are tested for the presence of major strain 2 or strain 13 specificities (a) with specific alloantisera and complement using the ^{51}Cr release assay, (b) by mixed leukocyte culture assay.

---

linked to *H-2* although in this case the precise location of the *Ir* gene in the *H-2* locus has not yet been ascertained.

Identical linkage between specific *Ir* gene and major histocompatibility specificities of the species has been demonstrated in guinea pigs in our laboratory with the added advantage that these studies could be extended to random-bred animals. The general approach employed in these experiments is shown in Table IV. In inbred strains the *PLL*, *GA*, and *BSA-1* genes were shown to be linked to the locus controlling the major histocompatibility specificities of strain 2 guinea pigs (Table III). The data establishing linkage between the *PLL* gene and the major histocompatibility locus of strain 2 guinea pigs are shown in Fig. 8 (Ellman *et al.*, 1970a). Similarly, the *GT* gene and the gene controlling responsiveness to limiting doses of DNP-GPA were found to be linked in strain 13 guinea pigs to the major *H* locus of this inbred strain as shown in Table V (Bluestein *et al.*, 1971c; Green *et al.*, 1972).

V. The Linkage of Specific Ir Genes with Major Strain 2 or
Strain 13 Histocompatibility Specificities in
Random-Bred Guinea Pigs

The issue must be considered whether the specific *Ir* genes of guinea pigs which we are discussing are identical with genes controlling major histocompatibility specificities, or, if they are closely linked with them, how close indeed is the linkage. This question has, so far, been explored only with the *PLL* gene and the *GT* gene, taking advantage of the fact that these genes are expressed both in inbred and also in some random-bred Hartley guinea pigs. To investigate these possibilities, 78 random-bred Hartley guinea pigs (42 PLL responders and 36 nonresponders) have been tested for the presence of strain 2 specificities on their lymphocytes with anti-strain 2 alloantisera prepared in strain 13 guinea pigs. The results of these experiments are found in Table VI. In each of these animals, without exception, possession of the *PLL* gene was always associated with

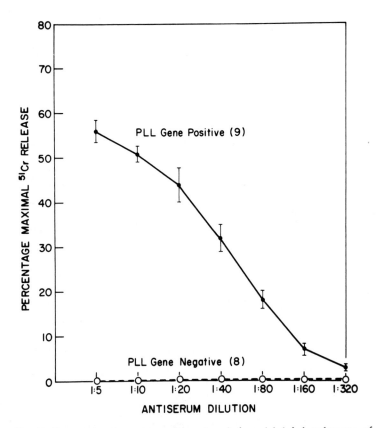

Fig. 8. Percentage of maximum ^{51}Cr released from labeled lymphocytes of $(2 \times 13)F_1 \times 13$ backcross guinea pigs exposed to varying concentrations of anti-strain 2 isoantiserum and complement. The vertical bars represent the standard errors of values obtained from nine responders and eight nonresponder offspring. From Ellman *et al.* (1970a), by permission of The National Academy of Sciences, Washington, D.C.

TABLE V

A. Relationship between GT Responsiveness and the Presence of Major Strain 13 Histocompatibility Antigens in $(2 \times 13)F_1$ Backcross Progeny

Number $(2 \times 13)F_1 \times 2$ backcross	Cellular and humoral anti-GT response	Anti-strain 13 cytotoxicity[a] (% ^{51}Cr release)
9	++++	32.8
8	—	3.5

B. Relationship between Anti-DNP Antibody Response to 1 µg DNP_6-GPA and the Presence of Major Strain 13 Histocompatibility Antigens in $(2 \times 13)F_1 \times 2$ Backcross Progeny

Number $(2 \times 13)F_1 \times 2$ backcross	% Binding DNP-3H-lysine by antiserum, (mean and SE)	Anti-strain 13 cytotoxicity[a] (% ^{51}Cr release)
7	85 ± 4	24.4 ± 2
7	7 ± 3	$1.2 \pm .6$

[a] Specific ^{51}Cr release from target lymph node cells incubated with strain 2 anti-strain 13 alloantiserum and complement.

TABLE VI

Relationship between Possession of the *PPL* Gene, as Shown by Responsiveness to DNP-PLL, and the Presence of Strain 2 Histocompatibility Specificities in Random-Bred Guinea Pigs

Hartley guinea pigs		NIH multipurpose guinea pigs	
Mean % ^{51}Cr release by $\frac{1}{5}$ anti-strain 2 alloantiserum and complement			
42 DNP-PLL responders	36 DNP-PLL nonresponders	1 DNP-PLL responder	14 DNP-PLL nonresponders
27.2	0.3	51	0.2

susceptibility to lysis of the cells by anti-strain 2 antisera and complement. In contrast, the cells from PLL negative animals were not susceptible to lysis by these antisera (Ellman *et al.*, 1971). With respect to the *GT* gene in random bred animals, the situation is more complex and also more interesting: the ability to respond to GT as shown in Table VII is associated with only some, but not all, of the strain 13 specificities detected in Hartley guinea pigs (Bluestein *et al.*, 1971d).

Thus, all the evidence in both mice and guinea pigs is compatible with the view that the histocompatibility-linked immune response genes map within the *H-2* locus in the mouse and are equally closely associated with the major histocompatibility locus in the guinea pig if not identical with genes coding for some of these specificities.

At this early stage, no simple explanation may be proposed to account for the relationship between *Ir* genes and the major histocompatibility loci of several species. Although this relationship is possibly fortuitous, in our opinion it is more reasonable, as well as more challenging, to consider it a fundamental feature of the immune mechanism and of its discriminating capacity, implying a fundamental relationship between individual specificity and the ability of a class of immunocompetent cells to recognize foreignness. We shall

TABLE VII

LINKAGE BETWEEN THE *GT* GENE AND THE LOCUS CODING FOR ONE OF THE MAJOR STRAIN 13 HISTOCOMPATIBILITY SPECIFICITIES IN HARTLEY GUINEA PIGS

GT status	Number of animals	Percent release ^{51}Cr[a]	
		Unabsorbed serum	Absorbed serum
Responder	25	56.1[b]	43.3
Nonresponder type I	8	0.84	0
Nonresponder type II	4	35.8	2.4

[a] The percent ^{51}Cr released by a 1–5 dilution of a strain 2 anti-strain 13 isoantiserum (unabsorbed serum) or by the same serum absorbed with spleen and lymph node cells from one of the type II GT nonresponders.

[b] Value expressed is the mean.

consider further the significance of this relationship when we discuss the process controlled by the *Ir* genes in the immune response.

However, the existence of genetic control of specific immune responses to a wide variety of antigens, all of which are linked to genes controlling major histocompatibility antigens, raises the possibility that this genetic control is, in fact, a manifestation of immunologic cross-reactivity between histocompatibility antigens and the foreign antigenic determinants under study, as well as the broader issue that the genetic control of immune responsiveness exemplified by the activity of *Ir* genes can be explained on the basis of tolerance to self-components related to the antigens studied.

I shall be unequivocal on this issue. There is a great deal of experimental evidence against this possibility and to date none in support of it. The observation that the F_1 between a responder and non-responder is a responder, although it possesses all the histocompatibility antigens of both parental strains, argues against the tolerance hypothesis. Furthermore, there are distinct examples of genetic control of immune responsiveness based on tolerance to self-components. These are all recessive, not dominant. For instance, guinea pigs genetically deficient in the C_4 component of complement will produce antibodies against this protein when immunized with antigen–antibody complexes and guinea pig complement. It is indeed this incidental finding which permitted the identification of C_4 deficient guinea pigs by Ellman *et al.* (1970b) in our laboratory and the development of the C_4 deficient line. The absence of C_4 as well as the ability to form antibodies against C_4 are recessive, not dominant, traits.

VI. The Cell Type Where Histocompatibility Linked *Ir* Genes Are Expressed

Let us consider now the cells where the class of *Ir* genes under discussion are expressed.

In the two systems most extensively studied, the *PLL* gene in guinea pigs and genes at the *Ir-1* locus in mice, responsiveness can be passively transferred to irradiated nonresponder recipient strains with immunocompetent cells from animals possessing the *Ir* genes, demonstrating that the genes are indeed expressed in cells which participate in the immune response. The adoptive transfer of the ability to mount both cellular and humoral immune responses to DNP-PLL to irradiated strain 13 guinea pigs (protected by strain 13 bone marrow) with responder (2 × 13)F₁ spleen and lymph node cells is illustrated in Fig. 9. It should be noted that, in these chimeras, the responding cells have been found to be of donor origin (Ellman *et al.*, 1970c). Thus, the *Ir* genes are expressed in immunocompetent cells. However, to identify the cell type involved, one must consider that the genetic complexities of the immune system have been magnified by the recent recognition of two pathways for the differentiation of antigen reactive cells. It is generally accepted nowadays that a class of lymphocytes from the bone marrow mi-

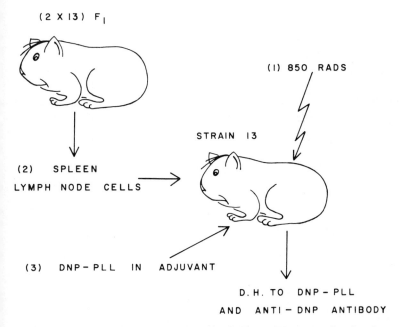

FIG. 9. Successful transfer of the ability to respond to DNP-PLL to irradiated strain 13 recipient guinea pigs protected by strain 13 bone marrow, with spleen and lymph node cells from normal (2 × 13)F₁ donors. The recipient animals developed both delayed hypersensitivity to DNP-PLL and high levels of anti-DNP antibodies. Control irradiated strain 13 recipients which received strain 13 cells did not respond.

grates to the thymus where the cells develop new surface antigens (Reif and Allen, 1964) and immunocompetence (Miller and Mitchell, 1969). These "thymus-derived" cells capable now of reacting specifically with antigen, migrate to the peripheral lymphoid tissues and recirculate in search of antigen through "thymus dependent" anatomical sites. These cells are responsible for the various phenomena of cell mediated immunity: delayed sensitivity, homograft and graft versus host reactions, etc., a major function of "thymus derived" lymphocytes or T cells being indeed the recognition of and reaction with histocompatibility antigens. "Thymus derived" lymphocytes are also concerned with the enhancement and regulation of the response to antigen by the other line of antigen-sensitive cells, the precursors of antibody secreting cells (Miller and Mitchell, 1970). This second lymphocyte cell line, which originates also in the bone marrow, settles directly in distinct anatomical sites in lymphoid tissues. These cells are usually referred to as "B cells." Thus, whereas phenomena of cellular immunity appear to depend exclusively upon "thymus derived" cells, specific antibody synthesis results, in large part, from the interaction of two specific cell types with antigen. The cooperation between "thymus derived" cells and B cells in antibody responses explains the fundamental observations of Landsteiner that antibodies may be produced against any structure or "hapten" provided it is bound to an immunogenic "carrier." In terms of the two-cell concept, now generally accepted, the "thymus derived" cell is the initial reactive cell which binds the carrier molecule (carrier function). As a result of this interaction the B cells bearing immunoglobulin receptors against the various determinants or "hapten" on the antigen are efficiently stimulated by the antigen (Katz and Benacerraf, 1972).

One may therefore conclude that the specificity of the two cell types need not be identical and that, whereas the specificity of the antibody-secreting cell precursor and the immunoglobulin nature of its receptors are easily identified from the product, the specificity of the "thymus derived" cell receptor has only been estimated indirectly from its reactivity to antigen. Moreover, the nature of the receptors on "thymus derived" cells is still a highly controversial problem. No convincing evidence has been produced as yet which identifies the receptors on "thymus-derived" cells as immunoglobulins whereas the receptors of the B lymphocytes have been easily identified as such. This uncertainty raises the possibility of a different class of receptors for antigen, distinct from immunoglobulin on thymus derived cells. This possibility becomes extremely relevant when considering the function of the histocompatibility linked *Ir* genes, which, as will be shown below, appear to be essentially concerned with immune phenomena attributed to "thymus derived" cells. This last statement is based on evidence from the guinea pig *Ir* genes and from the mouse *Ir-1* locus which display identical properties in every respect in both species. It is reasonable to conclude that this class of *Ir* genes controls the same process in the two species and that these genes may be considered models for other *Ir* genes similarly linked to histocompatibility genotype. First, in guinea pigs, those functions which are attributed essentially to the activity of "thymus derived" cells, such as cellular immunity and carrier function depend exclusively upon the presence of the relevant *Ir* gene. Thus, the reactions of cellular immunity to PLL, DNP-PLL, GA, and GT are totally under the control of the corresponding specific immune response genes. They are never observed in animals lacking the genes.

In addition, responsiveness to antigens under control of specific immune response genes is accompanied by antibody production to the haptens they bear. As illustrated in Table VIII, guinea pigs

TABLE VIII

Responses of Random-Bred Hartley Guinea Pigs to Immunization with Several Poly-l-Lysine Conjugates of Noncross-reacting Haptens

	Immune responses at 21 days			
Guinea pig No.	5-Dimethylamino 1-naphthalene sulfonyl-PLL	*p*-Toluene sulfonyl-PLL	2,4-Dinitrophenyl-PLL	Benzylpenicilloyl-PLL
1–11	Positive[a]	Positive	Positive	Positive
12–33	Negative	Negative	Negative	Negative

[a] A positive response is characterized by delayed sensitivity to 10 μg of hapten-PLL conjugates and by the production of antihapten antibodies.

capable of responding to DNP-PLL, because they possess the *PLL* gene, with the synthesis of anti-DNP antibodies, respond similarly to immunization with PLL conjugates of other noncross-reacting haptens, with vigorous antihapten synthesis. Guinea pigs lacking the *PLL* gene and incapable of responding to DNP-PLL are also incapable of responding to benzylpenecilloyl-PLL or to other un-

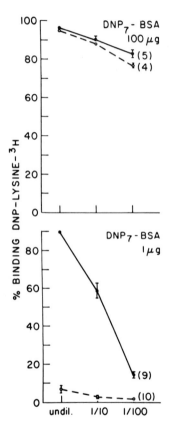

Fig. 10. Anti-DNP antibody response of strain 2 (●——●) and strain 13 (○ - - - ○) guinea pigs to 100 or 1 μg DNP$_7$-BSA. Data are expressed as percent binding of 0.1 ml 10^{-8} M DNP-lysine-^{3}H by globulin fraction of 0.1 ml of antiserum dilution. From Green and Benacerraf (1971), *J. Immunol.*, by permission of The Williams & Wilkins Co., Baltimore, Maryland.

related hapten PLL conjugates (Levine *et al.*, 1963b). This experiment indicates that the *PLL* gene is concerned with the specific recognition of the carrier molecules, which is known to be the function of thymus-derived cells. When sensitized T cells respond to the PLL carrier, the production of antibodies to the attached haptens by specific B cells is greatly enhanced.

A similar situation has been demonstrated in the genetic controls of the anti-DNP antibody responses to limiting doses of DNP_7-BSA or DNP_6-GPA (Figs. 10 and 11). As mentioned earlier (Table III), strain 2, but not strain 13, synthesizes anti-DNP antibodies when immunized with 1 μg DNP_7-BSA, whereas strain 13, but not strain 2, produces anti-DNP antibodies in response to 1 μg DNP_6-GPA (Green and Benacerraf, 1971). Furthermore, these anti-DNP responses are controlled by specific *Ir* genes linked to strain 2 H-specificity in the case of DNP_7-BSA and to strain 13 H-specificity in the case of DNP_6-GPA (Green *et al.*, 1972). The capacity to form anti-DNP antibody exists equally in both inbred strains, but it is determined by the genetically controlled recognition of the specificity of the carrier, again a function of thymus derived cells.

In other experiments use was again made of the cooperation between carrier-specific helper T cells and hapten specific cells, which is essential in the development of anti-hapten secondary antibody responses, to identify the cell type where the *Ir* gene is expressed. It is well established that optimal antihapten secondary responses require challenge with the hapten on the same carrier used for primary immunization. This requirement, which reflects the essential contribution of T and B cells, can, however, be obviated by supplemental immunization with an unrelated "immunogenic" carrier to stimulate the development of thymus derived cells specific for this second carrier, previous to challenge with the hapten-conjugate of this second carrier.

Such an experiment can be done using as the supplemental antigen GL, the response to which is under control of the *PLL* gene (Paul *et al.*, 1970). As shown in Fig. 12, DNP-ovalbumin (OVA) primed strain 2 and strain 13 guinea pigs received a supplemental immunization with GL in complete Freund's adjuvant and were challenged 3 weeks later with DNP-GL. Only strain 2 developed a secondary anti-DNP response. In contrast, strain 13 guinea pigs genetically

132 BARUJ BENACERRAF

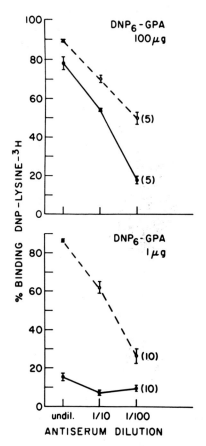

Fig. 11. Anti-DNP antibody in sera of strain 2 (●——●) and strain 13 (○ - - - ○) guinea pigs immunized with 100 or 1 μg DNP$_6$-GPA. Data are expressed as percent binding of 0.1 ml 10^{-8} M DNP-lysine-^{3}H by globulin fraction of 0.1 ml of antiserum dilution.

incapable of responding to GL showed a marked decrease in their serum level of anti-DNP antibodies after injection of DNP-GL.

This experiment establishes that GL can stimulate the development of GL specific helper cells only in strain 2 guinea pigs, which possess the *PLL* gene, but not in strain 13, which lack the gene. Thus, the activity of the *Ir* gene is essential for either the recognition of, or the response to, the carrier by specific thymus-derived helper cells, but not for the cells producing the specific antihapten antibody. If indeed the contribution of the genetically controlled helper cell is lacking, as in the nonresponder animal, the result is not only the absence of antihapten antibody synthesis, but rather the development of hapten-specific tolerance at the level of the antibody-secreting B cell precursors (Katz *et al.*, 1971).

The experiments discussed above and the conclusion we have reached of the necessary expression of the histocompatibility-linked *Ir* genes in T cells would lead one to predict that if a nonimmunogenic molecule such as DNP-PLL is administered to a nonresponder guinea pig, complexed with an immunogenic carrier which is able to stimulate thymus-derived cells specific for this carrier, an antibody response should be induced against DNP-PLL. This is precisely what

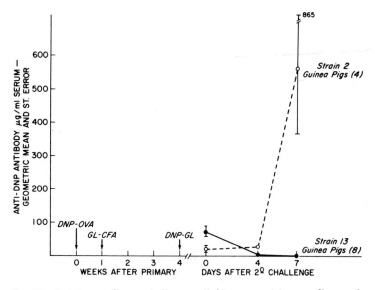

FIG. 12. Requirement for genetically controlled immunogenicity to mediate carrier function. Guinea pigs were primarily immunized with 3 mg of DNP-OVA intraperitoneally in saline. One week later, 100 μg of GL in complete Freund's adjuvant was administered. Three weeks later the animals were challenged with 1 mg of DNP_{20}-GL in saline. The numbers of animals in each group is shown in parentheses. From Paul *et al.* (1970), by permission of The Rockefeller University Press, New York.

happens when strain 13, or Hartley guinea pigs lacking the *PLL* gene, are immunized with DNP-PLL complexed with an immunogenic albumin, such as ovalbumin or acetylated bovine serum albumin, as shown in Table IX (Green *et al.*, 1966). Thus, DNP-PLL which is an immunogen in genetic responder animals may behave as a hapten in a nonresponder guinea pig. This experiment confirms that the genetic defect in nonresponder animals is not a result of the inability to synthesize antibodies to some determinants on the molecule. It may, however, be argued that these experiments have been done with antihapten antibodies. Similar data have also been obtained with carrier determinants, indicating that the capacity to form antibody against native determinants of genetically non-immunogenic molecules, although not detected, is potentially unimpaired in nonresponder animals. Thus, both genetic responder

TABLE IX

Anti-DNP Antibody Synthesis and Delayed Sensitivity to DNP-PLL in Responder and Nonresponder Hartley Guinea Pigs Immunized with DNP-PLL or with DNP-PLL Complexed with Immunogenic Albumins

Immunizing antigen in CFA	Number of animals	PLL genetic status	Delayed sensitivity	Anti-DNP antibody (mmoles hapten bound–ml serum $\times 10^{-10}$)[a]
100 μg DNP-PLL	6	Responders	Positive	36,700
	7	Nonresponders	Negative	370
100 μg DNP-PLL complexed with 80 μg ovalbumin	6	Responders	Positive	76,100
	4	Nonresponders	Negative	54,100
100 μg DNP-PLL complexed with 100 μg acet. BSA	10	Responders	Positive	88,400
	22	Nonresponders	Negative	111,500
Unimmunized controls	41			240

[a] Anti-DNP antibody was determined by equilibrium dialysis with DNP-EACA-^{3}H; 7.5 μg antibody may be bound by 1000 $\times 10^{-10}$ mM DNP hapten when both antibody sites are occupied.

mice and nonresponder mice to GAT were found by Dunham and Unanue in our laboratory to have similar numbers of lymphocytes in their spleen capable of binding ^{125}I-labeled GAT. In addition, Maurer and Merryman (1972) have also shown that GAT non-responder mouse strains may be stimulated to synthesize anti-GAT antibodies following immunization with GAT complexed with immunogenic methylated BSA.

Moreover, the recent findings of McDevitt and associates (presented in Fig. 13) on the cell type where the *Ir-1* genes are expressed are in complete agreement with the conclusion that histocompatibility linked genes are necessarily expressed in thymus-derived cells. Thus, responder and nonresponder strains form identical primary IgM antibody responses following immunization with (T,G)-A–L in saline. However, only the responder strains can synthesize IgG antibodies and develop secondary IgG responses (Grumet, 1972). Adult thymectomy does not affect the small IgM antibody synthesis to (T,G)-A–L by both strains, but completely suppresses the secondary IgG production of the responder strains. Thymectomy thus abolishes the genetic difference controlled by the *Ir-1* locus in the response to (T,G)-A–L (Mitchell *et al.*, 1972).

Convincing, although indirect, evidence has thus been obtained in both guinea pigs and mice for the necessary expression of histocompatibility-linked *Ir* genes in thymus-derived cells where they must perform a specific and essential function in the immune response. The issue whether *Ir* genes need to be expressed also in antibody-secreting cells has not been resolved as yet. It is clear, however, that H-linked *Ir* genes do not code directly for immunoglobulin sequences.

The critical question therefore is: What function do these H-linked *Ir* genes control in thymus derived cells? If the antigen receptors on T cells are not immunoglobulins, do the genes control another class of molecules responsible alone for the specificity of this type of lymphocyte? If, alternatively, T cells bind antigen through immunoglobulin receptors, do *Ir* genes control an additional though less specific level of interaction with protein antigens, required for these cells to be stimulated?

The possibility that histocompatibility linked *Ir* genes code in some way for antigen receptors of thymus derived cells, distinct

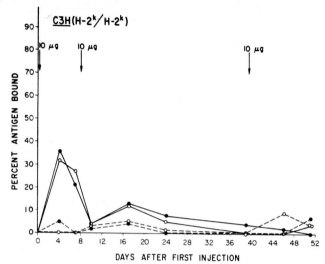

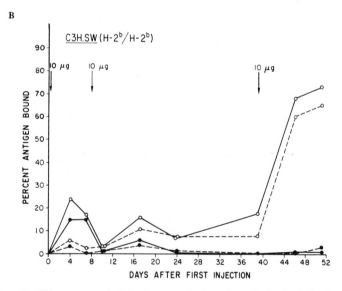

Fig. 13. The response of adult thymectomized or sham-thymectomized mice to 10 μg of aqueous (T,G)-A–L given intraperitoneally at times indicated. (A) C3H nonresponder mice. (B) C3H SW responder mice. ○——○, sham-thymectomized total antibody; ○ - - - ○, 2 ME resistant antibody; ●——●, thymectomized total antibody; ● - - - ,● 2 ME resistant antibody; From Mitchell *et al.* (1972), by permission of The Rockefeller University Press, New York.

from immunoglobulins, must be seriously considered. We realize that this represents an extremely revolutionary view in modern immunology where the dogma is very strong that immunological specificity in all classes of lymphocytes is contributed by immunoglobulins. This dogma is strongly supported by the faith of many immunologists that nature did not need to evolve several molecular systems for immune recognition and that the genetic problems presented by the generation of diversity in immunoglobulins are of sufficient magnitude to render unlikely the development of an independent specificity system for cellular immunity on thymocytes. The recognition that the specificity of T cells for antigen is at least as great and diverse as the specificity of humoral antibody for antigen has also been considered indirect although extremely strong evidence for the dogma.

However, attempts by many laboratories to detect immunoglobulin receptors for antigen on thymocytes by direct technology have proved to be very frustrating. Several investigators (Unanue and Karnovsky, 1972; Vitteta *et al.*, 1972) could not demonstrate immunoglobulin on the surface of thymocytes with techniques capable of detecting 10^3 molecules per cell. The most reliable positive study to date by Nossal *et al.* (1972) reported only about 10^3 molecules per T cell, an amount found also on erythrocytes; this finding places some doubt on the significance of these immunoglobulins as the main antigen receptors of thymus-derived cells. In contrast, several studies have shown that B cells possess around 10^5 immunoglobulin surface receptors capable of binding antigen specifically (Rabellino *et al.*, 1971; Vitteta *et al.* 1972). These results indicate that the precise nature of the antigen receptors of thymus-derived cells remains unresolved.

However, a recent experiment of Shevag *et al.* (1972) on the nature of the guinea pig *Ir* gene product provides some evidence in favor of the hypothesis that H-linked *Ir* genes code for specific antigen receptors distinct from immunoglobulins on the surface of thymus-derived cells. Anti-strain 2 and anti-strain 13 alloantisera were prepared by immunizing guinea pigs of each strain with lymphocytes and other tissues of the opposite strain. Then $(2 \times 13)F_1$ guinea pigs were immunized simultaneously with DNP-GL, an antigen the response to which is controlled by a strain 2 *Ir* gene, and with GT an antigen the response to which is controlled by a strain 13 *Ir* gene.

The $(2 \times 13)F_1$ animals possessing both genes respond to DNP-GL and GT and their peritoneal exudates lymphocytes cultured *in vitro* are stimulated by both antigens to display marked increased DNA synthesis. The *in vitro* response of sensitized $(2 \times 13)F_1$ lymphocytes to DNP-GL was specifically suppressed by anti-strain 2 antisera but not by anti-strain 13 antisera, whereas the stimulation of DNA synthesis in these same cells elicited by GT was specifically suppressed by anti-strain 13 but not by anti-strain 2 antisera. The inhibitory effects of the anti-2 or anti-13 alloantisera on specific blast transformation by DNP-GL or GT, respectively, were observed in the absence of complement and could not be suppressed by absorption of the antisera with guinea pig immunoglobulin.

The allelic behavior of the inhibition by antihistocompatibility antisera on the response of the $(2 \times 13)F_1$ cells is a significant built-in specificity control and suggests the presence in the F_1 guinea pig of two independent antigen receptors on the surface of thymus-derived cells, controlled by the respective *Ir* genes. However, this experiment does not indicate whether these receptors are clonally expressed. We should also comment on the precise specificity of the antibodies in the anti-strain 2 and anti-strain 13 antisera responsible for the inhibition observed. These antisera contain antibodies against the major histocompatibility specificities of each of the 2 guinea pig inbred strains, but they may also contain antibodies against alloantigens on the surface of thymus-derived lymphocytes. Further experiments will be needed to resolve this issue, but it is our feeling that the experiments of Shevag, Paul, and Green provide a promising and valid approach to the nature of the product of the histocompatibility linked *Ir* genes on T cells as well as some evidence that this product is distinct from immunoglobulins.

If indeed the hypothesis presented here that the H-linked *Ir* genes code for a unique class of specific antigen receptors on T cells is correct, it is not surprising that these genes are not linked to immunoglobulin allotypes, and also that other *Ir* genes not linked to histocompatibility but linked to immunoglobulin allotypes are being discovered. This second class of *Ir* gene should be concerned with the specificity of the antibodies expressed on B cells, and should be considered true immunoglobulin variable region structural genes.

VII.   THE HISTOCOMPATIBILITY LINKED *Ir* GENES AND DISEASE

The significance for medicine of the H-linked immune response genes depends only in part on our understanding of the nature of the *Ir* gene product. Whether their function represents merely a property of known histocompatibility antigenic specificities, or whether it represents a new class of antigenic receptors of thymus-derived lymphocytes, which we favor, there is considerable reason to believe that this type of genetic control of specific immune responses may play an important role in susceptibility to a variety of diseases in both animals and man. The practical importance of the relationship between *Ir* genes and histocompatibility specificity is exemplified in the manner in which histocompatibility typing, as shown in our guinea pig experiments, allowed us to predict the capacity of individual animals to form certain specific immune responses in random-bred populations of guinea pigs.

A practical example of the significance of this relationship is the demonstration by Lilly (1971) that one of the two major genes controlling susceptibility to Gross murine leukemia is linked to the right-hand part of the *H-2* locus. Similarly, susceptibility to Friend virus leukemia is also linked to *H-2*. It is reasonable to consider that the mechanism of these associations is via the activity of immune response genes, as resistance is dominant, and no relationship has been shown by Lilly between susceptibility to leukemia and the presence of virus receptors on the cells. These findings have stimulated similar studies of relationship in man between incidence of individual HL-A specificities and susceptibility to diseases where the immune response may play a part.

I would like finally to conclude that our present concept of the function and significance of H-linked *Ir* genes is still incomplete. However, we are much heartened by the remarkable progress made by several laboratories in the past few years, which permits the hope that we will soon develop a better understanding of the precise role of these genes in specific immune responses, and more important, of the evolutionary significance of the close relationship between these two highly polymorphic specificity systems: the histocompatibility specificities and the immune response genes.

ACKNOWLEDGMENTS

Many of the experiments described in this lecture have been carried out in collaboration with Bernard Levine, Ira Green, William Paul, Harry Bluestein, and Leonard Ellman. It is a pleasure to acknowledge their important contributions. I owe also a considerable debt to Hugh McDevitt, whose valuable discussions have to a great extent permitted the formulation of our present views on the function of H-linked *Ir* genes.

REFERENCES

Benacerraf, B., and McDevitt, H. O. (1972). *Science* **175,** 273.

Bluestein, H. G., Green, I., and Benacerraf, B. (1971a). *J. Exp. Med.* **134,** 458.

Bluestein, H. G., Green, I., and Benacerraf, B. (1971b). *J. Exp. Med.* **134,** 471.

Bluestein, H. G., Ellman, L., Green, I., and Benacerraf, B. (1971c). *J. Exp. Med.* **134,** 529.

Bluestein, H. G., Green, I., and Benacerraf, B. (1971d). *J. Exp. Med.* **134,** 1538.

Cohn, M. (1972). Personal communication.

Eichman, K., Brown, D., and Krause, R. (1971). *J. Exp. Med.* **134,** 48.

Ellman, L., Green, I., Martin, W. J., and Benacerraf, B. (1970a). *Proc. Nat. Acad. Sci. U.S.* **66,** 322.

Ellman, L., Green, I., and Frank, M. (1970b). *Science* **170,** 74.

Ellman, L., Green, I., and Benacerraf, B. (1970c). *Cell. Immunol.* **1,** 445.

Ellman, L., Green, I., and Benacerraf, B. (1971). *J. Immunol.* **107,** 382.

Gasser, D. L., and Silvers, W. K. (1971). *J. Immunol.* **106,** 875.

Green, I., and Benacerraf, B. (1971). *J. Immunol.* **107,** 374.

Green, I., Paul, W. E., and Benacerraf, B. (1966). *J. Exp. Med.* **123,** 859.

Green, I., Inman, J. K., and Benacerraf, B. (1970). *Proc. Nat. Acad. Sci. U.S.* **66,** 1267.

Green, I., Paul, W. E., and Benacerraf, B. (1972). *J. Immunol.* **109,** 457.

Grumet, F. C. (1972). *J. Exp. Med.* **135,** 110.

Katz, D. H., and Benacerraf, B. (1972). *Advan. Immunol.* **15,** 1.

Katz, D. H., Davie, J. M., Paul, W. E., and Benacerraf, B. (1971). *J. Exp. Med.* **134,** 201.

Levine, B. B., Ojeda, A., and Benacerraf, B. (1963a). *J. Exp. Med.* **118,** 953.

Levine, B. B., Ojeda, A., and Benacerraf, B. (1963b). *Nature (London)* **200,** 544.

Lieberman, R., and Humphrey, W., Jr. (1971). *Proc. Nat. Acad. Sci. U.S.* **68,** 2510.

Lieberman, R., and Humphrey, W., Jr. (1972). *J. Exp. Med.* **136,** 1222.

Lilly, F. (1971). *Proc. 2nd Convocation Immunol. Buffalo, 1970,* p. 103. Karger, New York.

McDevitt, H. O., and Benacerraf, B. (1969). *Advan. Immunol.* **11,** 31.

McDevitt, H. O., and Chinitz, A. (1969). *Science* **163,** 1207.

McDevitt, H. O., and Sela, M. (1965). *J. Exp. Med.* **122,** 517.

McDevitt, H. O., Deak, B. D., Shreffler, D. C., Klein, J., Stimpfling, J. H., and Snell, G. D. (1972). *J. Exp. Med.* **135,** 1259.

Martin, W. J., Maurer, P. H., and Benacerraf, B. (1971). *J. Immunol.* **107,** 715.

Maurer, P. H., and Merryman, C. F. (1972). Personal communication.

Merryman, C. F., and Maurer, P. H. (1971). *Fed. Proc., Fed. Amer. Soc. Exp. Biol.* **30,** 470.

Merryman, C. F., Maurer, P. H., and Bailey, D. W. (1972). *Fed. Proc., Fed. Amer. Soc. Exp. Biol.* **31,** 777.

Miller, J. F. A. P., and Mitchell, G. F. (1969). *Transplant. Rev.* **1,** 3.

Miller, J. F. A. P., and Mitchell, G. F. (1970). *J. Exp. Med.* **131,** 675.

Mitchell, F. G., Grumet, F. C., and McDevitt, H. O. (1972). *J. Exp. Med.* **135,** 126.

Nossal, G. J. V., Warner, N. L., Heather, L., and Sprent, L. (1972). *J. Exp. Med.* **135,** 405.

Paul, W. E., Katz, D. H., Goidl, E. A., and Benacerraf, B. (1970). *J. Exp. Med.* **132,** 283.

Pinchuck, F., and Maurer, P. H. (1968). *In* "Regulation of the Antibody Response" (B. Cinader, ed.), p. 97. Thomas, Springfield, Illinois.

Rabellino, E., Colon, S., Grey, H. M., and Unanue, E. R. (1971). *J. Exp. Med.* **133,** 156.

Reif, A. E., and Allen, J. M. V. (1964). *J. Exp. Med.* **120,** 413.

Shevag, E., Paul, W. E., and Green, I. (1972). *J. Exp. Med.* **136,** 1207.

Unanue, E. R., and Karnovsky, M. (1972). *J. Exp. Med.* **136,** 907.

Vaz, N. M., and Levine, B. B. (1970). *Science* **168,** 852.

Vaz, N. M., Vaz, E. M., and Levine, B. B. (1970). *J. Immunol.* **106,** 875.

Vitteta, E. S., Bianco, C., Nussenzweig, V., and Uhr, J. (1972). *J. Exp. Med.* **136,** 81.

Vladiutiu, A. O., and Rose, N. R. (1971). *Science* **174,** 1137.

Wurzburg, V. (1971). *Eur. J. Immunol.* **1,** 496.

THE CHEMICAL SYNTHESIS OF AN ENZYME*

BRUCE MERRIFIELD

The Rockefeller University, New York, New York

I. Introduction

THE complexity of the proteins presents an unparalleled challenge to the synthetic chemist, and it is only recently that he has been in a position to respond in a meaningful way. Until now essentially all that has been learned about this class of compounds has come from studies on the naturally occurring proteins themselves. The accumulated body of knowledge is enormous, and very much is known about the composition and structure of the proteins and how they function. There are certain questions, however, which cannot be answered easily in this way and for these questions the synthetic approach should provide a valuable alternative. If we could learn how to synthesize proteins in the laboratory it should become possible to make specific, well defined changes in their structures which could give answers that are hard to derive from studies on the native molecules. In certain special cases, such as the unusually reactive residues at the active sites of enzymes, it has been possible to modify individual amino acid residues selectively, but suppose it were to become important to modify or replace one particular valine residue in the protein; methods simply are not available to carry out such changes in the presence of many other similar groups within the same very sensitive macromolecule.

The three-dimensional structure of a small protein, ribonuclease, is shown in Fig. 1 to illustrate the kind of molecule we are talking about and to illustrate the magnitude of the synthetic task. This crystalline molecule (Kunitz, 1940) contains 124 amino acids in a single polypeptide chain, cross-linked by four disulfide bonds, with 1852 atoms precisely arranged in space in a well defined three-dimensional structure. A chemical synthesis of ribonuclease A means,

* Lecture delivered November 18, 1971.

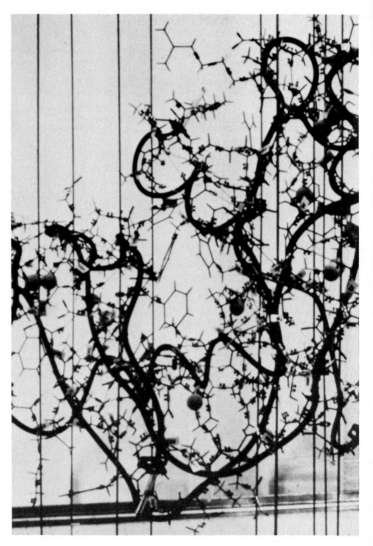

Fig. 1. The three-dimensional structure of bovine pancreatic ribonuclease. Taken from the model of RNase S by Wyckoff *et al.* (1967) which was deduced from X-ray diffraction data at 3.5 Å resolution and chemical sequence data. The heavy tubing outlines the general contours of the polypeptide backbone, and the fine wire structures show the positions of the amino acid side chains. Reproduced by permission of the American Society of Biological Chemists, Inc.

therefore, that each of these atoms must be assembled in the laboratory into exactly this same sequence and structure. An understanding of the problem can be greatly simplified, first, by looking at a two-dimensional picture in which the amino acid residues, rather than the individual atoms, are indicated as the basic units of the structure (Fig. 2) and, second, by recalling the important hypothesis of Anfinsen and his associates (White, 1961; Epstein et al., 1962) that the tertiary structure of this protein is determined by its primary structure. Thus, there was good reason to believe that if the amino acids could be assembled into the correct sequence the resulting molecule would direct its own folding and cross-linking to give the native protein, and a total synthesis of an enzyme would have been achieved.

In principle, a protein can be synthesized by either of two general approaches; by the classical method or by the solid phase method. The classical method (see Schröder and Lübke, 1965) involves the preparation of small peptides (fragments), the combination of these small fragments into larger peptides, and eventually the assembly of the larger fragments into the final protein molecule. All these reactions are carried out in homogeneous solution, and the essential feature of this technique is the opportunity to isolate and purify the product after each reaction. This helps to ensure high purity and careful identification of intermediates.

The most dramatic application of the classical technique to the synthesis of a protein occurred in the period between 1963 and 1965, with the nearly simultaneous synthesis of insulin by groups in Germany, the United States, and China (Meienhofer et al., 1963; Katsoyannis et al., 1964; Kung et al., 1965). At the present time, syntheses of proinsulin, ribonuclease T_1, staphylococcal nuclease, myoglobin, growth hormone and, no doubt, several other proteins are under way. As far as I know none of these has been completed, but two or three can be expected soon. The problems, of course, are enormous. Large numbers of synthetic reactions and purification steps are involved, and much time, expense, and manpower is required.

A variation of the strictly classical method, in which very rapid Leuchs anhydride couplings were employed, was applied successfully to the synthesis of S-protein (residues 21–124 of ribonuclease)

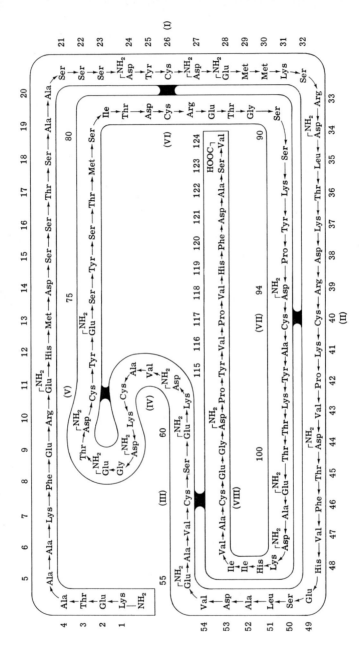

Fig. 2. The two-dimensional structure of bovine pancreatic ribonuclease A, showing the linear, 124 amino acid residue polypeptide chain cross-linked by the four disulfide bonds. The amino acids are indicated by their three-letter abbreviations. From Smyth *et al.* (1963), by permission of The American Society of Biological Chemists, Inc.

by Hirschmann *et al.* (1969). This accelerated technique eliminated the need for isolation of every intermediate, but permitted the isolation and purification of protected fragments. After noncovalent binding with S-peptide (residues 1–20) the resulting ribonuclease S possessed enzymatic activity.

The second general approach to the chemical synthesis of proteins is called solid phase peptide synthesis (Merrifield, 1963, 1969). The method was devised in our laboratory in an effort to overcome certain of the difficulties encountered with the classical methods. It is much faster and simpler to carry out and introduces sizable savings in manpower and materials. It has made possible our synthesis of ribonuclease A (Gutte and Merrifield, 1969, 1971). I would like to describe this technique in some detail and to discuss some of the difficulties and problems associated with it as well as some of the achievements.

II. SOLID PHASE PEPTIDE SYNTHESIS

The basic idea of the solid phase method is outlined in Fig. 3. It depends on the use of an insoluble solid support. The plan was to begin with an insoluble particle, indicated by the large circles, to functionalize it with a group, x, and to attach the first amino acid of the proposed peptide chain with a stable covalent bond by reaction at x. In practice we attach at the carboxyl of the amino acid (with the amino group protected), although in principle the attachment can also be at the amino group. The amino group is then deprotected, and the second amino acid is added to the first by a suitable peptide-forming reaction. In a similar way the subsequent amino acids are combined in a stepwise manner until the entire sequence has been assembled. Finally, the bond holding the peptide chain to the solid support is selectively cleaved, together with most side chain protecting groups, and the peptide is liberated into solution.

The advantage that I envisioned for this approach was the opportunity to purify intermediates after each reaction by simple, rapid washing procedures. Since the growing peptide chain would be completely insoluble as a consequence of its attachment to the large insoluble support, it could be filtered and washed with large volumes of solvents to remove reagents and by-products with no danger of losing the desired molecule. A related advantage, which was the real driving force behind the project, was the possibility that the

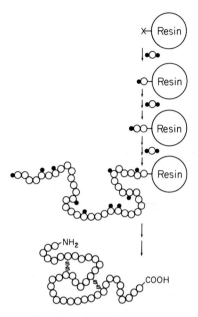

FIG. 3. The basic idea of solid phase peptide synthesis. The large circle represents the solid support, the small open circles represent amino acid residues, and the dark circles represent protecting groups and activating groups. From Merrifield, 1971, by permission of Gordon and Breach, New York.

process could be automated and thereby introduce further efficiency into the synthesis. It only remained to translate the general idea into a workable set of reactions.

The support which we have found to be most satisfactory is a copolymer of styrene and divinylbenzene, containing 1 or 2% of the cross-linking agent. The resulting beads are illustrated in Fig. 4. They are about 50 μm in diameter when dry and swell to nearly 8 times their volume in organic solvents such as the halogenated hydrocarbons. This means that the polystyrene chains are highly solvated during the chemical reactions and are readily accessible to diffusing reagents. The reactions occur not only at the surface of the bead, but, in major part, within the interior matrix of the bead. This could be readily demonstrated by autoradiography (Merrifield and Littau, 1968) of cross sections of beads containing a peptide in which tritiated proline had been incorporated. The gross distribution of peptide chains was quite uniform throughout the sections. The technique did not, however, have the resolving power to show the distribution at the molecular level and heterogeneity at that resolution is probable.

Many detailed chemical schemes have been devised to carry out solid phase synthesis. An early one which proved to be very useful is shown in Fig. 5. The aromatic rings of the styrene can be derivatized in several ways in order to provide an attachment site for the first amino acid. The first successful derivative was obtained by

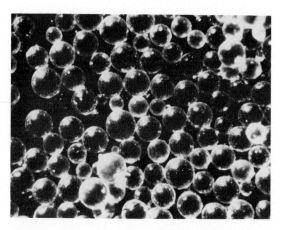

Styrene–divinylbenzene Copolymer

Fig. 4. The styrene-divinylbenzene copolymer support. The spheres average about 50 μm in diameter.

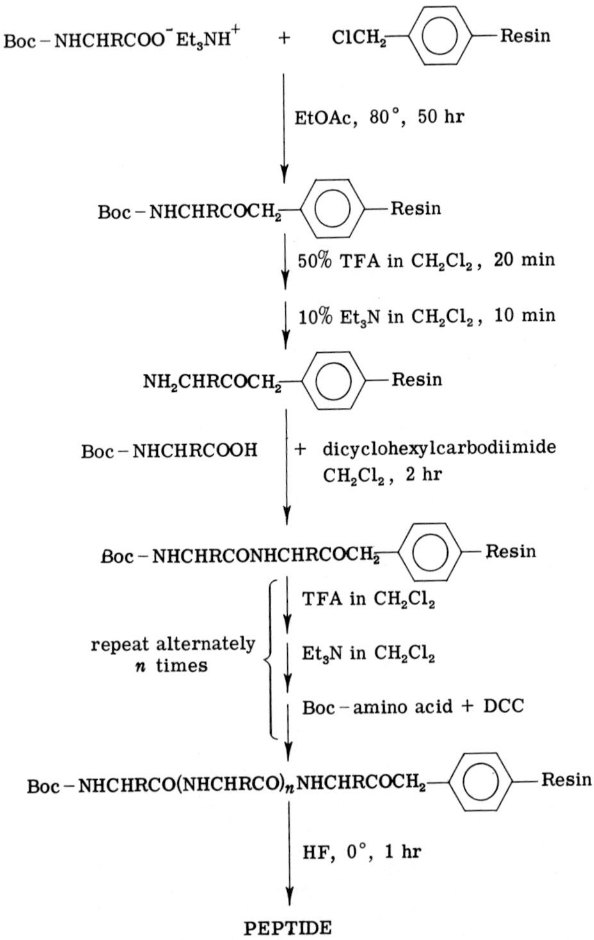

Boc − NHCHRCOO⁻ Et₃NH⁺ + ClCH₂−〈 〉−Resin

$$Boc-NHCHRCOO^- Et_3NH^+ \quad + \quad ClCH_2-\bigcirc-Resin$$

EtOAc, 80°, 50 hr

$$Boc-NHCHRCOCH_2-\bigcirc-Resin$$

50% TFA in CH_2Cl_2, 20 min

10% Et_3N in CH_2Cl_2, 10 min

$$NH_2CHRCOCH_2-\bigcirc-Resin$$

Boc − NHCHRCOOH + dicyclohexylcarbodiimide
CH_2Cl_2, 2 hr

$$Boc-NHCHRCONHCHRCOCH_2-\bigcirc-Resin$$

repeat alternately
n times

TFA in CH_2Cl_2

Et_3N in CH_2Cl_2

Boc − amino acid + DCC

$$Boc-NHCHRCO(NHCHRCO)_n NHCHRCOCH_2-\bigcirc-Resin$$

HF, 0°, 1 hr

PEPTIDE

Fig. 5. A scheme for solid phase peptide synthesis.

chloromethylation to give a substituted benzyl chloride which could be esterified by reaction with the triethylammonium salt of an N^α-protected amino acid. The resulting benzyl ester was carefully chosen because it is quite stable for the remainder of the synthesis but can be selectively cleaved at the end with strong anhydrous acid. In order to be compatible with the anchoring bond the amino protection should be relatively labile to acid, and the *t*-butyloxy-carbonyl (Boc) group is commonly employed for that reason. It can be removed by 1 N HCl or by 20% trifluoroacetic acid in methylene chloride, for example. The resulting amine salt is neutralized by a tertiary amine, such as triethylamine, and is then ready to couple to the next Boc-amino acid to form the first peptide bond. Any one of a number of peptide-forming reagents can be applied. We have found dicyclohexylcarbodiimide (Sheehan and Hess, 1955) to be especially useful. Subsequent amino acids are incorporated in exactly the same way by alternately repeating the deprotection and coupling reactions. The last step is the cleavage of the peptide from the resin by acidolysis of the anchoring benzyl ester bond. Hydrogen bromide in trifluoroacetic acid or hydrogen fluoride (Sakakibara *et al.*, 1967) are the methods of choice.

Each of the steps described here has been modified in several ways both in this laboratory and in others (see Marshall and Merrifield, 1971), and certain other changes are still necessary before the generally applicable, "ideal" system is evolved.

The reaction sequences just described can be illustrated by the synthesis of bradykinin, which is outlined in Fig. 6 (Merrifield, 1964). Bradykinin is a nonapeptide, derived from a plasma protein, with strong hypotensive and smooth muscle contracting properties. The solid phase synthesis began by attaching the protected C-terminal amino acid, Boc-nitroarginine, to the polystyrene support and proceeded by carrying out the three basic steps of deprotection, neutralization and coupling, alternately, eight times each until the final peptide sequence was assembled. The peptide was released from the resin by anhydrous HBr in trifluoroacetic acid, and at the same time some of the protecting groups were also removed. The remainder of the side chain protecting groups, in this case from the two nitroarginines, were removed by catalytic hydrogenation to give the crude bradykinin product. Purification by ion exchange chromatography finally gave analytically pure bradykinin, which was shown to have full biological activity when compared with the natural hormone.

Following this early synthesis large numbers of analogs of bradykinin (Stewart and Woolley, 1966) and several other small peptide

152   BRUCE MERRIFIELD

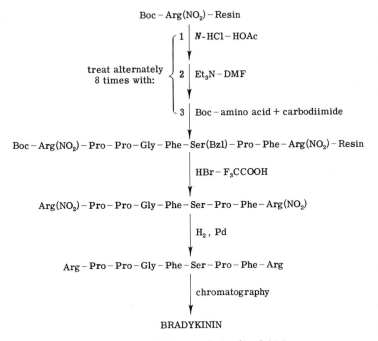

FIG. 6.   A solid phase synthesis of bradykinin.

hormones, such as angiotensin (Marshall and Merrifield, 1965) and oxytocin (Manning, 1968), have been synthesized by this same procedure and by various modifications of it. The method has been extended to insulin (Marglin and Merrifield, 1966) and to molecules such as ACTH, parathyroid hormone, secretin, valinomycin, trypsin inhibitor, several hormone-releasing factors, and a rather sizable number of model peptides for use in a variety of special problems.

The requirements for a successful synthesis by the solid phase method are: (1) rapid reactions, (2) quantitative reactions, (3) no side reactions. We can approach these requirements, but obviously we do not quite realize them even in the best case. In spite of the fact that these are heterogeneous reactions, they are very fast (Fig. 7), and there is no real problem in that regard. Some second-order rate constants for the coupling reaction have been measured which indicate that 99% of the reaction between the hindered amino acids isoleucine and valine required 140 seconds, while the coupling was 99% complete within 10 seconds for most unhindered amino acids.

At the moment the most pressing problem is to devise precise, sensitive, and rapid methods to monitor the coupling reaction, because an indication of quantitative bond formation is crucial to the success of the method. A number of techniques are at hand, but no one of them meets all the requirements satisfactorily. It is obviously not sufficient to measure the disappearance of the amino acid reagent because it is present in excess at the outset of the reaction and precision will only be of the order of a few percent, whereas we

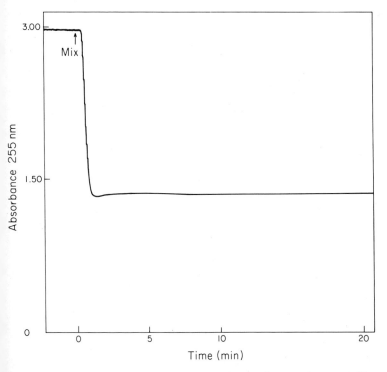

Fig. 7. A rate curve for the coupling reaction. Coupling reaction: Bpoc-Gly-anhydride $(1.6 \times 10^{-2} \ M)$ + Val-resin $(0.8 \times 10^{-2} \ M)$. $k_2 = 4.0$ liters/mole·sec. Bpoc = biphenylisopropyloxycarbonyl.

are looking for an accurate measure of the last tenths or even hundredths of a percent of the reaction. A more sensitive test is the determination of the amount of unreacted peptide chain, and several ways to measure the terminal amino group have been devised. It can be estimated by the ninhydrin reaction (Kaiser *et al.*, 1970) or, more quantitatively, by electrometric titration with perchloric acid (Brunfeldt *et al.*, 1969) or by titration of its hydrochloride (Dorman, 1969) or picrate salt (Gisin, 1972) or by conversion to a Schiff base and colorimetric assay of the aldehyde component (Esko *et al.*, 1968).

A second important and continuing effort is directed toward the identification and elimination of side reactions. Several have been examined in detail and can now be avoided, while others remain as special problems. Racemization, for example, has been the universal worry of peptide chemists since the time of Fischer. Loss of optical purity in a biologically active peptide usually will lead to an inactive molecule, and in all cases it will result in a diastereomeric mixture which is exceedingly difficult to purify. This area has received a great deal of attention, and both conventional and solid phase syntheses can be designed which result in a negligible degree of racemization. It is a remarkably fortunate circumstance that the urethane protecting groups for amino acids, which are among the best derivatives for synthetic reasons, also confer high resistance to racemization. The accumulated evidence from many syntheses confirms the belief that there is essentially no racemization by way of oxazolone intermediates in solid phase syntheses. It was discovered recently, however, that urethane-protected histidine derivatives can give rise to appreciable amounts of racemic products both by conventional couplings in solution and by solid phase couplings (Windridge and Jorgensen, 1971). The reaction probably proceeds by direct proton abstraction from the asymmetric α-carbon by the basic imidazole group, because the presence of an electron withdrawing substituent (dinitrophenyl) on the imidazole ring greatly reduced the effect. Work in our laboratory confirms their findings and shows that a *p*-toluene sulfonyl substituent on histidine essentially eliminates the racemization problem (Lin *et al.*, 1972).

Dr. Gisin has recently discovered another side reaction during a solid phase synthesis and, by studying its mechanism, has devised a way to eliminate it (Gisin and Merrifield, 1972). During the preparation of Boc-D-Pro-D-Val-L-Pro-resin it was observed that over 70% of the peptide had been lost from the resin. By examining each of the steps in the synthesis, it was found that the loss occurred during the customary 10-minute equilibration treatment of D-Val-L-Pro-resin with Boc-D-Val prior to addition of the coupling reagent. It was then shown that the product was D-Val-L-Pro-diketopiperazine and that its formation was strongly catalyzed by carboxylic acids—in this case by Boc-D-Pro (Fig. 8). Imino acid-containing dipeptides, such as those containing proline or N-methylalanine, are especially susceptible to the diketopiperazine formation because of the small energy difference between the cis and trans amide conformations. Once the problem was understood, a simple solution was forthcoming; the order of addition of reagents was reversed, the presence of free carboxylic acid was eliminated, and the catalysis of the ring closure was avoided. With this improvement Gisin has gone on to complete the stepwise solid phase synthesis of the very interesting valinomycin analog -[L-Val-D-Pro-D-Val-L-Pro]$_3$-. This

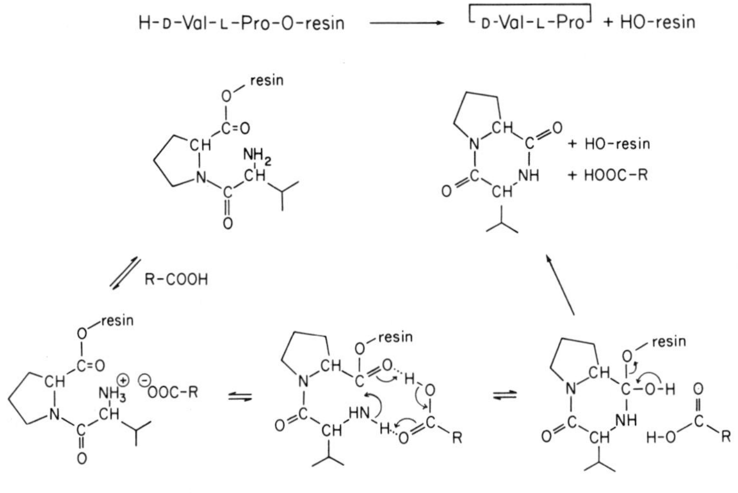

FIG. 8. The proposed mechanism for the acid-catalyzed formation of a diketo-piperazine. From Gisen and Merrifield (1972), by permission of the American Chemical Society, Washington, D.C.

is the first cyclic peptide composed entirely of amino acids that can selectively bind potassium and carry it from an aqueous solution into a hydrophobic organic phase.

Because the solid phase method in its usual form does not allow isolation of intermediates, some people feel that it can never be applied to the synthesis of high molecular weight products. I believe that it can be utilized for such problems at the present time and that, through the improvements which are constantly being made, the continuous, stepwise approach will eventually be the method of choice. For those who prefer to isolate protected intermediates, we have devised a new solid phase-fragment approach (Wang and Merrifield, 1969) in which small protected peptides are prepared on a resin support and, following cleavage and purification, are coupled in solution to give larger peptides. This technique, therefore, combines some of the best features of the solid phase and classical approaches into a unified procedure. In its initial and usual form, as already described here, the solid phase method produces partially

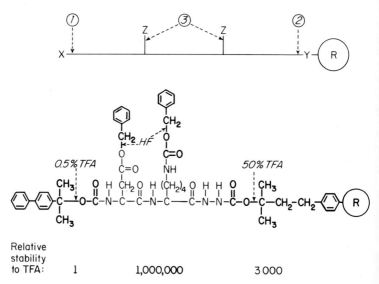

Fig. 9. A solid phase-fragment scheme. From Wang and Merrifield (1972), by permission of Munksgaard, Copenhagen.

or completely deprotected peptides following the cleavage step in strong acid. These products, of course, are not suited for further couplings because they contain functional side chains. To overcome the problem, three classes of protecting groups are needed which can be selectively removed, as illustrated in Fig. 9. The group on the α-amine must be readily removed at each step of the synthesis without loss of side chain protection or of the anchoring bond to the resin, and at the end of the synthesis it must be possible to cleave the anchoring bond without loss of side chain protection. Finally, after the intermediate protected peptide has been purified and coupled to other fragments it must be possible to completely deprotect the finished polypeptide. The scheme developed by Dr. Wang makes use of three greatly different degrees of acid stability. He uses the very labile biphenylisopropyloxycarbonyl (Bpoc) group of Sieber and Iselin (1968) for α-amine protection, relatively stable benzyl or tosyl groups for side chain protection, and a new linkage of intermediate stability for the carboxyl attachment. These groups differ by 3 and 6 orders of magnitude in their susceptibility to acid and, therefore, allow the satisfactory synthesis of protected fragments. A recent synthesis of an eledoisin analog will illustrate this general approach (Wang and Merrifield, 1972). The analog

$$Z-Lyx(Z)-Phe-Phe-Gly-O-\underset{\underset{CH_3}{|}}{\overset{\overset{CH_3}{|}}{C}}-CH_2-CH_2-\!\!\!\left\langle\bigcirc\right\rangle\!\!\!-Resin$$

was synthesized using Bpoc derivatives for the intermediate coupling steps and carbobenzoxy protection for the last step. The protected peptide was removed by 50% trifluoroacetic acid and was obtained as a pure crystalline product. It was coupled in solution with H-Leu-Met-OMe, crystallized, aminolyzed and finally deprotected to give H-Lys-Phe-Phe-Gly-Leu-Met-NH$_2$. The pure product showed the expected strong hypotensive action in the rat, which was equal to that of natural eledoisin itself.

Until now I have not discussed the mechanical aspects of this technique except to say that it was because of this potential feature that the solid phase method was developed in the first place. The ability to purify by simple filtration and washing and the fact that all reactions could be conducted within a single reaction vessel appeared to lend themselves ideally to a mechanized and automated process. Initially, a simple manually operated apparatus was constructed (Fig. 10), and later, together with Dr. Stewart, we designed and built the automated instrument shown in Fig. 11 (Merrifield *et al.*, 1966). The essential features were the reaction vessel containing the resin with its growing peptide chain and the necessary plumbing to enable the appropriate solvents and reagents to be pumped in, mixed, and removed in the proper sequence. The mechanical events were under the control of a simple stepping drum programmer and a set of timers. This instrument has been used for the synthesis of many small peptides and for the synthesis of ribonuclease A. In the past few years at least nine commercial instruments have been constructed in several countries. They differ considerably in detail, but are designed to carry out the same chemistry.

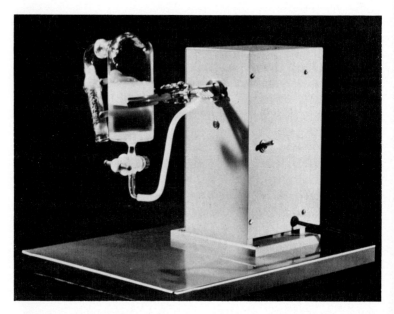

Fig. 10. A manually operated reaction apparatus, showing the glass reaction vessel with a fritted-glass filter disk and side arm. The resin is suspended by a rocking motion about the horizontal axis.

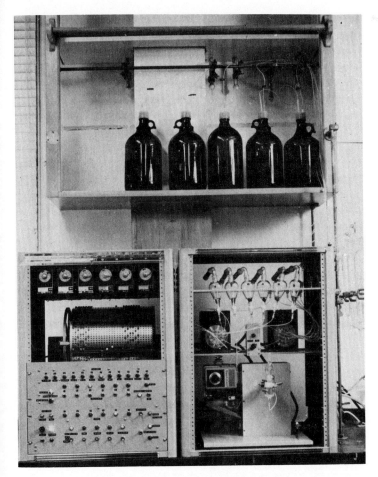

Fig. 11. The automated peptide synthesizer.

III. The Synthesis of Ribonuclease A

As a first step toward bringing to bear the synthetic approach to the study of enzymes we undertook the total synthesis of bovine pancreatic ribonuclease A (Gutte and Merrifield, 1969, 1971). This molecule, which has been so closely associated with this institution, was well suited for the synthetic work because it is small and

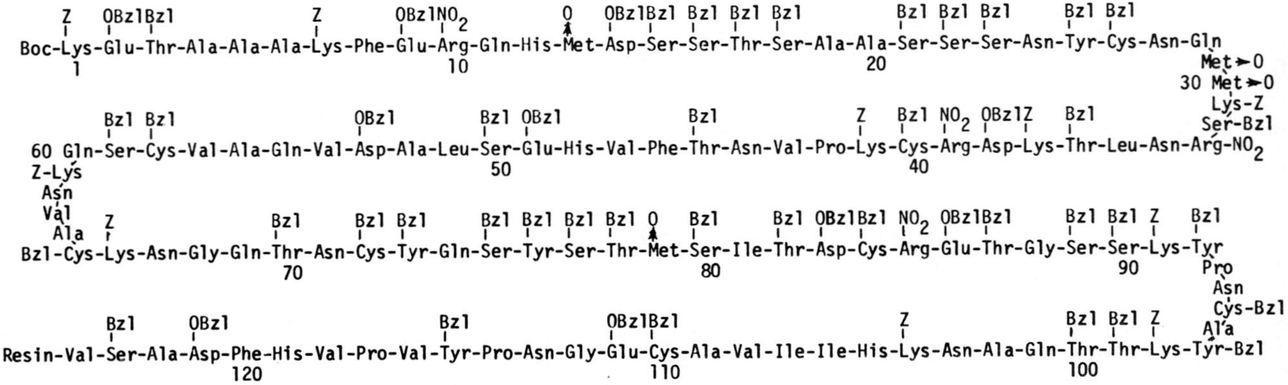

```
     Z       OBzlBzl               Z       OBzlNO2      O         OBzlBzl Bzl Bzl       Bzl Bzl
     |       |   |                 |       |   |        ‖         |    |   |   |         |   |
Boc-Lys-Glu-Thr-Ala-Ala-Ala-Lys-Phe-Glu-Arg-Gln-His-Met-Asp-Ser-Ser-Thr-Ser-Ala-Ala-Ser-Ser-Asn-Tyr-Cys-Asn-Gln
     1                                      10                        20                                        |
                                                                                                         Met —→ O
                                                                                                      30 Met —→ O
                                                                                                         Lys-Z
                                                                                                         Ser-Bzl
                                                                                                         |
            Bzl OBzl                          Bzl            Z     NO2 OBzlZ      Bzl               Ser-Bzl
            |   |                              |             |     |   |          |                    |
60 Gln-Ser-Cys-Val-Ala-Gln-Val-Ala-Asp-Ala-Leu-Ser-Glu-His-Val-Phe-Thr-Asn-Val-Pro-Lys-Cys-Arg-Asp-Lys-Thr-Leu-Asn-Arg-NO2
 |              50                                     40
Z-Lys
  |
 Asn
  |
 Val
  |
 Ala
  |
 Bzl      Z            Bzl         Bzl Bzl   O    Bzl              OBzlBzl1 NO2
  |       |            |           |   |     ‖    |                |    |   |
 Bzl-Cys-Lys-Asn-Gly-Gln-Thr-Asn-Cys-Tyr-Gln-Ser-Tyr-Ser-Thr-Met-Ser-Ile-Thr-Asp-Cys-Arg-Glu-Thr-Gly-Ser-Ser-Lys-Tyr
          70                       Bzl OBzl1 Bzl1       80         Bzl OBzl1Bzl1              Bzl Bzl Z  Bzl  |
                                                                                             90                Pro
                                                                                                                |
                                                                                                               Asn
                                                                                                                |
         Bzl  OBzl1Bzl1                       Z                      Bzl Bzl1 Z             Bzl            Cys-Bzl
         |    |    |                          |                      |   |    |             |              |
Resin-Val-Ser-Ala-Asp-Phe-His-Val-Pro-Val-Tyr-Pro-Asn-Gly-Glu-Cys-Ala-Val-Ile-Ile-His-Lys-Asn-Ala-Gln-Thr-Thr-Lys-Tyr-Bzl
          120                    110                                     100                              Ala
```

Fig. 12. Protected ribonuclease A.

stable and its amino acid sequence (Hirs *et al.*, 1960; Smyth *et al.*, 1963) and X-ray crystallographic structure were known (Kartha *et al.*, 1967; Wyckoff *et al.*, 1967, 1970).

The formula in Fig. 12 shows the protected derivative of ribonuclease which we wished to synthesize. It contains a total of 67 side chain protecting groups, largely based on benzyl derivatives for stability, and has a molecular weight of 19,791. The synthesis carried out by Dr. Gutte followed essentially the same procedure as that outlined in Fig. 5, while the workup, identification, and analysis of the product utilized a variety of techniques. The synthesis, which has already been described in complete detail (Gutte and Merrifield, 1971), is summarized in Table I. It shows that the overall yield was about 3%, i.e., of the first amino acid, valine, originally attached to the resin 3% was eventually recovered in the

TABLE I

Ribonuclease A Synthesis

Stage of synthesis	Overall yield	
	Mg	%
Boc-Val-Resin	2000	100
Deprotect ⎫		
Neutralize ⎬ Repeat 123 times		
Couple ⎭		
17% ↓		
Protected RNase-Resin	3430	17
Cleave and deprotect		
HF		
71% ↓		
Crude RNase (SH)$_8$	697	12
Sephadex G-75		
53% ↓		
RNase A (monomer fraction)	373	6.4
69% ⎮ Trypsin digestion		
↓ Sephadex G-50		
RNase A (Trypsin resistant fraction)	256	4.4
66% ↓ (NH$_4$)$_2$SO$_4$ fractionation		
RNase A	169	2.9

final purified protein. A large accumulated loss occurred during the synthesis itself. This means that the benzyl ester bond anchoring the peptide to the resin was not entirely stable to the repeated acidic conditions of the synthesis and was lost to the extent of about 1.4% at each cycle. I must emphasize that this has nothing to do with the individual coupling yields, which we believe were high. The cleavage step and the numerous workup steps taken together accounted for another 80% loss of material. The quantities of ribonuclease indicated in Table I are the calculated amounts of product that would have been obtained if all the material had been carried through all these steps. During this work the material was divided into many fractions in order to work out the best procedures and to obtain analytical samples, so that the most ribonuclease available at any time was of the order of 25 mg. When the crude HF-cleaved protein was oxidized and fractionated on an IRC-50 column in phosphate buffer it showed a large peak containing the enzymatic activity and two small inactive peaks. The specific activity could not be raised above 13% by recycling through this column. We then decided to take advantage of the known stability of ribonuclease A to trypsin digestion (Dubos and Thompson, 1938). The reasoning was that material with the correct structure would come through the treatment intact, while molecules with incorrect structures due to incomplete sequences or improper folding would give rise to a mixture of small molecules that could readily be separated from the native molecule (Fig. 13). To our great satisfaction the activity of a crude sample treated in this way increased from 8% to 61%, while only 25% of the protein was actually removed. A further purification step involved an ammonium sulfate fractionation in which some amorphous material could be separated, and a lyophilized preparation possessing nearly 80% specific activity was finally obtained. Table II summarizes the activity data obtained at various stages of purification of the synthetic enzyme. It also shows how the total number of units of RNase activity increased as the purification proceeded.

We interpret these data to mean that inhibitory peptides were present which were giving rise to low enzyme activity values and the crude preparation actually contained more enzyme than we had thought. The purified RNase A was then placed on a CM-cellulose

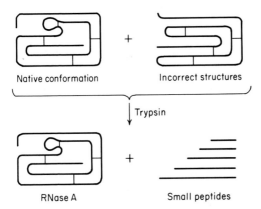

Native conformation   Incorrect structures

↓ Trypsin

RNase A   Small peptides

Fig. 13.   Schematic view of the purification of synthetic ribonuclease A by trypsin digestion.

column and compared with natural RNase A and reduced-reoxidized natural RNase A. They were identical by this criterion, which was the one first used by White (1961) to show that RNase A after reduction and reoxidation was indistinguishable from native RNase. His was the demonstration that led to the hypothesis that the primary structure of the protein determined its tertiary structure. Our synthesis provides a new kind of evidence for this hypothesis. The fact that the only information put into the synthesis was the linear sequence means that the primary structure must be sufficient

TABLE II

RIBONUCLEASE A ACTIVITY

Purification stage	Specific activity (%)	Total activity (mg RNase/2 gm resin)
HF cleavage	2	14
Sephadex G-75	9	33
IRC-50	13	53
Trypsin	61	156
$(NH_4)_2SO_4$	78	132

TABLE III

EVIDENCE FOR PURITY AND IDENTITY OF SYNTHETIC RNASE A

Technique	Conclusion
1. Gel filtration	Similar molecular size
2. Ion-exchange chromatography	Similar net charge
3. Paper electrophoresis	Similar charge and size
4. Amino acid analysis	Similar amino acid composition
5. Digested by papain + APM	No major racemization
6. Resistant to trypsin digestion	Compact folding
7. Fingerprint of tryptic digest of oxidized RNase	Similar amino acid sequence
8. Neutralization of antibody	Similar antigenic determinants
9. Enzymatic assay	High specific activity and similar substrate specificity

to direct the final folding of the molecule into its active tertiary structure. By starting with free amino acids any objections to the original experiments based on retention of some residual conformation after the reduction step which might serve to initiate the refolding are eliminated. The synthesis of an active enzyme containing no substituents except amino acids also provides a new proof for the now well-established belief that enzymatic activity can be a consequence of a simple protein and that no other components either known or unknown need be present. Not too many years ago such a view was vehemently opposed.

What we cannot claim is that this synthesis constitutes a proof of structure for ribonuclease A. Such a proof in the classical organic chemistry sense will be very difficult indeed because it is virtually impossible with present methods to establish absolute identity between two macromolecules of such complexity.

The various kinds of evidence that have been obtained to establish the identity and purity of the synthetic RNase A are listed in Table III. Clearly, each of these tests has limitations and we can only say that within these limits the synthetic preparation closely resembles native ribonuclease A in its chemical and physical properties, that it has a high specific activity and that it shows the expected substrate specificity.

IV. STRUCTURE FUNCTION STUDIES

As I indicated earlier, one of the prime objectives of synthetic work on proteins is to develop the methods and capability to investigate various questions that are not easy to examine by studies of the naturally occurring proteins themselves. The synthesis of ribonuclease A has provided answers to some rather fundamental questions, and we feel that it has laid a foundation for new studies on structure–function relations in enzymes. As a bare beginning, I would like to discuss two such studies.

In considering the well known S-peptide/S-protein system discovered by Richards (1955, 1958), in which these two inactive components can recombine noncovalently to produce a fully active enzyme, we wondered whether the recombination would occur if the protein component were shortened at its amino terminus by the removal of residues 21 through 25, and whether the complex would be enzymatically active. To test this question a sample of peptide-resin containing residues 25–124 was removed during the RNase synthesis, and another containing residues 21–124 was removed after the addition of 5 more residues (Fig. 14). These two synthetic proteins, corresponding to des-21–25 S-protein and to S-protein,

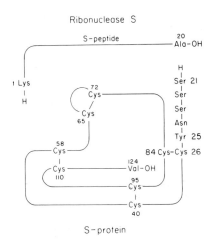

FIG. 14.   The S-peptide, S-protein, des 21–25 S-protein system. From Gutte and Merrifield (1970), by permission of The American Society of Biological Chemists, Inc.

were partially purified on Sephadex and then reduced at their 4 disulfide bonds. The resulting random coils were mixed with S-peptide (natural or synthetic), reoxidized and assayed for enzyme activity. The crude mixtures were both found to have approximately 25% as much activity as the product derived from native S-protein by the same treatment. From these data we can say, qualitatively, that the first five residues, 21–25, are definitely not necessary for the binding and reactivation to occur and, quantitatively, that there is probably no appreciable effect whether they are present or absent. Wyckoff and Richards had already predicted from their X-ray data that the three serines at positions 21, 22, and 23 would probably not be necessary since there was no indication of noncovalent interactions with other residues in the crystal. In contrast, asparagine 24 and tyrosine 25 appeared to be involved in a total of 5 hydrogen bonds, and it was reasonable to expect that they would be important in stabilizing the complex between S-peptide and S-protein and might be necessary for the formation of an active complex. Our data indicate that those bonds are not required either for binding or activity.

About 5 years ago I became interested in the question of whether or not a peptide component from the carboxyl end of ribonuclease might function in a manner analogous to that of S-peptide at the amino end. This was a good problem for synthesis because there was no enzyme available to make the necessary cleavage in the vicinity of residue 111. Consequently, Dr. Gutte synthesized the RNase 111–124 tetradecapeptide, H-Glu-Gly-Asn-Pro-Tyr-Val-Pro-Val-His-Phe-Asp-Ala-Ser-Val-OH, and obtained it in a high state of purity. To test its ability to bind and activate an inactive protein component he prepared N^1-carboxymethyl histidine-119-RNase. Many attempts to reactivate this protein by addition of the peptide met with uniform failure. It appeared that the peptide was unable to displace the tail of the protein and to bind in its place in a way that would place His^{119} in a proper position to function catalytically. The problem was set aside while the work on the total synthesis of RNase proceeded, but was resumed about two years later when Lin et al. (1968) succeeded in preparing a series of shortened RNases. They made RNase 1–120 by peptic digestion and RNase 1–119 and RNase 1–118 by further digestions with carboxypeptidase A. When

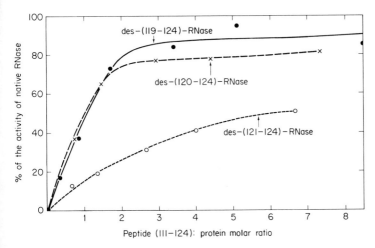

FIG. 15.   Enzymatic activity of the synthetic RNase 111–124 tetradecapeptide with shortened ribonucleases. From Lin *et al.* (1970), by permission of The American Society of Biological Chemists, Inc.

the synthetic peptide 111–124 was assayed in the presence of these inactive proteins, high enzymatic activity was regenerated (Fig. 15). Through a joint effort with Lin, Moore, Gutte, and Caldi, we have studied the combination of a number of carboxyl-terminal peptides with the shortened protein components and have been able to answer a number of interesting questions (Lin *et al.*, 1970, 1972; Gutte *et al.*, 1972). These experiments can be discussed best by referring to Fig. 16. This shows how we visualize the peptide inserting itself into the three-dimensional structure of the protein to produce an active enzyme. As can be seen there are 8–10 overlapping residues between the two components, and we naturally wondered how long a peptide was actually required to produce the effect. A series of C-terminal peptides was therefore synthesized and tested in the presence of RNase 1–118 (Table IV). With peptides containing 7 or 8 residues there was very little activity, but the addition of Val[116] made a dramatic increase to 60%. Further lengthening of the chain increased the binding gradually to a maximum of 98%. The role of Val[116] is now being examined in more detail to try to de-

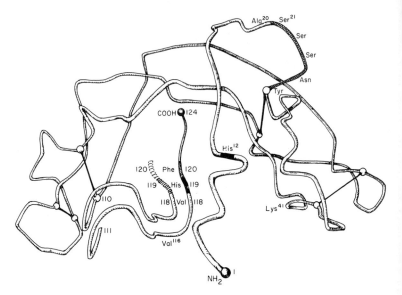

Fɪɢ. 16. Schematic representation of peptide-protein complexes in reconstituted ribonuclease. The drawing is based on the X-ray structure of RNase A by Kartha *et al.* (1967).

TABLE IV

Effect of Chain Length on Activation of
RNase 1–118 with COOH-terminal Peptides

Chain length	Peptide sequence	Activity[a] (%)
7	Val-His-Phe-Asp-Ala-Ser-Val	1
8	Pro-Val-His-Phe-Asp-Ala-Ser-Val	1.5
9	Val-Pro-Val-His-Phe-Asp-Ala-Ser-Val	60
10	Tyr-Val-Pro-Val-His-Phe-Asp-Ala-Ser-Val	70
11	Pro-Tyr-Val-Pro-Val-His-Phe-Asp-Ala-Ser-Val	80
12	Asn-Pro-Tyr-Val-Pro-Val-His-Phe-Asp-Ala-Ser-Val	90
14	Glu-Gly-Asn-Pro-Tyr-Val-Pro-Val-His-Phe-Asp-Ala-Ser-Val	98

[a] Maximum activity, in presence of excess peptide, relative to an equimolar amount of native RNase A. From Gutte *et al.* (1972), by permission of the Amerian Society of Biological Chemists, Inc.

termine whether it is simply a matter of peptide length or whether there is a unique function for valine itself.

Notice that in the combination of peptide 111–124 with protein 1–119 or protein 1–120 there is a His[119] in both components. Since His[119] is known to be involved in the catalytic mechanism of ribonuclease (Crestfield *et al.*, 1963) the question arose as to which of these residues was participating in the reconstituted complexes. Evidence was obtained by examining the alkylation pattern of the complexes after treatment with iodoacetate (Table V). Native ribonuclease alkylates either at His[12] or His[119], in a ratio of about 1 to 7, and the extent of alkylation correlates with the enzymatic activity of various derivatives of RNase; thus RNase 1–120 has very low activity and is poorly alkylated while RNase 1–119 is inactive and is not alkylated under these conditions. It was found that the complex between peptide 111–124 and RNase 1–120 was alkylated at His[119] of the protein component and also at His[119] of the peptide in a ratio of about 1 to 4, and the complex between peptide 111–124

TABLE V

ALKYLATION OF HISTIDINE RESIDUES IN THE RECONSTITUTED COMPLEXES

Components		Site of alkylation		
		His[12]	His[119]	
Protein	Peptide	Protein	Protein	Peptide
RNase 1–124 (native RNase A)		0.12	0.77	—
RNase 1–120		0.20	0.06	—
RNase 1–119		0	0	—
RNase 1–120 + RNase 111–114		0.14	0.24	0.06
RNase 1–119 + RNase 111–124		0.10	0.50	0.40
RNase 1–118 + RNase 111–124		0.10	—	0.70
RNase 1–118 + [Ile[120]]RNase 111–124		0.10	—	0.07

[a] Determined by measurement of the number of moles of N^3-His(Cm) or N^1-His(Cm) per mole of protein. The N^3-His(Cm) is assumed to occur only at His[12] of the protein and N^1-His(Cm) only at His[119] of the protein or peptide. From Gutte *et al.* (1972), by permission of The American Society of Biological Chemists, Inc.

and RNase 1–119 alkylated to nearly the same extent in both components. We interpret this to mean that these complexes exist in at least two conformations in which the peptide His[119] is functioning catalytically part of the time and the protein His[119] is functioning part of the time. Since dissociation constants could be measured, the two conformational forms must be in equilibrium with one another. In the case of peptide 111–124 and protein > 1–118 there is only one His[119], and all of the alkylation occurred in the protein.

A third question which we have studied by synthesis concerns the role of Phe[120]. This residue is known to stabilize ribonuclease and was expected to be involved in binding the synthetic peptides to the shortened RNase molecules. There is also evidence from X-ray and nuclear magnetic resonance studies that Phe[120] is located very close to the pyrimidine ring of the substrate and may be involved in binding substrate to RNase. We have obtained evidence on these points by synthesizing replacement analogs and combining them with RNase 1–118, (Table VI). Phe[120] in the peptide 111–124 was replaced by the hydrophobic but nonaromatic residues leucine and isoleucine and by the large aromatic residue tryptophan. It was found that the dissociation constant, K_d, increased by a factor of 12 when Leu[120] was present, by 20 when Ile[120] was present, and by

TABLE VI

EFFECT OF PHE[120] REPLACEMENTS ON THE DISSOCIATION CONSTANT OF THE
PEPTIDE–PROTEIN COMPLEXES AND ON THE MICHAELIS CONSTANT AND
INHIBITOR DISSOCIATION CONSTANT[a]

Components of the complex	K_d (M)	K_m for C > p (M)	K_i for 2' Cp (M)
RNase A	—	0.7×10^{-3}	0.9×10^{-5}
[Phe[120]]RNase 111–124 + RNase 1–118	2.0×10^{-7}	0.7×10^{-3}	—
[Leu[120]]RNase 111–124 + RNase 1–118	2.5×10^{-6}	1.0×10^{-3}	—
[Ile[120]]RNase 111–124 + RNase 1–118	4.0×10^{-6}	1.2×10^{-3}	1.1×10^{-5}
[Trp[120]]RNase 111–124 + RNase 1–118	3.5×10^{-5}	—	—

[a] From Lin et al. (1972), by permission of The American Society of Biological Chemists, Inc.

170 when Trp^{120} was present, suggesting a failure to fit properly into the hydrophobic pocket normally occupied by Phe^{120}. Furthermore, even when the peptide was present in saturating concentrations, full enzymatic activity could not be regenerated by these peptide analogs. It therefore appears that phenylalanine plays a very important role in binding the carboxyl end of ribonuclease to the remainder of the protein and in properly aligning the catalytic site.

To obtain information about the role of Phe^{120} in binding substrate, the Michaelis constant, K_m, for $2',3'$-cyclic cytidylic acid and the substrate inhibition constant, K_i, for $2'$-cytidylic acid were examined. These values are related to the strength of binding of substrate to the enzyme complex. Within the experimental error, K_m, was essentially the same for native RNase and for the complexes containing Phe, Leu, or Ile at position 120, indicating that phenylalanine had no unique role in binding substrate, and that if it played any part in the binding its role could be equally well assumed by leucine or isoleucine. A similar conclusion could be reached from the inhibition constant for $2'$-cytidylic acid which was nearly the same whether Phe^{120} or Ile^{120} was present.

The final experiment I would like to mention concerns the assembly of a three-component enzyme (Fig. 16). We discovered that S-peptide (1–20), containing His^{12}, and the C-terminal peptide (111–124), containing His^{119}, could be mixed in solution with RNase (21–118), containing Lys^{41}, and that they would bind noncovalently to produce a complex possessing about 30% specific activity. Thus, three separate peptides, each containing one of the amino acids known to function in the catalytic mechanism of ribonuclease, could reassociate in a very specific way to reconstitute the catalytic site and the substrate binding site and produce the active enzyme.

V. Conclusions

I have described a new approach to peptide synthesis, called solid phase peptide synthesis, and have indicated some of its virtues and some of the disadvantages and problems associated with it. The application of this technique to the synthesis of small peptides was described, and its use in the first total synthesis of an enzyme was discussed. Finally, some examples were presented to show how the synthetic approach can be used to answer questions about the structure and function of proteins.

It is now possible to synthesize true proteins with real enzymatic activity beginning with simple amino acids. I believe that in the years ahead we will see a great deal of progress in this area which will contribute in a significant way to our understanding of this very important class of compounds.

ACKNOWLEDGMENTS

I want to thank my friends who have worked with me during the past twelve years on the subject of this Harvey Lecture. The contributions of Bernd Gutte, although discussed in some detail, must be reemphasized here, and, especially, I wish to recall the help and guidance of Dr. D. W. Woolley. From its outset this research has been supported by Grant AM 1260 from the National Institutes of Health.

REFERENCES

Brunfeldt, K., Roepstorff, O., and Thomsen, J. (1969). *Acta Chem. Scand.* **23**, 2906.

Crestfield, A. M., Stein, W. H., and Moore, S. (1963). *J. Biol. Chem.* **238**, 2413.

Dorman, L. C. (1969). *Tetrahedron Lett.*, 2319.

Dubos, R. J., and Thompson, R. H. S. (1938). *J. Biol. Chem.* **124**, 501.

Epstein, C. J., Goldberger, R. F., Young, D. M., and Anfinsen, C. B. (1962). *Arch. Biochem. Biophys.*, Suppl. 1, 223.

Esko, K., Karlson, S., and Porath, J. (1968). *Acta Chem. Scand.* **22**, 3342.

Gisin, B. F. (1972). *Anal. Chim. Acta.* **58**, 248.

Gisin, B., and Merrifield, R. B. (1972). *J. Amer. Chem. Soc.* **94**, 3102.

Gutte, B., and Merrifield, R. B. (1969). *J. Amer. Chem. Soc.* **91**, 501.

Gutte, B., and Merrifield, R. B. (1971). *J. Biol. Chem.* **246**, 1922.

Gutte, B., Lin, M. C., Caldi, D. E., and Merrifield, R. B. (1972). *J. Biol. Chem.* **247**, 4763.

Hirs, C. H. W., Moore, S., and Stein, W. H. (1960). *J. Biol. Chem.* **235**, 633.

Hirschmann, R., Nutt, R. F., Veber, D. F., Vitali, R. A., Varga, S. L., Jacob, T. A., Holly, F. W., and Denkewalter, R. G. (1969). *J. Amer. Chem. Soc.* **91**, 507.

Kaiser, E., Colescott, R. L., Bossinger, C. D., and Cook, P. I. (1970). *Anal. Biochem.* **34**, 595.

Kartha, G., Bello, J., and Harker, D. (1967). *Nature (London)* **213**, 862.

Katsoyannis, P. G., Fukuda, K., Tometsko, A., Suzuki, K., and Tilak, M. (1964). *J. Amer. Chem. Soc.* **86**, 930.

Kung, Y. T., Du, Y. C., Huang, W. T., Chen, C. C., Ke, L. T., Hu, S. C., Jiang, R. Q., Chu, S. Q., Niu, C. I., Hsu, J. Z., Chang, W. C., Chen, L. L., Li, H. S., Wang, Y., Loh, T. P., Chi, A. H., Li, C. H., Shi, P. T., Yieh, Y. H., Tang, K. L., and Hsing, C. Y. (1965). *Sci. Sinica* **14**, 1710.

Kunitz, M. (1940). *J. Gen. Physiol.* **24,** 15.

Lin, M. C., Stein, W. H., and Moore, S. (1968). *J. Biol. Chem.* **243,** 6167.

Lin, M. C., Gutte, B., Moore, S., and Merrifield, R. B. (1970). *J. Biol. Chem.* **245,** 5169.

Lin, M. C., Gutte, B., Caldi, D. G., Moore, S., and Merrifield, R. B. (1972). *J. Biol. Chem.* **247,** 4768.

Manning, M. (1968). *J. Amer. Chem. Soc.* **90,** 1348.

Marglin, A., and Merrifield, R. B. (1966). *J. Amer. Chem. Soc.* **88,** 5051.

Marshall, G. R., and Merrifield, R. B. (1965). *Biochemistry* **4,** 2394.

Marshall, G. R., and Merrifield, R. B. (1971). *In* "Biochemical Aspects of Reactions on Solid Supports" (G. Stark, ed.), p. 111. Academic Press, New York.

Meienhofer, J., Schnabel, E., Bremer, H., Brinkhoff, O., Zabel, R., Sroka, W., Klostermeyer, H., Brandenburg, D., Okuda, T., and Zahn, H. (1963). *Z. Naturforsch. B* **18,** 1120.

Merrifield, R. B. (1963). *J. Amer. Chem. Soc.* **85,** 2149.

Merrifield, R. B. (1964). *Biochemistry* **3,** 1385.

Merrifield, R. B. (1969). *Advan. Enzymol.* **32,** 221.

Merrifield, R. B., and Littau, V. (1968). *In* "Peptides" (E. Bricas, ed.), p. 179. North-Holland Publ., Amsterdam.

Merrifield, R. B., Stewart, J. M., and Jernberg, N. (1966). *Anal. Chem.* **38,** 1905.

Richards, F. M. (1955). *Trav. Lab. Carlsberg* **29,** 322.

Richards, F. M. (1958). *Proc. Nat. Acad Sci. U.S.* **44,** 162.

Sakakibara, S., Shimonishi, Y., Kishida, T., Okada, M., and Sugihara, H. (1967). *Bull. Chem. Soc. Jap.* **40,** 2164.

Schröder, E., and Lübke, K. (1965). "The Peptides." Academic Press, New York.

Sheehan, J. C., and Hess, G. P. (1955). *J. Amer. Chem. Soc.* **77,** 1067.

Sieber, P., and Iselin, B. (1968). *Helv. Chim. Acta* **51,** 622.

Smyth, D., Stein, W. H., and Moore, S. (1963). *J. Biol. Chem.* **238,** 227.

Stewart, J. M., and Woolley, D. W. (1966). *In* "Hypotensive Peptides" (E. G. Erdos, N. Back, and F. Sicuteri, eds.), p. 23. Springer-Verlag, Berlin and New York.

Wang, S. S., and Merrifield, R. B. (1969). *J. Amer. Chem. Soc.* **91,** 6488.

Wang, S. S., and Merrifield, R. B. (1972). *Int. J. Peptide Protein Res.* **4,** 309.

White, F. H., Jr. (1961). *J. Biol. Chem.* **236,** 1353.

Windridge, G. C., and Jorgensen, E. C. (1971). *Intra-Sciences Chem. Rep.* **5,** 375.

Wyckoff, H. W., Hardman, K. D., Allewell, N. M., Inagami, T., Johnson, L. N., and Richards, F. M. (1967). *J. Biol. Chem.* **242,** 3984.

Wyckoff, H. W., Tsernoglou, D., Hanson, A. W., Knox, J. R., Lee, B., and Richards, F. M. (1970). *J. Biol. Chem.* **245,** 305.

THE FATE OF NORADRENALINE IN THE SYMPATHETIC NEURONE*

JULIUS AXELROD

Laboratory of Clinical Science, National Institute of Mental Health, Bethesda, Maryland

I. Introduction

THE striking similarity between the actions of extracts of the adrenal medulla and those produced by sympathetic nerve stimulation was recognized more than 70 years ago. Elliot (1905), a research student at Cambridge University, observed that the active principle of the adrenal medulla, adrenaline, produced physiological responses similar to those obtained after stimulation of the sympathetic nerves. As a result of these findings he proposed a brilliant and germinal hypothesis that sympathetic nerves liberate a chemical similar to adrenaline which was responsible for the physiologic responses of nerve stimulation. It was not until 1921 that Loewi, in an elegant experiment, demonstrated that inhibitory and excitatory compounds were released from the frog heart when its nerves were stimulated electrically. It was initially believed that the substance discharged from sympathetic nerves was adrenaline, but small differences between the responses after nerve stimulation and administered adrenaline indicated that the neurotransmitter was a compound resembling adrenaline. The neurotransmitter in sympathetic nerves was definitely identified as noradrenaline by von Euler in 1946.

During the past decade, there were rapid advances in our knowledge concerning the disposition of catecholamines and the anatomy of the sympathetic neurone. This was due mainly to the development of specific and sensitive methods for the measurement of catecholamines (von Euler and Floding, 1955), the availability of radioactive noradrenaline of high specific activity (Axelrod *et al.*,

---

* Lecture delivered December 16, 1971.

175

1959), the use of sophisticated histofluorescent techniques (Carlsson *et al.*, 1962), electron microscopic observations (Wolfe *et al.*, 1962), and adrenergic drugs (Hertting *et al.*, 1961). The sympathetic neurone consists of a cell body, long axon, and high branched nerve terminals. These terminals have a beaded appearance due to swellings or varicosities which lie in close proximity to effector cells (Hillarp, 1959). This type of structural organization is present in the peripheral and central nervous systems. Noradrenaline is stored primarily in the varicosities of the nerve terminals, and when released it acts locally on postsynaptic cells. Adrenaline is highly concentrated in the adrenal medulla and acts on distant target organs when it is discharged into the bloodstream. Another important catecholamine is dopamine. It serves as a precursor of noradrenaline and appears to have synaptic transmitter functions in the striatum of the brain.

II. Biosynthesis of Catecholamine and Its Regulation

Catecholamine biosynthesis proceeds as shown in Fig. 1. Tyrosine enters the sympathetic nerve terminal, cell body, or chromaffin cell of the adrenal medulla, where it is hydroxylated to 3-(3,4-di-hydroxyphenyl)alanine (dopa) by the enzyme tyrosine hydroxylase. Tyrosine hydroxylase requires tetrahydropteridine as a cofactor, and Fe^{2+} and O_2 are necessary for maximum activity (Nagatsu *et al.*,

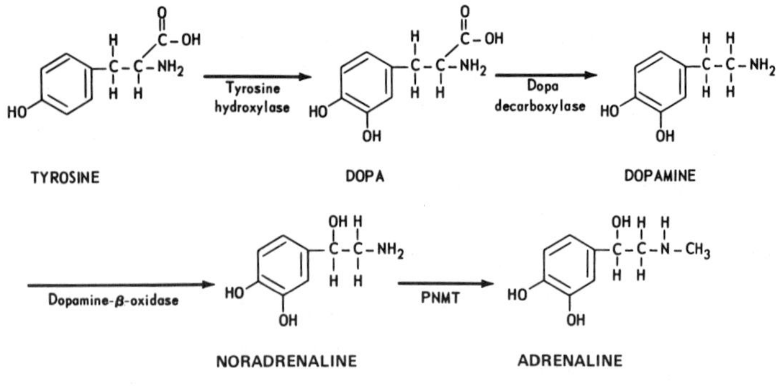

Fig. 1. Biosynthesis of catecholamines.

1964). This enzyme is inhibited by catecholamines, and it is believed that this inhibition is important in the regulation of the biosynthesis of noradrenaline in sympathetic nerves and the adrenal medulla (Nagatsu *et al.*, 1964). Inhibition of tyrosine hydroxylase by catecholamines is competitive with reduced pteridine cofactor rather than its substrate, tyrosine (Ikeda *et al.*, 1966). The enzymatically formed dopa is rapidly decarboxylated by aromatic amino acid decarboxylase to form dopamine (Holtz *et al.*, 1938). This enzyme requires pyridoxal phosphate, is widely distributed, and can decarboxylate a wide variety of aromatic amino acids. The dopamine enters the specific storage vesicles in nerve terminals or chromaffin granules in the adrenal medulla, where it is β-hydroxylated by the enzyme dopamine-β-hydroxylase to form noradrenaline. Dopamine-β-hydroxylase, like tyrosine hydroxylase, is a mixed function oxidase but requires ascorbic acid and O_2 (Levin *et al.*, 1960) and is highly localized in saclike vesicles in the sympathetic nerves (Potter and Axelrod, 1963) and chromaffin granules (Kirshner, 1957) in the adrenal medulla. Noradrenaline formed by dopamine-β-hydroxylase is then stored in the vesicle where it is made. In the adrenal gland, noradrenaline undergoes an additional biosynthetic step, N-methylation, to form adrenaline. This step is catalyzed by the enzyme phenylethanolamine-N-methyltransferase (Axelrod, 1962). The enzyme requires S-adenosylmethionine as the methyl donor (Kirshner and Goodall, 1957) and is highly localized in the cytoplasmic fraction of the adrenal medulla. Phenylethanolamine-N-methyltransferase N-methylates phenylethanolamines, but not phenylethylamines (Axelrod, 1962). It can also methylate secondary amines.

III. Regulation of the Biosynthesis of Catecholamines

The sympathetic nervous system is in a state of flux, yet its catecholamine content remains constant. The amount of noradrenaline in the nerves is hardly changed even under marked increase or decrease in sympathetic nerve activity. This is due to a precise control of the biosynthesis of catecholamines by nervous and hormonal mechanisms. There are at least two types of neuronal control of catecholamine formation; one is rapid, taking place in seconds, and the other is slower and is apparent only many hours later.

Alousi and Weiner (1966) observed that there was an increased synthesis of noradrenaline-^{14}C from tyrosine-^{14}C in the vas deferens when its hypogastric nerve was stimulated. However, no such increase in noradrenaline-^{14}C formation was found when dopa-^{14}C was used as the precursor. This indicated that nerve stimulation specifically increased the rate of conversion of tyrosine to dopa. There was no change in the activity of tyrosine hydroxylase, the enzyme responsible for this reaction. When noradrenaline was added to the vas deferens preparation, the increased formation of nor-adrenaline-^{14}C from tyrosine-^{14}C after nerve stimulation was blocked (Weiner and Rabadjija, 1968). Previous work had shown that catecholamines inhibit the activity of tyrosine hydroxylase (Uden-friend et al., 1965). It appears that increased nervous activity re-duces the level of noradrenaline in the axoplasm and this allows the conversion of tyrosine to dopa to proceed at a more rapid rate. On the other hand, elevation of noradrenaline levels by giving mono-amine oxidase inhibitors or exogenous noradrenaline leads to a decrease of formation of catecholamines from tyrosine but not from dopa (Spector et al., 1967).

A gradual increase in catecholamine biosynthesis can be caused by a prolonged increase in the activity of sympathetic nerves. The administration of reserpine, phenoxybenzamine, or 6-hydroxydopa-mine, drugs which lower blood pressure via a carotid sinus reflex, results in an increased firing of sympathetic nerves (Iggo and Vogt, 1960). These drugs were found to increase the activity of tyrosine hydroxylase (Mueller et al., 1969a,b) (Table I), dopamine-β-hydroxylase (Molinoff et al., 1970) and phenylethanolamine-N-methyltransferase (Mueller et al., 1969a) in the adrenal gland. Simi-lar increases in the catecholamine biosynthetic enzymes were also found after different types of stress such as immobilization (Kvetnansky et al., 1970, 1971), cold, psychosocial stimulation (Thoenen, 1970; Axelrod et al., 1970), and insulin shock (Viveros et al., 1969). In rats with elevated enzyme levels there was an increase in the formation of noradrenaline-^{14}C (Dairman and Uden-friend, 1970) from tyrosine-^{14}C in the adrenal gland.

The repeated administration of reserpine also elevated tyrosine hydroxylase (Mueller et al., 1969b) and dopamine-β-hydroxylase (Molinoff et al., 1970) activity in sympathetic nerve cell body

TABLE I

Transsynaptic Induction of Tyrosine Hydroxylase and Dopamine-β-Hydroxylase

Tissue	Treatment	Tyrosine hydroxylase units[a]	Dopamine-β-hydroxylase units[a]
Adrenal	None	4 ± 0.5	14.2 ± 0.13
Adrenal	Reserpine	12.2 ± 1.3^b	33.9 ± 0.5^b
Adrenal denervation	Reserpine	4.8 ± 0.7^b	—
Superior cervical ganglia	None	0.036 ± 0.003	11.6 ± 0.16
Superior cervical ganglia	Reserpine	0.076 ± 0.004^b	20.1 ± 0.14^c
Superior cervical ganglia denervation	Reserpine	0.033 ± 0.004^b	9.1 ± 0.1^c

[a] 1 unit = 1 nmole of product formed per adrenal or milligram of protein in ganglia.

[b] Reserpine 5 mg/kg was given subcutaneously 48 and 24 hours before animals were killed, and 3 days after splanchnic nerve denervation.

[c] Reserpine 2.5 mg/kg was given subcutaneously on alternate days for 7 days. Treatment began 6 days after decentralization.

(stellate and celiac and superior cervical ganglia), axon, nerve terminal, and brainstem (Table I). There was a delay of 2 days in the increased activity of tyrosine hydroxylase in the nerve terminal suggesting a proximodistal axoplasmic transport of the induced enzyme from the cell body to the nerve terminal (Thoenen et al., 1970a). This is supported by the observation that after reserpine administration there was an increase in tyrosine hydroxylase in the proximal segments of the axon followed by an increase in the activity of the enzyme in the distal segments.

The increase in enzyme activity could be due to changes in its conformation or in an increase in the amount of enzyme. The administration of a protein synthesis inhibitor, cycloheximide, blocked the increase in tyrosine hydroxylase (Mueller et al., 1969c) and dopamine-β-hydroxylase (Molinoff et al., 1972). These results indicated that the elevation in enzyme activity after increased nerve activity was due to the formation of new protein molecules. Additional evidence to support this was obtained by immunoabsorption techniques (Hartman et al., 1970). After the repeated administration of reserpine, there was an increased incorporation of leucine-^{3}H into dopamine-β-hydroxylase. With the use of protein synthesis inhibitors, it was possible to measure the turnover of dopamine-β-hydroxylase in the cell body. It was found to be rapid, with a half-life of 17 hours, possibly reflecting the transport of this enzyme from the cell body to the nerve terminals (Molinoff et al., 1972).

The most likely possibilities that cause an increase in catecholamine biosynthetic enzymes are blood-borne factors, adrenocorticoids for example, or changes in nervous activity. To establish the latter possibility, the splanchnic nerve innervating the adrenal medulla was cut on one side and tyrosine hydroxylase (Thoenen et al., 1969a), dopamine-β-hydroxylase (Patrick and Kirshner, 1971; Thoenen et al., 1970b) and phenylethanolamine-N-methyltransferase were measured after giving reserpine. There was the expected elevation of tyrosine hydroxylase, dopamine-β-hydroxylase, and phenylethanolamine-N-methyltransferase activity in the innervated adrenal, but no increase in the denervated adrenal (Table I). Similar experiments were carried out in the sympathetic ganglia (Thoenen et al., 1969b; Molinoff et al., 1970). The superior cervical ganglia was cut preganglionically on one side and reserpine was administered. The increase in both tyrosine hydroxylase and dopamine-β-hydroxylase activity was blocked on the denervated side (Table I). Inhibiting nerve transmission by ganglionic blocking agents also prevented the rise of these enzymes after increasing nervous activity with reserpine (Mueller et al., 1970a). These observations clearly indicated a transsynaptic induction of the biosynthetic enzymes for catecholamines.

Increased nervous activity is necessary for enzyme induction. This would imply that acetylcholine released from preganglionic nerves causes a depolarization of the postganglionic nerve. It was observed that adrenal gland treated with acetylcholine and eserine showed an increase in tyrosine hydroxylase in the intact and denervated gland (Patrick and Kirshner, 1971). It was also found that dopamine-β-hydroxylase can be induced in rat ganglia in organ culture when they are depolarized with high levels of potassium (Silberstein et al., 1972). Acetylcholine and depolarization would be expected to release noradrenaline from postganglionic nerves and thus reduce its level. This would suggest that a decrease of noradrenaline would stimulate the increase in enzyme protein. Conversely, elevation of noradrenaline levels should inhibit induction of its biosynthetic enzymes. When the noradrenaline-depleting action of reserpine was blocked with monoamine oxidase inhibitors, the rise in ganglia tyrosine hydroxylase and dopamine-β-hydroxylase was markedly slowed (Molinoff et al., 1972). Similar results were obtained when the catecholamine levels were elevated by the administration of its precursor L-dopa. All these results suggested that noradrenaline represses the formation of its own biosynthetic enzymes.

6-Hydroxydopamine destroys sympathetic nerve terminals but leaves cell body and adrenal gland morphologically intact (Tranzer and Thoenen, 1968). As shown above, it also induces catecholamine biosynthetic enzymes in the adrenal gland but leads to a decrease in dopamine-β-hydroxylase in sympathetic ganglia. Pretreatment of rats with 6-hydroxydopamine or surgical destruction of postganglionic fibers prevented the induction of dopamine-β-hydroxylase and tyrosine hydroxylase in sympathetic ganglia (Brimijoin and Molinoff, 1971). This indicates that nerve terminals can influence induction of enzymes in the cell body.

The catecholamine biosynthetic enzymes in the adrenal gland are also controlled by hormones. Removal of the pituitary gland caused a decrease in phenylethanolamine-N-methyltransferase in the adrenal medulla (Fig. 2), a fall in its adrenaline content (Wurtman and Axelrod, 1966) and secretion of this catecholamine resulting from hypoglycemia by insulin (Wurtman et al., 1967). Phenylethanolamine-N-methyltransferase activity can be restored by large doses of glucocorticoids or by ACTH (Wurtman and Axelrod, 1966; Wurtman, 1966) (Fig. 2). The amount of glucorticoids necessary to increase enzyme activity in a hypophysectomized rat was similar to that delivered to the adrenal medulla from the cortex via the adrenal portal circulation. The increase in phenylethanolamine-N-methyltransferase activity by ACTH was blocked when protein synthesis was inhibited by puromycin or actinomycin D, suggesting that this enzyme is induced by these hormones. Phenylethanolamine-N-methyltransferase and adrenaline are absent in newborn rats if they are hypophysectomized in utero (Margolies et al., 1966). When

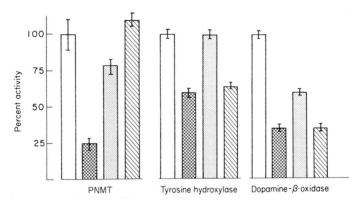

Fig. 2. Hormonal control of catecholamine biosynthetic enzymes in the adrenal. Rats were hypophysectomized for about 6 days and then given dexamethasone (1 mg) or ACTH. □, Normal; ▨, hypophysectomy; ⊞, hypophysectomy + ACTH; ◩, hyphophysectomy + dexamethasone.

corticoids or ACTH are given to the mothers of hypophysectomized fetuses, the activity of phenylethanolamine-N-methyltransferase is restored to normal.

Hypophysectomy also reduced the activity of dopamine-β-hydroxylase (Weinshilboum and Axelrod, 1970) and tyrosine hydroxylase (Mueller et al., 1970b) in the adrenal medulla (Fig. 2). The decrease in tyrosine hydroxylase and dopamine-β-hydroxylase in the adrenal gland was elevated by ACTH, but not by glucocorticoids, sufficient to restore phenylethanolamine-N-methyltransferase (Fig. 2). This points to a direct action of ACTH on these enzymes.

Recent experiments showed that the administration of dexamethasone can induce the formation of phenylethanolamine-N-methyltransferase in ganglia of newborn rats (Ciaranello, et al., 1973). This enzyme is not normally present in ganglia. The ability to induce phenylethanolamine-N-methyltransferase by glucorticoids disappears 1 week after birth. This suggests that some factor(s) present soon after birth prevents the elaboration of the adrenaline-forming enzyme normally present in adrenal medullary cells.

There are negligible amounts of phenylethanolamine-N-methyltransferase and adrenaline in fetal extrachromaffin tissue in the organ of Zuckerkandl. The administration of glucocorticoids or ACTH to newborn rats can induce the formation of the adrenaline-forming enzyme in this tissue (Roffi, 1968).

A. Metabolism

The metabolic pathway of noradrenaline and other catecholamines was elucidated as a result of the discovery of the enzyme catechol-O-methyltransferase (Axelrod, 1957). It was observed that a large amount of 3-methoxy-4-hydroxymandelic acid (VMA) was excreted in the urine of subjects with adrenaline-forming tumors (Armstrong et al., 1957). Following this the O-methylated catecholamines normetanephrine, metanephrine, and methoxytyramine were found in the urine, especially after the administration of catecholamines (Axelrod et al., 1958). These findings suggested that catecholamines are metabolized via two pathways: O-methylation and deamination. The enzymes concerned with these metabolic transformations are catechol-O-methyltransferase and monoamine oxidase. The metabolism of catecholamines are shown in Fig. 3.

Catechol-O-methyltransferase was isolated and partially purified from rat liver, and its properties were studied (Axelrod and Tomchick, 1958). S-Adenosylmethionine serves as the methyl donor, and there is an absolute requirement for Mg^{2+}. Other divalent ions (Ca^{2+}, Co^{2+}, Zn^{2+}, and Mn^{2+}) can substitute for Mg^{2+}. The enzyme can O-methylate catechols, but not monophenols. Normally occurring substrates for catechol-O-methyltransferase are adrenaline, noradrenaline, dopamine, dopa, 3,4-dihydroxymandelic acid, 3,4-dihydroxyphenylacetic acid (Axelrod and Tomchick, 1958), 3-hydroxyestradiol (Knuppen et al., 1969), and ascorbic acid (Blaschke and Hertting, 1970). The enzyme can also O-methylate foreign catechols and polyphenols in the body. O-Methylation of catecholamines in vivo occurs mainly on the meta position. In vitro catechol-O-methyltransferase can methylate hydroxy group on both the para and meta position depending on the polarity of the substrate and the pH at which the enzyme reaction is carried out (Senoh et al., 1959).

Catechol-O-methyltransferase is inhibited by sulfhydryl binding

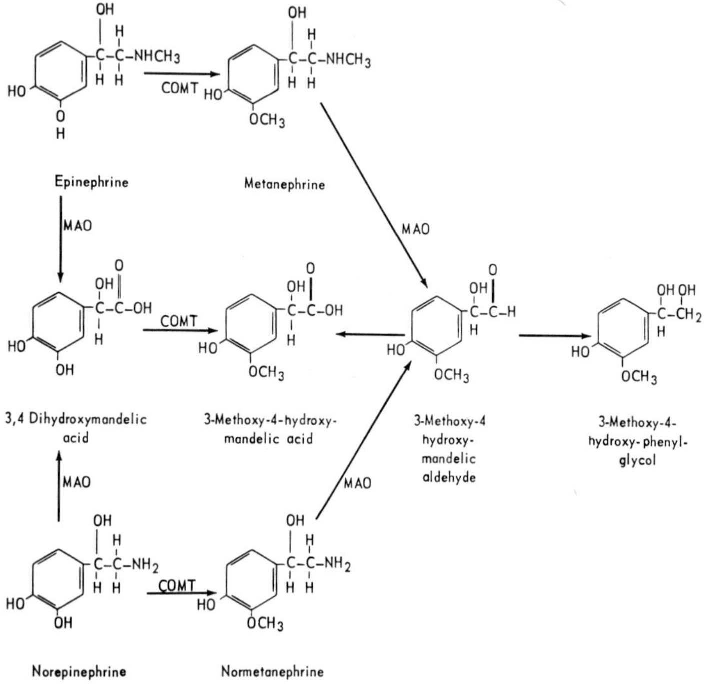

FIG. 3. Metabolism of noradrenaline (norepinephrine) and adrenaline (epinephrine). COMT, catechol-0-methyltransferase; MAO, monoamine oxidase.

reagents, polyphenols (Axelrod and Laroche, 1959), substituted 3,5-dihydroxy-4-methoxybenzoic acid (Nikodijevic *et al.*, 1970), and tropolone (a metal chelating agent) (Belleau and Burba, 1963). A normally occurring compound that inhibits O-methylation both *in vitro* and *in vivo* is 3-hydroxyestradiol (Knuppen *et al.*, 1969).

The O-methylating enzyme has been highly purified (450-fold) and has a molecular weight of about 24,000 (Anderson and D'Iorio, 1968; Assicot and Bohuon, 1970). With starch block electrophoresis two separate forms of catechol-0-methyltransferase have been found with the same substrate specificity but different heat stabilities and K_m values (Axelrod and Vesell, 1970).

Catechol-0-methyltransferase is widely distributed in mammalian tissues but the highest activity is found in liver and kidney (Axelrod and Tomchick, 1958). It is present in different areas of brain in unequal concentrations (Axelrod *et al.*, 1959). It acts mainly outside the sympathetic neurone while monoamine oxidase metabolizes noradrenaline in the neurone (Kopin, 1964). Catechol-0-methyltransferase metabolizes noradrenaline and other catecholamines released into the circulation. It also serves to inactivate the neurotransmitter noradrenaline in tissues with sparse adrenergic innervation (Levin and Furchgott, 1970).

Monoamine oxidase is an important enzyme in regulation of levels of noradrenaline in nerves (Spector *et al.*, 1960). It metabolizes noradrenaline that leaks out of the storage vesicles in nerve terminals to form a physiologically inactive metabolic product (Kopin, 1964). A large fraction of tissue monoamine oxidase is present in nerves of heavily innervated tissues such as the pineal gland (Snyder *et al.*, 1965), iris, and vas deferens. Monoamine oxidase can be almost completely and irreversibly inhibited by hydrazine derivatives (Zeller and Barsky, 1952). The administration of monoamine oxidase inhibitors elevates endogenous tissue levels of noradrenaline, dopamine, octopamine, serotonin, and tryptamine (Spector *et al.*, 1960).

B. *Uptake and Inactivation*

Neither catechol-0-methyltransferase nor monoamine oxidase is responsible for the rapid inactivation of noradrenaline. When both enzymes are inhibited, the action of noradrenaline is only slightly prolonged (Crout, 1961). A novel mechanism for terminating the action of the neurotransmitter noradrenaline was uncovered in studies involving the physiological disposition of noradrenaline-^{3}H and adrenaline (Axelrod *et al.*, 1959; Whitby *et al.*, 1961). The intravenous administration of noradrenaline-^{3}H resulted in the retention of the unchanged catecholamine long after its physiological effects are dissipated. This suggested that the catecholamine was taken up in tissues and bound in such a way as to make it unavailable to enzymatic attack. To examine whether the uptake and binding sites were the sympathetic nerve terminals, the superior cervical ganglia of cats were removed unilaterally and the nerves were allowed to degenerate (Hertting *et al.*, 1961a). After the administration of noradrenaline-^{3}H the radioactive amine was taken up and stored only in the innervated tissues. Similar results were obtained when sympathetic neurones were destroyed immunologically with anti-nerve growth factor (Iversen *et al.*, 1966) or chemically with 6-hydroxydopamine (Thoenen and Tranzer, 1968). The ability of noradrenaline-^{3}H to be taken up by sympathetic nerve terminals made possible a study of its subcellular site of storage. Noradrenaline-^{3}H was injected intravenously, and the pineal gland (an organ rich in sympathetic nerve terminals) was prepared for radioautography and examined with the electron microscope (Wolfe *et al.*, 1962). Almost all the photographic grains were present over nonmyelinated axons which contained dense-core vesicles of about 500 Å.

The fate of the radioactive neurotransmitter was studied in splenic nerves of the cat, which were previously labeled with noradrenaline-^{3}H (Hertting and Axelrod, 1961). Stimulation of the splenic nerve caused a sharp increase in the venous outflow of noradrenaline-^{3}H. There was also a small release of normetanephrine, the O-methylated metabolite of noradrenaline, but no increase in deaminated metabolites. The uptake and release of noradrenaline-^{3}H was also examined in the vascular bed of the dog gracilis muscle *in situ* (Rosell *et al.*, 1963). Perfusing this muscle with noradrenaline-^{3}H resulted in the uptake and retention of noradrenaline-^{3}H and stimulation of the vasomotor nerves caused an elevation of venous outflow of the radioactive amine. When the dog was pretreated with phenoxybenzamine, a compound which was previously shown to inhibit uptake of noradrenaline by sympathetic neurones, there was an increased outflow of noradrenaline-^{3}H after vasomotor stimulation. These experiments demonstrated that reuptake by neuronal membrane of sympathetic nerves and subsequent retention in storage vesicles is the principal means for terminating the action of the neurotransmitter (Fig. 4). Other mechanisms for inactivating noradrenaline are O-methylation by catechol-O-methyltransferase, deamination by monoamine oxidase, physical removal by the circulation (Fig. 4) or by an extraneural uptake process. The relative importance of these latter processes depends on the sparsity of nerve terminals or the size of the synaptic cleft. Noradrenaline liberated into the bloodstream is ultimately

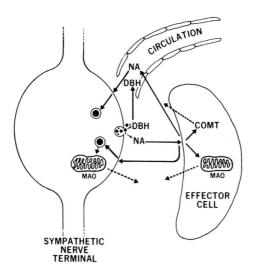

Fig. 4.   Fate of the neurotransmitter at sympathetic nerve terminal. NA, nor-adrenaline; DBH, dopamine-β-hydroxylase; MAO, monoamine oxidase; COMT, catechol-O-methyltransferase.

metabolized by catechol-O-methyltransferase and/or monoamine oxidase in liver and kidney.

Studies on the uptake of noradrenaline-^{3}H by isolated heart and brain slices show that it obeys saturation kinetics of the Michaelis-Menten type with a high affinity and involves active transport (Iversen, 1967). It also requires sodium ions in the external medium, and it is a temperature-dependent process. The neuronal uptake shows stereoselectivity and it can be utilized by other amines structurally related to noradrenaline, e.g., adrenaline, dopamine, tyramine, α-methylnoradrenaline, metaraminol, and amphetamine. An uptake process similar to noradrenaline has also been described for other putative neurotransmitters, serotonin, γ-aminobutyric acid (Iversen, 1971), glutamate, aspartate, and glycine (Logan and Snyder, 1971). Such a high affinity neuronal uptake might be a general mechanism for the rapid inactivation of most neurotransmitters.

C.   Effect of Drugs on Uptake

The accumulation of noradrenaline by sympathetic nerves of tissues made it possible to examine the effect of drugs in blocking its uptake. In these experiments rats were pretreated with drugs and then noradrenaline-^{3}H was administered (Hertting *et al.*, 1961b; Axelrod *et al.*, 1962). The tissue (heart) level of noradrenaline-^{3}H was measured shortly afterward. The following drugs were found to block the uptake of noradrenaline: cocaine, imipramine (an antidepressant drug), sympathomimetic amines (amphetamine, tyramine), and phenoxybenzamine. The pharmacological consequence of blocking neuronal uptake is to increase the actions of noradrenaline by blocking inactivation by neuronal uptake (Fig. 5).

D.   Octopamine as a Putative Neurotransmitter

Using phenylethanolamine-N-methyltransferase and S-adenosylmethionine-methyl-^{14}C, octopamine (*p*-hydroxyphenylethanolamine) was found to occur normally in tissues in nanogram amounts (Molinoff *et al.*, 1969). It also showed an unequal localization in different brain areas (Molinoff and Axelrod, 1972). When sympathetic nerves were denervated chemically with 6-hydroxydopamine or surgically, octopamine disappeared from tissues together with noradrenaline (Molinoff and Axelrod, 1969). Octopamine had a similar subcellular localization as noradrenaline. Electrical stimulation of splenic nerves resulted in a release of octopamine

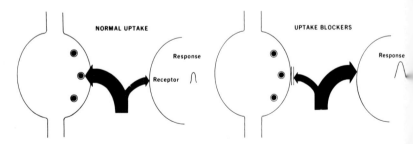

FIG. 5.   Effect of drugs that block uptake of noradrenaline at the sympathetic nerve membrane.

together with noradrenaline (Molinoff and Kopin, unpublished observations). These observations indicated that octopamine might serve as a neurotransmitter and that more than one neurotransmitter can be discharged from the same nerve.

The biosynthesis and metabolism of octopamine was found to occur as follows: tyrosine → tyramine → octopamine → p-hydroxymandelic acid. The first step is catalyzed by aromatic amino acid decarboxylase, the second by dopamine-β-hydroxylase, and the third by monoamine oxidase. A minor metabolic pathway for the formation of octopamine occurs via the dehydroxylation of dopa and/or dopamine (Brandau and Axelrod, 1972).

The physiological role of octopamine is difficult to assess. However, relatively large amounts of octopamine are present in crustacean central nerve cord (1 μg) (Molinoff and Axelrod, 1972), nerves of *Octopus vulgaris* (10 μg) (Juorio and Molinoff, unpublished observations). It might be the neurotransmitter in these species where tyrosine hydroxylase is absent. Although the concentration of octopamine is about one-tenth that of noradrenaline, its turnover rate is about six times more rapid. Thus the synthesis rate of octopamine constitutes approximately one-third of the biogenic amines found in the adrenergic neurone of many tissues. This is supported by the high excretion rate of its deaminated metabolite, p-hydroxymandelic acid (Armstrong *et al.*, 1956).

E.   *Storage*

Noradrenaline is stored in the sympathetic nerve terminal in membrane-bound dense-core vesicles of about 400–600 Å (Fig. 4) (Wolfe *et al.*, 1962). Attempts to purify these vesicles by centrifugation techniques have met with only partial success (Potter and Axelrod, 1963). In addition to noradrenaline the storage vesicles in sympathetic neurones contain dopamine-β-hydroxylase, other proteins called chromogranins (Geffen *et al.*, 1969), and relatively large amounts of ATP. Most of the dopamine-β-hydroxylase present in the storage granules exists in a bound form (about 90%). Uptake of noradrenaline into granules isolated from splenic nerves requires ATP and Mg^{2+} (von Euler and Lishajko, 1963). The storage vesicles of sympathetic nerve terminals can take up and store other structurally related amines such as adrenaline, dopamine, α-methylnoradrenaline, octopamine, and metaraminol (Musacchio *et al.*, 1966). These compounds can displace noradrenaline from its storage granules, and upon nerve stimulation they are released from the nerve terminal as false neurotransmitters.

Drugs such as reserpine (Carlsson *et al.*, 1957) and guanethidine (Cass *et al.*, 1960) prevent the storage of noradrenaline and related amines and serve as useful agents in lowering blood pressure. When reserpine releases the noradrenaline it is deaminated within the neurone by monoamine oxidase, and the neurotransmitter leaves the nerve as a physiologically inactive compound (Fig. 6C). Sympathomimetic amines such as tyramine and amphetamine can release noradrenaline from the storage granule in a physiologically active form (Fig. 6B), and thus raise blood pressure by releasing the neurotransmitter in a physiologically active form (Burn and Rand, 1958). Many compounds related in structure to noradrenaline can be stored in sympathetic nerve granules and released together with the catecholamine. These compounds, called "false neurotransmitters," have less pressor activity and they lower blood pressure by decreasing the effects of the normal transmitter (Fig. 6D). Monoamine oxidase inhibitors lower blood pressure by elevating

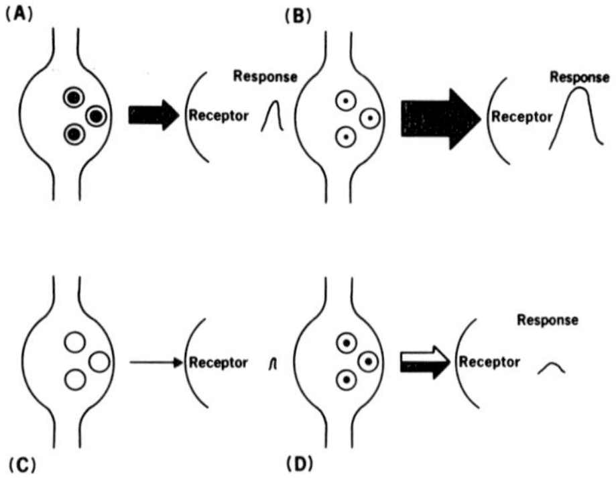

Fig. 6.   Effect of drugs that release noradrenaline from sympathetic nerve terminal. (A) Normal release; (B) releasing agents; (C) agents interfering with normal storage; (D) false neurotransmitters. From Axelrod and Weinshiboum (1972), by permission of the Massachusetts Medical Society, Boston, Massachusetts.

octopamine levels (Kopin *et al.*, 1964). Octopamine is then released together with noradrenaline, and this dilutes the actions of the catecholamine.

F. *Release of Noradrenaline*

Noradrenaline in the sympathetic nerve is stored as a membrane-bound vesicle. Its release upon nerve stimulation could occur through a variety of mechanisms, such as a discharge from vesicle into the axoplasm followed by passage through the neural membrane, fusion of vesicle with neuronal membrane and then by diffusion through both vesicle and neural membrane, by fusion of vesicle with neuronal membranes followed by an opening whereby noradrenaline is discharged from the vesicle into the exterior of the cell together with the soluble contents of the vesicle (exocytosis). When the adrenal medulla is stimulated chemically or electrically, there is a release of catecholamines together with ATP (Douglas and Rubin, 1961), soluble proteins, chromogranins, as well as dopamine-β-hydroxylase (Kirshner *et al.*, 1966).

These results together with microscopic evidence indicated that the secretion of catecholamines in the adrenal medulla occurs by a process of exocytosis. Stimulation of splenic nerves releases both dopamine-β-hydroxylase (an enzyme highly localized in the adrenergic storage vesicles) and noradrenaline (Geffen *et al.*, 1969). For dopamine-β-hydroxylase and noradrenaline to be liberated by exocytosis it should be shown that the ratio of noradrenaline to enzyme released is similar to the ratio present in the storage vesicle. However, it had been reported that the noradrenaline to dopamine-β-hydroxylase ratio is many times higher than that found in vesicles from splenic nerves (DePotter *et al.*, 1969). The development of a sensitive enzymatic assay to measure dopamine-β-hydroxylase and the means to stabilize this enzyme once it is released made possible a quantitative study of the mechanism of release of the neurotransmitter (Weinshilboum *et al.*, 1971b). Vasa deferentia of guinea pigs and attached hypogastric nerves were placed in a bath containing Ca^{2+} and albumin to protect released dopamine-β-hydroxylase. Electrical stimulation of the hypogastric nerve resulted in a liberation of both noradrenaline and dopamine-β-hydroxylase into the bath fluid. The ratio of noradrenaline to dopamine-β-hydroxylase present in the bath fluid was similar to that present in the vas deferens. These experiments demonstrate that noradrenaline and dopamine-β-hydroxylase, and presumably the other soluble contents of the vesicle, are released from nerve terminals by exocytosis (Fig. 7).

Drugs and ions were found to affect the release of noradrenaline and dopamine-β-hydroxylase from sympathetic nerves. Phenoxybenzamine and pentolamine (alpha adrenergic blocking agents), enhance the release of noradrenaline and dopamine-β-hydroxylase after nerve stimulation. High concentrations of Ca^{2+} (7.5 mM) also resulted in a marked increase in release of both noradrenaline and dopamine-β-hydroxylase (Johnson *et al.*, 1971). The increased release of dopamine-β-hydroxylase and noradrenaline by 7.5 mM Ca^{2+} or phenoxybenzamine was reversed by prostaglandin E_2. It appears that blocking action of prostaglandin might be due to its interference with availability of Ca^{2+} necessary for release.

Nerves are rich in microtubules, cellular elements (Shelanski and Taylor, 1967) involved in the proximodistal transport in axon in the cell body to the nerve terminals (Dahlstrom, 1968). Microtubules have also been shown to be necessary for the release of intracellular stored products such as insulin from beta cells of the pancreas (Lacy *et al.*, 1968), thyroid-stimulating hormone induced release of [131]I

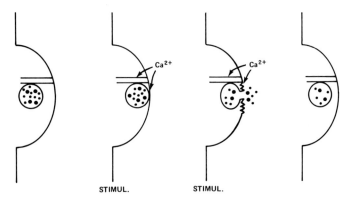

Fig. 7. A possible mechanism for release of noradrenaline (•) and dopamine-β-hydroxylase (●) by exocytosis (see text for explanation).

(Williams and Wolff, 1970) histamine from mast cells (Gillespie *et al.*, 1968) and catecholamines from the adrenal medulla (Poisner and Bernstein, 1971). Alkaloids such as colchicine (Shelanski and Taylor, 1967) and vinblastine can disaggregate microtubules. When either colchicine or vinblastine were added to the organ bath and the hypogastric nerve was stimulated, the release of dopamine-β-hydroxylase and noradrenaline from the vas deferens was inhibited (Thoa *et al.*, 1972). The addition of cytocholasin B to the bath also prevented the release of dopamine-β-hydroxylase and noradrenaline after nerve stimulation. Cytocholasin B is a fungal metabolite that disrupts the function of contractile filaments in cells (Carter, 1967). It has also been reported that microfilaments are activated by calcium in nonmuscle cells (Wessells *et al.*, 1971). Microtubules are believed to function as a cytoskeleton and nerve depolarization might activate this cellular component in such a manner as to bring the vesicle to the proper site on the neuronal membrane from which release occurs (Fig. 7). There also might be a contractile microfilament on the neuronal membrane which is activated by Ca^{2+} thus making an opening in the membrane large enough to allow the soluble contents of the vesicle to be discharged (Fig. 7).

G. Plasma Dopamine-β-Hydroxylase

The release of dopamine-β-hydroxylase from the sympathetic neurone suggested that it might appear in the blood (Fig. 4). When a sensitive enzymatic assay was used for this enzyme, it was found to be present in the plasma of man as well as a number of mammalian species (Weinshilboum and Axelrod, 1971a). Plasma dopamine-β-hydroxylase had the same cofactor requirements as the adrenal enzyme (ascorbic acid, fumarate), K_m for substrate, and electrophoretic mobility. Man had the highest plasma dopamine-β-hydroxylase activity, about 50 times that of most laboratory species. To determine whether the plasma dopamine-β-hydroxylase comes from sympathetic nerve terminals and/or adrenal gland, rats were treated with 6-hydroxydopamine (Weinshilboum and Axelrod, 1971b), a drug which destroys sympathetic nerve terminals. This resulted in a sharp fall in plasma dopamine-β-hydroxylase. Removal of adrenal gland had no effect on the plasma enzyme suggesting that it arises from the sympathetic nerve terminals. In rats subjected to repeated stress by immobilization there was an increase in plasma dopamine-β-hydroxylase (Weinshilboum *et al.*, 1971a). This increase was found even after adrenal gland demedullation, indicating that increased enzyme activity present after stress comes mainly from sympathetic nerves.

Plasma dopamine-β-hydroxylase was also examined in several neurological diseases. It was found that in children with familial dysautonomia, a disease characterized by symptoms of altered autonomic nervous system function and sensory deprivation, there was a reduced plasma dopamine-β-hydroxylase (Weinshilboum and Axelrod, 1971c). About 25% of patients with dysautonomia had no detectable plasma enzyme, and the mothers of patients without blood dopamine-β-hydroxylase had a decreased enzyme activity in plasma.

REFERENCES

Alousi, A., and Weiner, N. (1966). *Proc. Nat. Acad. Sci. U.S.* **56,** 1491.
Anderson, P. J., and D'Iorio, A. (1968). *Biochem. Pharmacol.* **17,** 1943.
Armstrong, M. D., Shaw, K. N., and Wall, P. E. (1956). *J. Biol. Chem.* **218,** 293.
Armstrong, M. D., McMillan, A., and Shaw, K. N. (1957). *Biochim. Biophys. Acta* **25,** 422.
Assicot, M., and Bohuon, C. (1970). *Eur. J. Pharmacol.* **12,** 490.
Axelrod, J. (1957). *Science* **126,** 400.
Axelrod, J. (1962). *J. Biol. Chem.* **237,** 1657.
Axelrod, J., and Laroche, M. J. (1959). *Science* **130,** 800.
Axelrod, J., and Tomchick, R. (1958). *J. Biol. Chem.* **233,** 702.
Axelrod, J., and Vesell, E. S. (1970). *Mol. Pharmacol.* **6,** 78.
Axelrod, J., Senoh, S., and Witkop, B. (1958). *J. Biol. Chem.* **233,** 697.
Axelrod, J., Albers, W., and Clemente, C. D. (1959). *J. Neurochem.* **5,** 68.
Axelrod, J., Hertting, G., and Potter, L. (1962). *Nature (London)* **194,** 297.
Axelrod, J., Mueller, R. A., Henry, J. P., and Stephens, P. M. (1970). *Nature (London)* **225,** 1059.
Axelrod, J., Weil-Malherbe, H., and Tomchick, R. (1959). *J. Pharmacol. Exp. Ther.* **127,** 251.
Belleau, B., and Burba, J. (1963). *J. Med. Chem.* **6,** 755.
Blaschko, H., and Hertting, G. (1970). *Arch. Exp. Pathol. Pharmakol.* **266,** 296.
Brandau, K., and Axelrod, J. (1972). *Naunyn-Schmiedebergs Arch. Pharmakol.* **273,** 123.
Brimijoin, S., and Molinoff, P. B. (1971). *J. Pharmacol. Exp. Ther.* **178,** 417.
Burn, J. H., and Rand, M. J. (1958). *J. Physiol. (London)* **144,** 314.
Carlsson, A., Rosengren, E., Bertler, A., and Nilsson, J. (1957). *In* "Psychotropic Drugs" (S. Garattini and V. Ghetti, eds.), p. 363. Elsevier, Amsterdam.

Carlsson, A., Falck, B., and Hillarp, N. A. (1962). *Acta Physiol. Scand.* **56,** Suppl. 196.

Carter, S. B. (1967). *Nature* **213,** 261.

Cass, R., Kuazman, R., and Brodie, B. B. (1960). *Proc. Soc. Exp. Biol. Med.* **103,** 871.

Ciaranello, R., Jacobowitz, D., and Axelrod, J. (1973). *J. Neurochem.* in press.

Coyle, J. T., and Snyder, S. H. (1969). *J. Pharmacol. Exp. Ther.* **170,** 221.

Crout, J. R. (1961). *Proc. Soc. Exp. Biol. Med.* **108,** 482.

Dahlstrom, A. (1968). *Eur. J. Pharmacol.* **5,** 111.

Dairman, M., and Udenfriend, S. (1970). *Mol. Pharmacol.* **6,** 350.

DePotter, W. P., DeSchaepdryver, A. F., Moerman, E. J., and Smith, A. D. (1969). *J. Physiol. (London)* **204,** 102P.

Douglas, W. W., and Rubin, R. P. (1961). *J. Physiol. (London)* **159,** 40.

Elliott, T. R. (1905). *J. Physiol. (London)* **32,** 401.

Geffen, L. B., Livett, B. G., and Rush, R. A. (1969). *J. Physiol. (London)* **204,** 593.

Gillespie, E., Levine, R. J., and Malawista, S. E. (1968). *J. Pharmacol. Exp. Ther.* **164,** 158.

Hartman, B. K., Molinoff, P. B., and Udenfriend, S. (1970). *Pharmacologist* **12,** 470.

Hertting, G., and Axelrod, J. (1961). *Nature (London)* **192,** 172.

Hertting, G., Axelrod, J., Kopin, I. J., and Whitby, L. G. (1961a). *Nature (London)* **189,** 66.

Hertting, G., Axelrod, J., and Whitby, L. G. (1961b). *J. Pharmacol. Exp. Ther.* **134,** 146.

Hillarp, N. A. (1959). *Acta Physiol. Scand.* **46,** Suppl. 157.

Holtz, P., Heise, R., and Ludtke, K. (1938). *Naunyn-Schmiedebergs Arch. Exp. Pathol. Pharmakol.* **191,** 87.

Iggo, A., and Vogt, M. (1960). *J. Physiol. (London)* **150,** 114.

Ikeda, M., Fahien, L. A., and Udenfriend, S. (1966). *J. Biol. Chem.* **241,** 4452.

Iversen, L. L. (1967). "The Uptake and Storage of Noradrenaline in Sympathetic Nerves." Cambridge Univ. Press, London and New York.

Iversen, L. L. (1971). *Brit. J. Pharmacol.* **41,** 571.

Iversen, L. L., Glowinski, J., and Axelrod, J. (1966). *J. Pharmacol. Exp. Ther.* **151,** 273.

Johnson, D., Thoa, N. B., Weinshilboum, R. M., Axelrod, J., and Kopin, I. J. (1971). *Proc. Nat. Acad. Sci. U.S.* **68,** 2227.

Kirshner, N. (1957). *J. Biol. Chem.* **226,** 821.

Kirshner, N., and Goodall, M. (1957). *Biochim. Biophys. Acta* **24,** 658.

Kirshner, N., Sage, H. J., Smith, W. J., and Kirshner, A. G. (1966). *Science* **154,** 529.

Knuppen, V. R., Höller, M., Tilmann, D., and Breuer, H. (1969). *Hoppe Seylers Z. Physiol. Chem.* **350,** 1301.

Kopin, I. J. (1964). *Pharmacol. Rev.* **16,** 179.

Kopin, I. J., Fischer, J. E., Musacchio, J. M., and Horst, W. D. (1964). *Proc. Nat. Acad. Sci. U.S.* **52,** 716.

Kvetnansky, R., Weise, V. K., and Kopin, I. J. (1970). *Endocrinology* **87,** 744.

Kvetnansky, R., Gewirtz, G. P., Weise, V. K., and Kopin, I. J. (1971). *Mol. Pharmacol.* **7,** 81.

Lacy, P. E., Howell, S. L., Young, D. A., and Fink, C. J. (1968). *Nature (London)* **219,** 1177.

Levin, J. A., and Furchgott, R. F. (1970). *J. Pharmacol. Exp. Ther.* **172,** 320.

Levin, E. Y., Levenberg, B., and Kaufman, S. (1960). *J. Biol. Chem.* **235,** 2080.

Loewi, O. (1921). *Pfluegers Arch. Gesamte Physiol. Menschen Tiere* **189,** 239.

Logan, W. J., and Snyder, S. H. (1971). *Nature (London)* **234,** 297.

Margolies, F. L., Roffi, J., and Jost, A. (1966). *Science* **154,** 275.

Molinoff, P. B., and Axelrod, J. (1969). *Science* **164,** 428.

Molinoff, P. B., and Axelrod, J. (1972). *J. Neurochem.* **19,** 157.

Molinoff, P. B., Landsberg, L., and Axelrod, J. (1969). *J. Pharmacol. Exp. Ther.* **170,** 253.

Molinoff, P. B., Brimijoin, W. S., Weinshilboum, R. M., and Axelrod, J. (1970). *Proc. Nat. Acad. Sci. U.S.* **66,** 453.

Molinoff, P. B., Brimijoin, S., and Axelrod, J. (1972). *J. Pharmacol. Exp. Ther.* **182,** 116.

Mueller, R. A., Thoenen, H., and Axelrod, J. (1969a). *Science* **163,** 468.

Mueller, R. A., Thoenen, H., and Axelrod, J. (1969b). *J. Pharmacol. Exp. Ther.* **169,** 74.

Mueller, R. A., Thoenen, H., and Axelrod, J. (1969c). *Mol. Pharmacol.* **5,** 463.

Mueller, R. A., Thoenen, H., and Axelrod, J. (1970a). *Eur. J. Pharmacol.* **10,** 51.

Mueller, R. A., Thoenen, H., and Axelrod, J. (1970b). *Endocrinology* **86,** 751.

Musacchio, J. M., Fischer, J. E., and Kopin, I. J. (1966). *J. Pharmacol. Exp. Ther.* **152,** 51.

Nagatsu, T., Levitt, M., and Udenfriend, S. (1964). *J. Biol. Chem.* **239,** 2910.

Nikodijevic, B., Senoh, S., Daly, J. W., and Creveling, C. R. (1970). *J. Pharmacol. Exp. Ther.* **174,** 83.

Patrick, R. L., and Kirshner, N. (1971). *Mol. Pharmacol.* **7,** 87.

Poisner, A. M., and Bernstein, J. (1971). *J. Pharmacol. Exp. Ther.* **177,** 102.

Potter, L. T., and Axelrod, J. (1963). *J. Pharmacol. Exp. Ther.* **142,** 299.

Roffi, J. (1968). *J. Physiol. (Paris)* **60,** 455.

Rosell, S., Kopin, I. J., and Axelrod, J. (1963). *Amer. J. Physiol.* **205,** 317.

Senoh, S., Daly, J., Axelrod, J., and Witkop, B. (1959). *J. Amer. Chem. Soc.* **81,** 6240.

Shelanski, M. L., and Taylor, E. W. (1967). *J. Cell Biol.* **34,** 549.

Silberstein, S. D., Brimijoin, S., Molinoff, P. B., and Lemberger, L. (1972). *J. Neurochem.* **19,** 919.

Snyder, S. H., Fischer, J. E., and Axelrod, J. (1965). *Biochem. Pharmacol.* **14,** 363.

Spector, S., Shore, P., and Brodie, B. B. (1960). *J. Pharmacol. Exp. Ther.* **128,** 15.

Spector, S., Gordon, R., Sjoerdsma, A., and Udenfriend, S. (1967). *Mol. Pharmacol.* **3,** 549.

Thoa, N. B., Wooten, G. F., Axelrod, J., and Kopin, I. J. (1972). *Proc. Nat. Acad. Sci. U.S.* **69,** 520.

Thoenen, H. (1970). *Nature (London)* **228,** 861.

Thoenen, H., and Tranzer, J. P. (1968). *Naunyn-Schmiedebergs Arch. Pharmakol. Exp. Pathol.* **261,** 271.

Thoenen, H., Mueller, R. A., and Axelrod, J. (1969a). *J. Pharmacol. Exp. Ther.* **169,** 249.

Thoenen, H., Mueller, R. A., and Axelrod, J. (1969b). *Nature (London)* **221,** 1264.

Thoenen, H., Mueller, R. A., and Axelrod, J. (1970a). *Proc. Nat. Acad. Sci. U.S.* **65,** 58.

Thoenen, H., Mueller, R. A., and Axelrod, J. (1970b). *Biochem. Pharmacol.* **19,** 669.

Tranzer, J. P., and Thoenen, H. (1968). *Experientia* **24,** 155.

Udenfriend, S., Zaltzman-Nirenberg, P., and Nagatsu, T. (1965). *Biochem. Pharmacol.* **14,** 837.

Viveros, O. H., Arqueros, L., Connett, R. J., and Kirshner, N. (1969). *Mol. Pharmacol.* **5,** 69.

von Euler, U. S. (1946). *Acta Physiol. Scand.* **12,** 73.

von Euler, U. S., and Floding, I. (1955). *Acta Physiol. Scand.* **33,** Suppl. 118, p. 57.

von Euler, U. S., and Lishajko, F. (1963). *Acta Physiol. Scand.* **59,** 454.

Weiner, N., and Rabadjija, M. (1968). *J. Pharmacol. Exp. Ther.* **160,** 61.

Weinshilboum, R., and Axelrod, J. (1970). *Endocrinology* **87,** 894.

Weinshilboum, R., and Axelrod, J. (1971a). *Circ. Res.* **28,** 307.

Weinshilboum, R., and Axelrod, J. (1971b). *Science* **173,** 931.

Weinshilboum, R., and Axelrod, J. (1971c). *N. Engl. J. Med.* **285,** 938.

Weinshilboum, R., Kvetnansky, R., Axelrod, J., and Kopin, I. J. (1971a). *Nature (London) New Biol.* **230,** 287.

Weinshilboum, R., Thoa, N. B., Johnson, D., Kopin, I. J., and Axelrod, J. (1971b). *Science* **174,** 1349.

Wessells, N. K., Spooner, B. S., Ash, J. F., Bradley, M. O., Luduena, M. A., Taylor, E. L., Wrenn, J. T., and Yamada, K. M. (1971). *Science* **171,** 135.

Whitby, L. G., Axelrod, J., and Weil-Malherbe, H. (1961). *J. Pharmacol. Exp. Ther.* **132,** 193.

Williams, J. A., and Wolff, J. (1970). *Proc. Nat. Acad. Sci. U.S.* **67,** 1901.

Wolfe, D. E., Potter, L. T., Richardson, K. C., and Axelrod, J. (1962). *Science* **138,** 440.

Wurtman, R. J. (1966). *Endocrinology* **79,** 608.

Wurtman, R. J., and Axelrod, J. (1966). *J. Biol. Chem.* **241,** 2301.

Wurtman, R. J., Casper, A., Axelrod, J., and Bartter, F. (1967). *J. Clin. Invest.* **46,** 1135.

Zeller, E. A., and Barsky, J. (1952). *Proc. Soc. Exp. Biol. Med.* **81,** 459.

HEROIN ADDICTION—AN EPIDEMIC DISEASE*

VINCENT P. DOLE

The Rockefeller University, New York, New York

I. Introduction

EIGHT years ago Dr. Nyswander and I admitted two heroin addicts for metabolic studies into the Hospital of Rockefeller University. Both of these men had been heroin "mainliners" for several years. When we first saw them, they were waiting for admission to another hospital for detoxification—not with any hope of cure, since they had been detoxified many times before, but simply to reduce their narcotic habits to manageable size.

We wanted to observe in some detail the pharmacological effects of known doses of narcotics in addicts. Although this drug study seemed radical when first proposed, the Research Committee of the Hospital and President Bronk of the University recognized that it would not expose the subjects to any new hazards since their bodies had long been habituated to intake of narcotics. Indeed, the patients would be far better off during the projected few months of the study receiving controlled doses of chemically pure drugs in a hospital than they would be on the street using contaminated mixtures of heroin. For their part, the subjects were delighted at the prospect of what they saw as a free ride on drugs with rest and good food. We promised to detoxify them before discharge, but otherwise did not offer any rehabilitative services and certainly could not hold out any hope of curing their addiction.

As it worked out, both patients after discharge from the hospital stayed with us as outpatients and are now normal members of society. The younger patient returned to high school during the first year of treatment, and then completed college with a degree in aeronautical engineering. Both are now employed in responsible jobs. I would like to tell you how this unforeseen result came about.

* Lecture delivered January 20, 1972.

We launched these studies out of dissatisfaction with the older psychological theories of narcotics addiction. According to these theories, all addictions were psychiatric problems, character weaknesses marked by the addict's desire to escape reality. Physical dependence on narcotic drugs and the punishing symptoms of abstinence when drug intake is suddenly stopped were recognized as factors that reinforced the drug-taking habit—but the root of the disease, according to the traditional theory, was psychological and therefore the treatment had to be psychotherapeutic. The difficulty with this old theory was its lack of cures. Fifty years of psychotherapy, group therapy, psychoanalysis, hypnosis, persuasion, vocational training, and confinement in prisons had failed to stop more than a small number of addicts from using heroin, perhaps no more than would have stopped without treatment.

On the other hand, the pharmacological aspects of addiction seemed neglected. Although addicts had been given morphine and other narcotics for periods of months at the Addiction Research Center (Lexington, Kentucky) for the purpose of assaying the addiction potential of different drugs, there had been no systematic study of the functional state of addicts receiving different narcotic drugs in various dosages, or of the potential for rehabilitation when patients were maintained on narcotic drugs outside of a prison environment. Moreover, research in this direction was actively discouraged by both medical authorities and regulatory bureaus. The reason cited for opposing this research was that ambulatory clinics had attempted to maintain addicts with morphine in the early 1920's and had failed. Nevertheless, with support from the Health Research Council, New York City, we launched the studies.

Our first experiment—an attempt to maintain two hospitalized patients with morphine—made us sympathize with the operators of the early clinics. After a few days of morphine injections the patients began to complain that the dose was insufficient. By the end of the sixth week, at which time we halted this experiment, the total daily dose had reached the astronomical level of 500 mg per day. It appeared that the authorities were right in saying that narcotic maintenance was impractical. Of course if the patients had been locked in a prison, we could have maintained them on a fixed dose and injection schedule like laboratory animals, but with patients free to leave we had to retain their cooperation, and this was not easy. Despite the large doses given, the patients were not happy with the experiment. Their periods of sedation and euphoria after each dose became shorter; within an hour or two after each injection they were anxiously watching the clock, waiting for the next dose. Each morning they would awaken with abstinence symptoms.

But morphine was only one of the narcotic drugs in the planned study. Although oxycodone, like morphine, was disappointing, the third drug tested—methadone—showed quite different effects. Gradually we became aware of a change in behavior of the two patients. The daily dosage of methadone became stabilized. No longer were the patients watching the clock, waiting for the next injection; no longer were they sedated after receiving a dose, or awakening sick in the morning. They became interested in art and craft work provided by the occupational therapist (Ann Morris), and they even initiated a plan of going to night school while the experiments continued. Had these patients become acclimated to the therapeutic environment of our metabolic ward, or did methadone, given on the schedule that we had stumbled into, have effects so different from those of morphine?

To answer this question we brought in four more addict patients, and with Dr. Mary Jeanne Kreek (who had joined us as a visiting investigator) began a systematic study of the effects of methadone at different dosage levels. We found that with a gradual increase in daily ration the patients remained alert and in good function. As the dose was increased they became progressively more refractory to the euphoriant action of heroin and other narcotic drugs given as intravenous challenges, without showing narcotic effects from the methadone. Their preoccupation with narcotic drugs was markedly reduced on the stabilized methadone schedule, and three of the patients sought and were given permission to take outside jobs on days when injection experiments were not being conducted. The route of administration of methadone was changed from intra-muscular or oral, and the frequency from twice daily to once daily, with improvement in result. The patients on this schedule appeared to be entirely normal individuals, without drug hunger. Methadone had brought about a dramatic change in behavior without producing narcotic effects. We verified the patients' claim that they were not feeling any narcotic sensations by making substitutions with the narcotically inactive isomer, *d*-methadone. None of the patients detected the change from active to inactive medication when one-day substitutions were made in double-blind experiments. At a later stage, when the inactive isomer was continued for 36–48 hours, they gradually developed withdrawal symptoms.

The most important difference between morphine and methadone is the much longer period of action of methadone on the once-daily, oral schedule. Unlike methadone, morphine and oxycodone had failed to stabilize the patients pharmacologically. The addict on the street using heroin (which is rapidly converted into morphine in the body) oscillates between sedation and sickness, both of which conditions incapacitate him for normal life (Fig. 1). Methadone, presumably because it establishes a steadier depot in the tissue and because its effects are further smoothed by oral administration, maintains the patient in pharmacological stability. Given in a steady maintenance dose, it extinguishes the abnormal drug hunger of narcotics addicts and maintains a high tolerance against the narcotic effects of injected narcotic drugs without producing euphoria (Fig. 2).

There is thus a marked difference in the pharmacological properties of heroin and methadone on chronic administration (Table I).

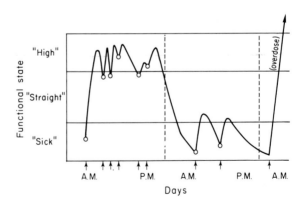

FIG. 1.   Period of action of heroin.

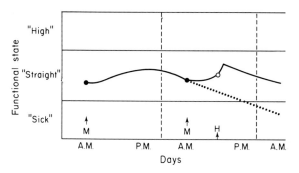

Fᴉɢ. 2.   Period of action of steady maintenance dosage of methadone.

Previous work, showing a similarity of these drugs when assayed by single, intravenous injections given to ex-addicts, had obscured the critically important differences in effect of heroin and methadone on chronic administration. With these findings, it became reasonable to consider long-term maintenance treatment with methadone.

We brought these preliminary results to Dr. Ray Trussell, then Commissioner of Hospitals, New York City, and were invited by him to try a demonstration on a larger scale in the ward of a general hospital. He was particularly struck by the fact that four of the six patients were working at jobs outside the hospital, in addition to having stopped their use of heroin. We had the very good fortune to be given space at the Manhattan General Hospital, which later became the Bernstein Institute division of Beth Israel Medical

TABLE I

Hᴇʀᴏɪɴ ᴠꜱ. Mᴇᴛʜᴀᴅᴏɴᴇ[a]

	Heroin	Methadone
Mode of administration	IV	Oral
Onset of action	Immediate	30 Minutes
Duration of action	3–6 Hours	24–36 Hours
Euphoria	First 1–2 hours	None
Withdrawal symptoms	After 3–4 hours	After 24 hours

[a] Effects of high dosages in tolerant individuals.

204   VINCENT P. DOLE

Center. The courageous administrative support of this medical center made possible the emergence of methadone maintenance treatment as a large-scale program. Following on the model developed at Beth Israel Medical Center, successful methadone programs are now operating in major cities of United States and Canada. All the programs that have adopted the Beth Israel procedure have had comparable success: retention of 80% or more of the patients and reduction in crime to less than 5% of the pretreatment rate (Fig. 3).

II.   Heroin Addiction as a Disease

Implicit in the maintenance programs is an assumption that heroin addiction is a metabolic disease, rather than a psychological prob-

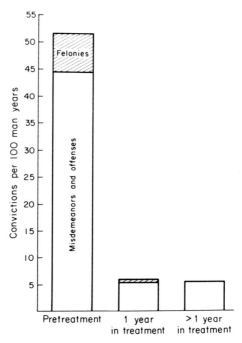

Fig. 3.   Conviction record of 912 former heroin addicts before treatment and after one year and over one year of methadone maintenance treatment.

lem. Although the reasons for taking the initial doses of heroin may be considered psychological—adolescent curiosity or neurotic anxiety—the drug, for whatever reason it is first taken, leaves its imprint on the nervous system. This phenomenon is clearly seen in animal studies: A rat, if addicted to morphine by repeated injections at 1–2 months of age and then detoxified, will show a residual tolerance and abnormalities in brain waves in response to challenge doses of morphine for months, perhaps for the rest of its life. Simply stopping the drug does not restore the nervous system of this animal to its normal, preaddictive condition. Since all studies to date have shown a close association between tolerance and physical dependence, and since the discomfort of physical dependence leads to drug-seeking activity, a persistence of physical dependence would explain why both animals and men tend to relapse to use of narcotics after detoxification. This metabolic theory of relapse obviously has different implications for treatment than the traditional theory that relapse is due to moral weakness.

Whatever the theory, all treatments should be measured by results. The main issue, in our opinion, is whether the treatment can enable addicts to become normal, responsible members of society, and if a medication contributes to this result it should be regarded as useful chemotherapy. Methadone, like sulfanilamide of the early antibiotic days, undoubtedly will be supplanted by better medications, but the success of methadone maintenance programs has at least established the principle of treating addicts medically.

Maintenance is not indicated for every heroin user. For rational treatment, we must distinguish early and late stages of narcotics addiction:

Stage I is the initial, experimental stage of exposure to heroin (usually by sniffing) beginning with curiosity or peer group pressure.

Stage II is a social interlude of 6–12 months, in which the drug is used occasionally with a group for excitement and pleasure.

Stage III is the end point of true pharmacological addiction. The addict will become abstinent if he does not have a dose of narcotic every few hours. In the argot of the addicts, he is "hooked"; in that of the pharmacologists, he is physically dependent.

All the addicts seen in Stage III obviously have passed through I and II, but it is possible that many persons who experimented with narcotics, or even used narcotic drugs socially for a time, have stopped before reaching the terminal stage. There are no statistics on this. Quite certainly, however, if a person exposes himself to enough narcotic he will become addicted. The usual history of the Stage III addict is that he had used narcotics intermittently under the illusion of taking the drug or not as he chose, and then woke up sick one morning with the realization that he was hooked. He needed a shot to relieve his sickness, and from that time was a slave to this need

Maintenance with methadone should be considered only for addicts in Stage III, and not for every one of these. For Stages I and II, the treatment is indirect—diminishing the availability of drugs, and relieving the social conditions that make drug use attractive. To be a suitable candidate for chemotherapy, a Stage III addict also must want this treatment. If he is motivated toward a drug-free program, every effort should be made to find a proper placement.

III. HEROIN ADDICTION AS AN EPIDEMIC

The large numbers of heroin addicts in New York City (over 150,000), and the mode of spread from areas of high drug usage (Fig. 4) with the addicts serving as carriers to infect susceptibles, are typical of an epidemic. The loss of property (over a billion dollars per year), the destruction of families and neighborhoods, and the danger of the streets add up to economic disaster for New York City. Seen in the perspective of epidemiology, the problem of heroin addiction goes beyond the treatment of isolated cases. What is needed is a comprehensive approach, with strong leadership, in which we use all that we know about prevention and treatment of this disease.

Reducing the availability of heroin is a key to prevention. Here (despite much adverse publicity) the enforcement agencies have been quite effective, as shown by the high price and poor quality of heroin on the black market today, compared with the more potent supply available fifteen years ago. The fallacy in the enforcement approach, however, is the assumption that the epidemic of heroin use could be stopped by enforcement alone. With large numbers of Stage III addicts in the city, a shortage of heroin increases their desperation. What is needed is a combination of enforcement activities to limit

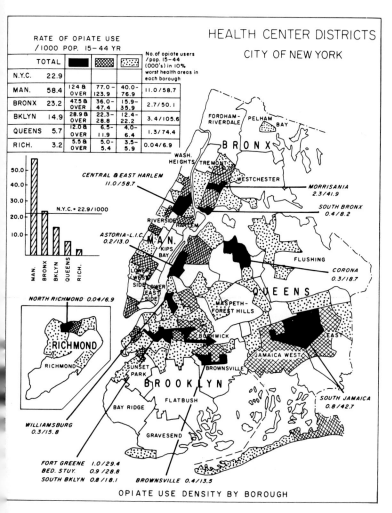

Fig. 4.   Data showing mode of spread from areas of high drug usage with addicts as carriers.

the supply of drug, with effective treatment programs to deal with persons already addicted. Enforcement and treatment are complementary, and both essential, if the epidemic is to be controlled.

For young people in Stages I and II, it is also essential that the social conditions favoring drug use be remedied. Adolescents need alternatives to drugs—recreation, wholesome challenges, job opportunities, hope for the future, adults that they can respect and imitate, understanding, and counseling. Few, if any, adolescents are helped by sermonizing or prison.

The immediate problem in the New York City epidemic is to treat the vast number of Stage III addicts. Unless a significant fraction of them are brought under control, the epidemic will continue unchecked. They will continue to support the market for heroin, whatever the price. We must bring effective treatment to at least 50,000 of these addicts in the near future, and the only possibility of achieving this is through large-scale methadone maintenance programs. Therapeutic communities conceivably might expand to hold 7500 ex-addicts, but even this optimistic projection would account for only 5% of the number of addicts now known to the Narcotics Registry.

Every treatment program that can remove any addict from the census should be supported (providing that it keeps objective records), but at present the only alternative to large-scale methadone maintenance is to leave the majority of the addicts untreated. Future research no doubt will yield better medicines than methadone (what we need is something as effective as methadone in stopping heroin addiction, but nontoxic when misused and entirely safe for general distribution), but to wait for the appearance of this ideal medicine would be a prescription for doing nothing about the epidemic.

IV. HEROIN ADDICTION AND THE CRIMINAL JUSTICE SYSTEM

We must also undo the mistakes of our criminal justice system, which have complicated the problem of dealing with addicts. Although it is frequently said that addicts must be treated as sick people, in practice we put them in jail. Even the civil commitment programs, which started with the high purpose of providing treatment as an alternative to punishment, became in practice another kind of prison, and so failed to solve the heroin problem. One lesson that should be learned from the expensive failures of the New York State civil commitment program, the California commitment program, the Federal jail hospitals at Lexington and Forth Worth, and the New York City civil commitment program at Riverside Hospital is that prisons, even when called hospitals, do not cure addicts.

A second lesson is that prisons cannot be used for removal of addicts from the streets. There are too many addicts. There is not enough space in prison, and we could not build enough prisons to solve the problem by removal. If all the space in all the jails of New York were to be used only for segregation of addicts, 10% of the addicts would be removed from the streets. The remaining 90% would be left in the community, using heroin and committing crimes.

Let us look at our present policy of criminalizing addiction (Fig. 5). We circulate the addicts through the police stations, arraignment courts, houses of detention, trial courts, prisons, and back again to the streets, finally releasing them worse than when they were arrested. No one in this present cycle has responsibility to ask *why* the person committed the crime that led to his arrest. There is

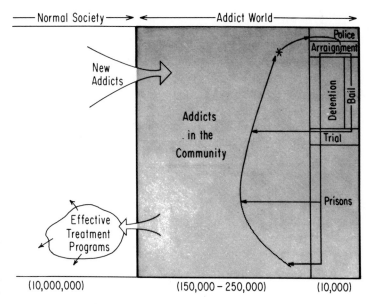

FIG. 5. Present management of addiction.

at present no systematic effort to place the addict in a treatment program that could deal with the cause of his criminal activity, namely his addiction. As a result, the machine grinds on, making the problem worse. Addicts are created in ghettos; they commit crimes to support the drug habit and are punished for the crimes they commit without treatment for the addiction. How much longer can we support such an irrational system?

The alternative is to transform the Houses of Detention into diagnostic clinics. Everyone who arrives in a detention jail has a problem. For some detainees, the immediate problem is to hold on to their family and job; they should be returned home as soon as possible and managed as outpatients. But for others with intractable addiction, a thorough medical and social workup could be the beginning of a new life. If effective treatment programs are available, the criminal addict has a chance to become a normal citizen.

This alternative approach to detention is outlined in Fig. 6. The emphasis in the new approach is motion of addicts into treatment.

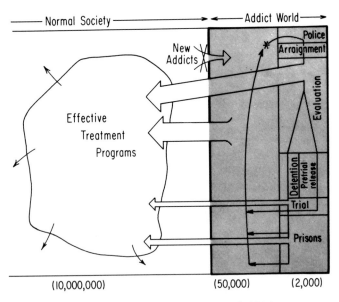

FIG. 6. Alternative future management of addiction.

Only by effective treatment of the addicts in community programs can we break the cycle of crime-jail-crime-jail.

Perhaps, if we in normal society are capable of learning, addicts will teach us a generally important lesson about human behavior. Whenever a person deviates from social standards, there has to be a cause. Someone in the criminal justice system should have the responsibility to ask what it is, knowing that society's interest in crime is to prevent a recurrence of the offense, not to avenge it. Addicts have shown us the futility of punishment in prevention of crime, and this lesson forces us to the general question of what prisons are for. Many nonaddict prisoners are also deteriorating in jail.

With addicts we now have the means to make a new start. We can reform the criminal justice system to provide medical treatment for them as an alternative to jail. We must not stop until diagnosis and nonpunitive therapy are also available for rehabilitation of other offenders. Confinement of criminals, like banishment of lepers, is the last resort of a desperate society that has no effective ways to treat behavioral disease. It is our duty as physicians to find these treatments.

ANTIGEN DESIGN AND IMMUNE RESPONSE*†

MICHAEL SELA

*Department of Chemical Immunology,
The Weizmann Institute of Science,
Rehovot, Israel*

I. Introduction

IMMUNOLOGY has been an art since time immemorial, and a science for approximately one hundred years. It is a branch of life sciences dealing not only with immunity, but also with such disparate medical aspects as allergy, organ transplantation, auto-immune diseases, and cancer. The main interest of the immunologist today is to elucidate the basic molecular and cellular events which are common to the manifold immunological phenomena. The materials leading to an immune response are called antigens, and the body reacts to them either by producing antibodies or by a cellular immunological reaction. The antigens used in medicine and in research were of a natural (animal, vegetal, microbial, etc.) origin until a dozen years ago, when synthetic antigens were first described (for earlier literature, see Sela, 1969). The notion of antigen encompasses two distinct properties, namely, its immunogenicity and antigenic specificity. Immunogenicity is the capacity to provoke an immune response and is independent of the specificity of the antibodies formed. Antigenic specificity is reflected in the nature of the antibody combining site and is defined as the capacity of a molecule, or small portions of it, to react with antibodies, already formed.

The synthetic approach offers the advantage that, once the immunogenicity of one synthetic material has been unequivocally demonstrated, many analogs may be prepared and tested. If the "antigen design" is known, it seems possible, through a study of

* Lecture delivered February 17, 1972.

† The work from our laboratory was supported by Agreements 06-010 and 06-035 with the National Institutes of Health, U.S. Public Health Service, and a grant from Minerva Foundation.

compounds showing only limited variations in their chemical formulas, to arrive at conclusions concerning the role of various structural features in their antigenic function. Indeed, this approach has been very helpful in reaching a better understanding of the molecular basis of antigenicity (Sela, 1966, 1969). Among the problems which have been considered, I would like to mention the roles of shape, size, and composition of the immunogenic macromolecule, of the locus within the molecule of the areas important for immunogenicity and for specificity, of the optical configuration of its component amino acids, and of its electrical charge. I shall discuss in this lecture the role of steric conformation in antigenicity, and the use of model antigens in the elucidation of this problem.

In many of our immunological studies, my colleagues and I have used not only linear synthetic polypeptides but also branched amino acid copolymers, denoted "multichain polyamino acids" (Sela *et al.*, 1956). One example, namely, multi-copoly (Tyr, Glu)-polyDLAla—polyLys, abbreviated to (T, G)-A—L (Sela *et al.*, 1962), is shown in Fig. 1. Besides synthetic antigens composed exclusively of amino acids, immunogenic macromolecules have also been prepared that are capable of provoking antibodies reacting specifically with sugars, lipids, nucleosides, vitamins, etc. As a matter of fact it seems possible to prepare antibodies of almost any specificity desired provided the antigen is designed properly.

A fascinating observation largely due to the use of synthetic antigens is the inverse relationship between the net electrical charge on an immunogen and that on its specific antibodies. It led me to the conclusion that an immunogen is much more than an antigenic determinant attached to an inert carrier (Sela, 1967). The antigenic carrier is of paramount importance both in influencing the chemical nature of the antibodies formed and in controlling the antibody biosynthesis. I shall describe here some recent experiments on the cellular nature of the inverse relationship between the net charge of immunogens and of antibodies elicited, taking into consideration the cooperation between cells derived from the thymus and those derived from the bone marrow.

This cooperation between the so-called T and B cells, while valid for most antigens investigated, does not seem to hold for some antigens. We have now studied carefully designed immunogens,

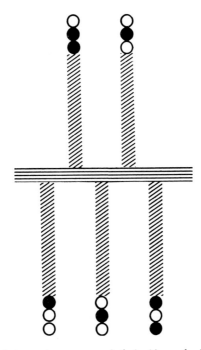

Fig. 1. A multichain copolymer composed of a backbone of poly-L-lysine to which are attached side chains of poly-DL-alanine, elongated with peptides of L-tyrosine and L-glutamic acid. The polymer is denoted multi-copoly(Tyr, Glu)-polyDLAla—polyLys, and abbreviated as (T, G)-A—L.

identical in their chemical structure and differing only in the optical configuration of the amino acids composing them. I shall discuss here these results, leading to the conclusion that difficultly metabolizable antigens seem to be thymus independent.

Synthetic antigens have been helpful in elucidating many immunological phenomena, but nowhere has the progress been as striking as in the understanding of the genetic control of immune response (McDevitt and Benacerraf, 1969). I shall describe here some of the most interesting results in this fascinating area of immunology. Thus, it is my intention to discuss in this lecture several recent examples from my laboratory, illustrating the effect of antigen structure both on the nature of the antibodies formed

and on the antibody production itself. While some of these studies
are largely on a chemical (molecular) level, it became apparent
recently that many cellular immunological phenomena became
prone for a molecular attack, and that the use of the proper antigen
design may help toward their elucidation.

II. ROLE OF STERIC CONFORMATION IN ANTIGENICITY

A. Recognition on Molecular Level

The interaction of the determinant group on the antigen with the
combining site on the antibody represents a uniquely specific pattern
of recognition on a molecular level, and it involves two macromolecules. One of these molecules is the antibody, and we know
today that the specificity of its combining sites results from a unique
conformation, controlled by the amino acid sequence of its component polypeptide chains, i.e., by its primary structure. This has
been concluded from studies in which all the disulfide bridges in
antibody fragments (Haber, 1964; Whitney and Tanford, 1965) or
in the complete antibody molecule (Freedman and Sela, 1966b)
have been opened under denaturing conditions, with concurrent
loss of the native tertiary structure and biological activity, and
have been reformed to restore to a large extent the original antibody
activity. These studies support the hypothesis that no other genetic
information is required to specify the three-dimensional structure
of a protein molecule beyond that which codes for the amino acid
sequence of the nascent polypeptide chain (Sela *et al.*, 1957; Anfinsen,
1967), and they demonstrate that the specificity of antibodies is
not an exception to this rule.

The three-dimensional structure of the antigen may also be of
utmost importance for its immunogenicity and for the antigenic
specificity of its determinants. In protein and polypeptide antigens
it is possible to distinguish between "sequential" determinants and
conformation-dependent determinants (Sela *et al.*, 1967; Sela, 1969).
I would like to call a sequential determinant one due to an amino
acid sequence in a random coil form, and antibodies to such a determinant are expected to react with a peptide of identical, or
similar, sequence. On the other hand, a conformational determinant

results from the steric conformation of the antigenic macromolecule, and leads to antibodies that would not necessarily react with peptides derived from that area of the molecule. It seems that antibodies to native proteins are directed mostly against conformational rather than sequential determinants. Similar argumentation makes it possible to distinguish between sequential and conformational determinants in other macromolecules, such as nucleic acids.

Many studies of the immunological properties of native proteins have shown conclusively that the antibodies obtained are directed mostly, and in several well-documented cases exclusively, against conformation-dependent determinants. Thus, for example, antisera produced with native bovine pancreatic RNase do not react with the denatured, open-chain RNase, in which all the disulfide bridges were severed, nor do antibodies against the open chain react with the native enzyme (Brown, 1963). Rabbit immunoglobulin G may serve as another example. Antibodies prepared in goat are not able to react with a derivative in which all the disulfide bridges in the immunoglobulin G were opened (Freedman and Sela, 1966a; Sela et al., 1967).

B. Collagenlike Immunogen

In recent years we have tried to obtain a better understanding of the role of conformation in antigenicity by building appropriate synthetic models. The investigation of the immunological properties of a collagenlike synthetic polypeptide may serve as one example (Borek et al., 1969). A synthetic polypeptide $(\text{LPro-Gly-LPro})_n$ with an ordered sequence, previously shown to have physical properties similar to those of collagen was found to be immunogenic in guinea pigs and rabbits. Guinea pigs, immunized with $(\text{LPro-Gly-LPro})_n$, produced antibodies which cross-reacted by passive cutaneous anaphylaxis with a random copolymer of similar composition, poly(L-Pro^{66}, Gly^{34}). Skin cross-reactions in guinea pigs were also observed between $(\text{LPro-Gly-LPro})_n$ and fish, rat, Ascaris, and guinea pig collagens (Borek et al., 1969; Maoz et al., 1972). As demonstrated in Table I, guinea pigs immunized with the collagenlike polymer gave delayed type skin reactions with several natural collagens. No cross-reactions between poly(L-Pro^{66}, Gly^{34}) and collagens, or

TABLE I

Skin Cross-Reactions in Guinea Pigs Immunized with
(LPro-Gly-LPro)$_n$ 10 Days after Immunization[a]

	Skin reactions[b]	
Test antigen	Immediate (2 hours)	Delayed (24 hours)
(L-Pro-Gly-L-Pro)$_n$	3/8 (13)[c]	8/8 (12)
(L-Pro^{66}, Gly^{34})$_n$	0/3	8/8 (6)
Guinea pig skin collagen	0/3	8/8 (7)
Reduced and carboxymethylated *Ascaris* cuticle collagen	0/3	8/8 (10)
Rat tail tendon collagen	0/3	8/8 (6)

[a] From Maoz *et al.* (1972).

[b] Reactions with an average diameter of 5 mm or less were considered negative. Control animals that were injected with buffered saline and complete Freund's adjuvant gave negative reactions with all the test antigens.

[c] Ratio of responders to total number of animals. Numbers in parentheses give the average reaction diameter in nanometers.

between gelatin and the synthetic polypeptides were observed. Thus, the polymer of ordered sequence cross-reacts immunologically with collagen by virtue of the triple helix conformation common to both substances. This cross-reactivity at the cellular level shows that it is possible to provoke a cross-reacting immune response to an autologous protein by immunization with a synthetic antigen.

C. Transconformation of a Polypeptide upon Interaction with Related Antibodies

In contrast to antibodies against sequential determinants [e.g., alanine peptides in polyalanyl proteins (Clerici *et al.*, 1970; Schechter *et al.*, 1970)], antibodies against conformation-dependent determinants usually do not react with small peptides derived from the same area of the molecule but devoid of the characteristic conformation. The same tripeptide, Tyr-Ala-Glu, may be either attached to a branched polymer of alanine (and then it behaves as a sequential determinant) or may be polymerized to yield a high molecular weight periodic polymer which exists in an α-helical form under physiological conditions (Sela *et al.*, 1967; Sela, 1969; Schechter *et al.*, 1971b). The two polymers are denoted, respectively, TAG-A—L and $(TAG)_n$ (Fig. 2). There is no immunological cross-precipitation between the two polymeric systems. The peptides Tyr-Ala-Glu and $(Tyr-Ala-Glu)_2$ are efficient inhibitors of the TAG-A—L homologous system, but not of the $(TAG)_n$ system. Even $(Tyr-Ala-Glu)_3$ is a poor inhibitor of the reaction of $(TAG)_n$ with anti-$(TAG)_n$ antibodies, whereas $(Tyr-Ala-Glu)_7$ and $(Tyr-Ala-Glu)_9$ are effective inhibitors of this system. It has to be assumed that only those peptides of $(Tyr-Ala-Glu)_n$ structure that can fold themselves into an q-helical conformation will react with anti-$(TAG)_n$ antibodies. This may mean that either these peptides possess, under physiological conditions, a structure similar to that of $(TAG)_n$ or that they are devoid of such structure, but capable of acquiring it upon interaction with the specific combining site on the antibody.

Circular dichroic studies (Fig. 3) showed clearly that the peptides with $n=7$ and $n=9$ possess very little α-helical conformation (Schechter *et al.*, 1971a), and led to the conclusion that a trans-

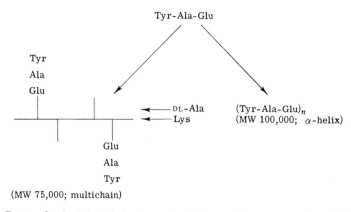

FIG. 2. Synthetic branched polymer in which peptides of sequence Tyr-Ala-Glu are attached to the amino termini of polymeric side chains in multi-poly-DL-alanyl—poly-L-lysine (left) and a periodic polymer of the tripeptide Tyr-Ala-Glu (right).

220 MICHAEL SELA

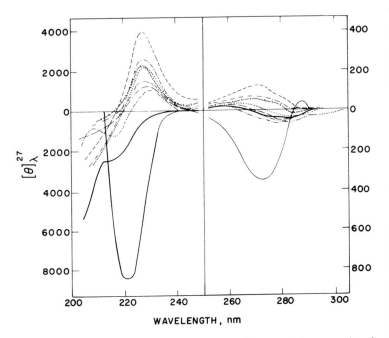

Fig. 3. Circular dichroic spectra of the peptides (Tyr-Ala-Glu)$_n$, $n = 1$ (– – –), 2 (–·–·), 3 (—ı—ı—), 4 (· · · ·), 7 (–· · ·—· · ·), 9 (— — —), 13 (–· ·—· ·), the random copolymer (TAG)$_r$, and the high molecular weight polymer (TAG)$_n$ ($n = 200$), in 0.15 M sodium chloride–0.002 M sodium phosphate buffer, pH 7.4. From Schechter *et al.* (1971a), by permission of The Rockefeller University Press, New York.

conformation into the correct antigenic determinant occurs in these peptides only upon reaction with antibodies, most probably due to the decrease in entropy, accompanying the antibody–peptide reaction. We have now examined this problem experimentally by checking whether the addition of Fab fragments derived from anti-(TAG)$_n$ antibodies to the peptide (Tyr-Ala-Glu)$_{13}$—which has a very low helical content but is able to form precipitates with anti-(TAG)$_n$ antibodies—could transconform this oligopeptide into a structure more similar to the high molecular weight polymer (Schechter *et al.*, 1971c). The circular dichroic measurements illustrated in Fig. 4 detected profound changes upon the interaction of (Tyr-Ala-Glu)$_{13}$ with the Fab fragment of antibodies against the helical (TAG)$_n$. No such changes occurred upon reacting tetra-L-alanine with antibodies against a nonhelical short poly-L-alanyl segment, nor were any changes in ellipticity observed upon mixing (Tyr-Ala-Glu)$_{13}$ with the Fab fragment of normal IgG. The difference spectrum observed with a mixture of (Tyr-Ala-Glu)$_{13}$ and anti-(TAG)$_n$-Fab shows a large peak at 278 nm corresponding to the ellipticity band of (Tyr-Ala-Glu)$_{13}$ (Fig. 4). When Fab and (Tyr-Ala-Glu)$_{13}$ were mixed in a molar ratio of 1 to 6, a 3-fold increase in the ellipticity value of (Tyr-Ala-Glu)$_{13}$ at 278 nm was observed. At a ratio of 1 to 1.6 a 6-fold increase was observed.

The difference spectrum observed could be due to an effect of Fab on (Tyr-Ala-Glu)$_{13}$ or vice versa. It seems very unlikely, however, that if a tyrosine chromophore of Fab was affected by binding to (Tyr-Ala-Glu)$_{13}$ the change in the resultant circular dichroism spectrum would be so large, precisely at the ellipticity band of (Tyr-Ala-Glu)$_{13}$ and in the direction of more ordered (Tyr-Ala-Glu)$_n$. For this reason it was concluded that the ellipticity changes

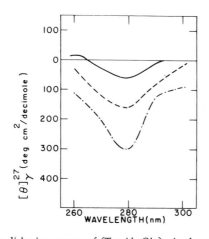

FIG. 4. Circular dichroism spectra of (Tyr-Ala-Glu)$_{13}$ in the presence and in the absence of Fab fragments derived from anti-(TAG)$_n$ antibodies in 0.15 M sodium chloride–0.02 M sodium phosphate, pH 7.4. The ellipticity values of the Fab fragment were subtracted from those of the mixture. ————, (Tyr-Ala-Glu)$_{13}$ alone; – – – –, (Tyr-Ala-Glu)$_{13}$ with Fab in a ratio of 6 to 1 (mole/mole); –·–, (Tyr-Ala-Glu)$_{13}$ with Fab in a ratio of 1.6 to 1 (mole/mole). From Schechter *et al.* (1971c), by permission of The Rockefeller University Press, New York.

shown in Fig. 5 are mainly due to an increase in the helical content of (Tyr-Ala-Glu)$_{13}$. Thus, antibodies against a helical structure may induce the helical tendency of a polypeptide which is largely in a random coil form when in free solution. This has been concluded also by Crumpton and Small (1967) for a peptide derived from myoglobin which, although in a random coil form, was capable of reacting with antibodies against a helical segment within this protein. The experiments described here are among the first examples showing by physicochemical measurements an induced fit occurring upon the interaction of two specific sites present on two biologically active macromolecules.

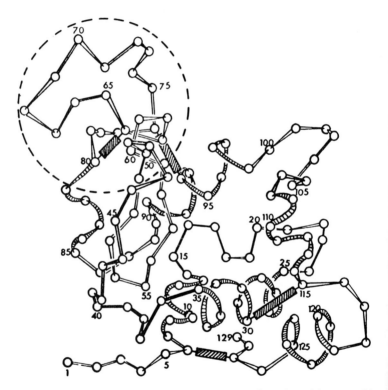

FIG. 5. Schematic drawing of the main chain conformation of hen egg-white lysozyme. The area encompassing the "loop" peptide is encircled. From Blake *et al.* (1965), from *Nature (London)*, by permission of Macmillan, London.

In a separate study, we have shown recently that the "arsanil" hapten attached to the periodic polymer (Tyr-Ala-Glu)$_n$ is hidden and incapable of provoking a specific immune response. Nevertheless, it is capable of interacting with anti-arsanil antibodies (Conway-Jacobs et al., 1970). The arsanilated polymer has a characteristic positive ellipticity in the region of arsanil absorption, which is converted into a negative ellipticity upon the reaction with Fab of an anti-arsanil antibody. In other words, the Fab may "suck out" the arsanil moiety from its conformation within the ordered copolymer and convert it into another conformation, recognized by Fab.

Both the reaction of an arsanilazo helical conjugate with anti-arsanilazo antibodies described here, and the above-mentioned reaction of (Tyr-Ala-Glu)$_{13}$ with anti-(TAG)$_n$, are examples of a *conformational change induced with antibodies on a "cross-reacting" antigen*. To the same category belongs the reaction of a myoglobin segment with antimyoglobin (Crumpton and Small, 1967), the reaction of metmyoglobin with anti-apomyoglobin (Crumpton, 1966), the reaction of a β-galactosidase mutant with anti-wild-type β-galactosidase (Rotman and Celada, 1968), stabilization of mutant catalase by complex formation with antibody to normal catalase (Feinstein et al., 1971), and the increase in ribonuclease enzymatic activity upon adding anti-RNase antibodies to a mixture of S-protein and S-peptide, the two moieties obtained from RNase upon the cleavage of a single peptide bond by subtilisin (Cinader et al., 1971). Of interest in this connection is also the recent study of Liberti et al. (1971), who have shown a correlation between the ability of calcium ions to induce conformational changes in linear synthetic polypeptides containing glutamic acid and their respective ability to induce calcium-dependent antibodies in sheep.

D. Antibodies Reactive with a Native Protein Elicited with a Synthetic Antigen

I would now like to give an example of antigen design, where the purpose was to prepare antibodies capable of reacting with conformational determinants on a native protein. Antiprotein sera usually contain mixtures of antibodies against different determinants on the protein. As the determinants of globular proteins are mostly conformation dependent, their elucidation clearly requires a detailed knowledge of both the amino acid sequence and the three-dimensional structure of the protein. Three years ago Dr. Ruth Arnon and I showed that antibodies reacting with a natural protein may be obtained upon immunization with a synthetic antigen conjugate (Arnon and Sela, 1969). A peptide containing the sequence 60–83 of hen egg white lysozyme (Jollès et al., 1963; Canfield, 1963), and denoted the "loop" peptide since it still contains one disulfide bridge (Fig. 5), was attached to multichain poly-DL-alanine (multi-poly-DL-alanyl—poly-L-lysine). The resulting synthetic conjugate elicited in rabbits and goats the formation of antibodies with specificity directed against a unique region in native lysozyme. This was shown by the capacity of lysozyme to inhibit the homologous antigen–antibody reaction as followed by either precipitin or passive cutaneous anaphylaxis techniques. Antiloop antibodies obtained with the synthetic conjugate were isolated immunospecifically on a lysozyme immunoadsorbent. Similarly, antiloop antibodies provoked upon immunization with lysozyme could be isolated immunospecifically on a loop immunoadsorbent.

The capacity of the antiloop antibodies to distinguish between the loop peptide, containing a disulfide bridge, and the open-chain peptide derived from it, suggested that they are directed against a conformation-dependent determinant. More recently, the specificity of antiloop antibodies was investigated making use of bacteriophage coated chemically either with lysozyme or with loop (Maron et al., 1971). The closed loop was an efficient inhibitor of the inactivation of the modified bacteriophages by antiloop antibodies. Unfolding of the loop peptide, achieved by either reduction and alkylation or by performic acid oxidation, resulted in a drastic decrease in the reactivity with the specific antibodies. These findings are indicative of the decisive role played by the spatial conformation in the antigenic specificity of this unique region in the lysozyme molecule.

The antibodies to the loop region, prepared according to the two approaches, described above, showed restricted structural heterogeneity as compared to the totality of antilysozyme antibody population, as manifested both in the acrylamide electrophoresis of their respective light chains and in the isoelectric focusing of the intact antibodies (Maron *et al.*, 1971). The restricted functional hetero-geneity of antiloop antibodies obtained with the synthetic conjugate is apparent from equilibrium dialysis studies (Pecht *et al.*, 1971). In one experiment the association constant calculated was 3.0×10^6 M^{-1}, and the slope in a Sips plot was 1.02 ± 0.05. Similar results (3.2×10^6 M^{-1} and 0.98 ± 0.05) were obtained when the binding and homogeneity parameters of the loop–antiloop interaction were calculated from fluorescence measurements. In this case, the loop peptide was labeled with the dansyl (1-dimethylaminonaphthalene-5-sulfonyl) group. The binding of the labeled peptide to the antiloop antibodies led to a specific excitation energy transfer from the antibody to the dansyl group on the hapten.

We have more recently synthesized by the solid-phase technique (Merrifield, 1965) a loop peptide which is different from the natural loop of lysozyme in position 76, in which alanine replaces half-cystine (Arnon *et al.*, 1971). The peptide synthesized corresponds to the sequence 64 to 82 in the amino acid sequence of lysozyme. The oxidized peptide possesses a disulfide bridge between half-cystines 64 and 80. The scheme of synthesis is given in Fig. 6. Closure to form a larger loop, containing two or more peptide units, con-nected through disulfide bonds, was ruled out by ultracentrifugal analysis which showed that the molecular weight of the synthetic loop is equal to that of the performic acid-oxidized peptide. Thus, the synthetic loop consists of a cyclic monomer and closely re-sembles the loop that occurs in native lysozyme. The synthetic loop was attached to multichain poly-DL-alanine, and the resulting syn-thetic macromolecule led to the formation of antiloop antibodies in rabbits and goats, cross-reacting efficiently with lysozyme. The antibodies were very similar to those obtained upon immunization with conjugates of the natural loop and multichain poly-DL-alanine, as apparent from inhibition experiments carried out with both anti-body populations (Fig. 7). As seen in the figure, the closed loops are in both cases very efficient inhibitors of the homologous reactions, whereas the open loops do not react at all with the respective anti-loop antibodies. Thus, the above experiments show that it is pos-sible to prepare a *completely synthetic macromolecule* which may elicit in experimental animals antibodies directed against a conformation-dependent determinant of a native protein.

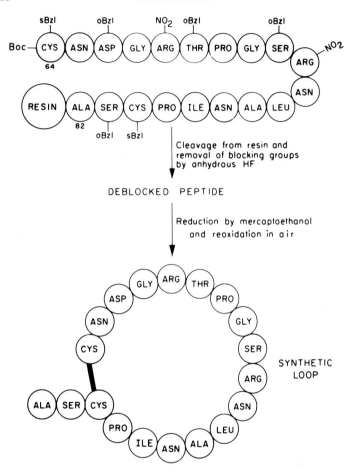

Fig. 6. Scheme of solid-phase synthesis of the loop peptide of lysozyme, residues 64–82 (cysteine residue 76 is replaced by alanine). The abbreviations used for the protecting groups are as follows: Boc-N^α-t-butyloxycarbonyl; oBzl-benzyl ester of the β position in aspartic acid, or the benzyl ether of threonine or serine; sBzl-benzyl group attached to the sulfhydryl group of cysteine; NO_2-nitroguanido group of arginine. From Arnon *et al.* (1971), by permission of The National Academy of Sciences, Washington, D.C.

The synthetic approach has been recently extended to several synthetic analogs of the loop peptide (Teicher *et al.*, 1972). The derivatives in which either leucine at position 75 or isoleucine at position 78 were replaced by alanine were almost indistinguishable from the original synthetic loop peptide. However, replacing one proline at position 79 brought about a drastic decrease in antigenic reactivity. Another analog, in which the two arginine residues (positions 68 and 73) were replaced with alanine, lacked completely the ability to bind to antiloop antibodies.

The experiments described here show clearly the importance of the steric conformation of antigens in the definition of the specificity of the antibodies obtained. It is evident that no significant splitting by proteolytic enzymes may occur between the moment an immunogen is administered and the moment it is being recognized at the

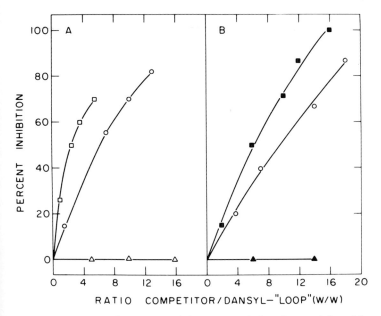

Fig. 7. Inhibition of the enhanced fluorescence of the mixture of dansyl loop ($4 \times 10^{-6} M$) and (A) antiloop antibodies obtained with the conjugate of natural loop with multichain poly-DL-alanine ($0.6 \times 10^{-6} M$); and (B) antiloop antibodies obtained with the conjugate of the synthetic loop with multichain poly-DL-alanine ($1.8 \times 10^{-6} M$); by varying concentrations of the natural loop peptide (□), synthetic loop peptide (■), hen egg-white lysozyme (○), and the open-chain peptide obtained by reduction and carboxymethylation of the natural loop peptide (△), and of the synthetic loop peptide (▲). From Pecht *et al.* (1971) and Arnon *et al.* (1971), by permission of *European Journal of Biochemistry* and the National Academy of Sciences, Washington, D.C.

biosynthetic site. Such proteolysis would have to result in the destruction of the conformation of most protein determinants. It seems, therefore, that if proteolytic destruction of the antigen plays a role in controlling antibody formation, it would have to occur after the determinant has been "recognized" at the site of biosynthesis. Studies on the role of the optical configuration in determining the antigenicity of synthetic polymers are in agreement with this interpretation (Sela, 1969). Namely, the destruction of the immunogenic macromolecule, or at least of its antigenic determinants, may be necessary to prevent the overwhelming of the immune system with excess antigen which may obstruct antibody synthesis. It should nevertheless be stressed that the *recognition* of the antigenic determinant occurs while the immunogenic molecule is still intact.

As seen in Fig. 5, the "loop" area occupies a protruding corner of native lysozyme. From the few immunological studies on proteins whose three-dimensional structure is known, it seems that, as a general rule, the "corners" represent the most immunopotent areas of the molecule. Thus, whereas X-ray crystallography sees best what is inside a protein, the immunological techniques recognize mainly the hydrophilic periphery of the molecule. In this connection it is pertinent to mention the studies of Arnon and Maron (1970, 1971) on an immunological approach to the structural relationship between hen egg-white lysozyme and bovine α-lactalbumin, two proteins similar in amino acid sequence (Brew *et al.*, 1967) and probably also in conformation (Browne *et al.*, 1969). No immunological cross-reaction was found between native lysozyme and native lactalbumin, but definite cross-reactivity has been observed between the reduced and carboxymethylated derivatives of hen egg-white lysozyme and bovine α-lactalbumin, i.e., between the unfolded peptide chains devoid of the native structural features (Fig. 8).

III. Net Charge of Immunogens

The role of conformation in antigenicity, illustrated in the examples described above, suggests strongly that the antigenic determinants on an immunogenic macromolecule are recognized while the antigen is still intact. An additional argument for the intactness of the immunogenic molecule at the moment of recognition comes from a study on the role of net electrical charge of the complete

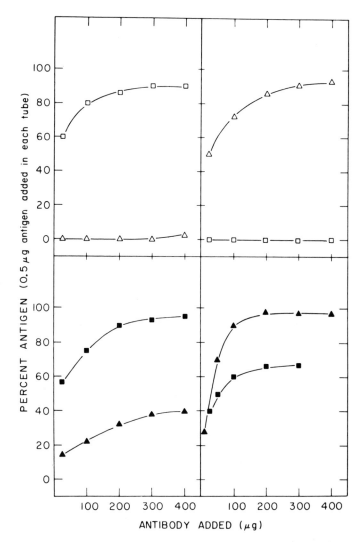

FIG. 8. Antigen-binding capacity of native and open-chain hen egg-white lysozyme and bovine α-lactalbumin by isolated antibodies against native lysozyme (upper left), native lactalbumin (upper right), reduced and carboxymethylated lysozyme (lower left), and reduced and carboxymethylated lysozyme (lower right). The antigens are: □, native lysozyme; △, native lactalbumin; ■, reduced and carboxymethylated lysozyme; and ▲, reduced and carboxymethylated lactalbumin. From Arnon and Maron (1970, 1971), by permission of Academic Press, New York.

antigen in determining the chemical nature of anti-p-azobenzene-arsonate antibodies (Rüde *et al.*, 1968). This study shows clearly that the inverse correlation, observed between the charge of the immunogen and the charge of the antibodies elicited, depends on the net electric charge of the intact immunogen, not on the net charge within a limited area around the antigenic determinant.

The inverse relationship between the net electric charge of immunogenic macromolecules and the net charge of antibodies provoked by them has been demonstrated for antibodies produced in rabbits, mice, goats, and humans, and is valid for antibodies of IgG, IgM, and IgE class (for literature, see Sela, 1971). Thus, e.g., antibodies to the acidic diphtheria toxoid and to negatively charged synthetic copolymers of amino acids appear mainly under the first peak upon fractionation on DEAE-Sephadex, whereas antibodies to the basic lysozyme and positively charged amino acid copolymers appear predominantly, or exclusively, under the second peak (Sela and Mozes, 1966; Sela, 1967).

Haptens such as the dinitrophenyl group or a peptide of D-alanine will lead to antibodies fractionating under the first or under the second peak, depending on whether they are attached to a negatively or positively charged carrier. The antihapten antibodies produced upon immunization with such conjugates differ in their net electric charge, but not in their specificity or affinity, as measured by means of small molecules related chemically to the original haptens (Licht *et al.*, 1971). The great similarity of the antigenic specificity and, under controlled conditions, of the affinity of the various anti-polyalanyl antibody preparations suggests that the differences are contained mainly in areas of the immunoglobulin other than the combining sites proper.

We have recently established that the net charge correlation has a cellular basis, making use of spleen cell fractionation on glass beads (Sela *et al.*, 1970). If a population of potentially immunocompetent cells exists that can select immunogens on the basis of net antigenic charge, in addition to recognition based on determinant specificity, then more positively charged immunocompetent precursor cells would be expected to react preferentially with more acidic immunogens. Should the above assumption be correct, one would predict that more acidic immunocompetent cells will be more readily eluted from columns of glass beads, since glass is acidic, whereas more basic cells should adhere to such surfaces. Consequently, cells collected after glass bead filtration should be preferentially stimulated by the more positively charged immunogen.

Thus glass bead columns were used to reduce the number of immunocompetent spleen cells preferentially reactive with more acidic immunogens. After a single immunization, titers of antibodies to the acidic dinitrophenyl (DNP)-901, poly(Tyr, Glu, Lys) elicited in recipient mice by filtered spleen cells were significantly lower than those generated by unfiltered cells. After secondary stimulation, the majority of the antibodies provoked by the acidic antigen was found in the more acidic fraction eluted from DEAE-Sephadex, in contrast to the more basic antibodies, of the same specificity, generated by unfiltered spleen cells. Limiting dilution transfers of spleen cells were made in irradiated (BALB/c × C57BL/6)F$_1$ mice injected with graded numbers of syngeneic spleen cells (Mozes et al., 1970). Recipients were immunized either with acidic dinitrophenyl-901, poly(Tyr, Glu, Lys) or basic dinitrophenyl-912, poly(Tyr, Glu, Lys). Two weeks later, the mice were bled and their sera were assayed for anti-DNP activity by passive hemagglutination. A 2-fold but insignificant difference was detected in the frequencies of precursors stimulated by the two immunogens. When spleen cells filtered on glass bead columns were used, depletion in the number of precursor cells reactive with the dinitrophenyl hapten on the acidic 901, poly(Tyr, Glu, Lys) was observed, whereas no change was found in the response to DNP on the basic 912, poly(Tyr, Glu, Lys) (Sela et al., 1970).

We have now used glass beads coated with the basic poly-L-lysine, in order to reverse their net electrical charge (Karniely et al., 1972). In contrast to uncoated glass beads, which appear to bind the more basic cells, polylysine-coated glass beads were expected to bind selectively the more acidic cells, i.e., those reactive with basic antigens. Indeed, fractionation of spleen cells on polylysine-coated columns, followed by their inoculation with antigens into irradiated mice, resulted in a marked reduction in the percentage of responders immunized with the basic DNP-912, poly(Tyr, Glu, Lys), whereas no change was observed in response to the acidic DNP-901, poly(Tyr, Glu, Lys). It has been suggested previously that charged antigens preferentially select populations of cells synthesizing antibodies of opposite charge (Benacerraf *et al.*, 1969). The data described here provide direct experimental evidence for the cellular basis of net charge correlation between immunogens and the antibodies produced.

In accord with presently accepted views on the role of cell co-operation in immune response, and I am referring to the cooperation between T (thymus-derived) and B (bursa analog-derived, or bone marrow-derived) cells (Claman *et al.*, 1966; Mitchell and Miller, 1968; Rajewsky *et al.*, 1969; Mitchison, 1971), we have found that, for successful transfer experiments into irradiated mice, both T cells and B cells are needed in order to provoke antibody formation with the synthetic antigens mentioned above. It was thus possible to enquire which of the two cell types is mainly responsible for the net charge effect (Karniely *et al.*, 1973). Similarly to the results obtained with spleen cells, it was observed that cell suspensions containing a mixture of thymocytes fractionated on glass beads and unfractionated marrow cells showed a reduction in the capacity to respond to the dinitrophenyl group on the acidic immunogen, but not on the basic immunogen (Table II). In contrast, no reduction was detected in the ability of cell mixtures containing fractionated bone marrow and unfractionated thymus cells to respond to DNP on either copolymer.

Similar experiments carried out with T cells and B cells fractionated on polylysine-coated glass beads are also summarized in Table II. In this case, using cell mixtures of fractionated thymocytes and unfractionated marrow cells, a reduction was obtained in percentage of responders to the basic immunogen, but not to the acidic one. Again, no reduction in the response frequency to DNP on either carrier was obtained when mixtures of fractionated marrow cells and unfractionated thymocytes were used. In conclusion, relevant cells may be fractionated either on negatively or on positively charged columns. The results obtained with them verify and extend the cellular basis for the inverse net charge phenomenon, and raise the possibility that populations of thymocytes may exist which recognize immunogens on the basis of their overall electrical charge. This may not be surprising as the net charge effect is a typical "carrier" effect, i.e., it does not involve the nature of the antibody

TABLE II

Percent of Syngeneic Irradiated Mice[a] Producing Anti-DNP Antibodies[b]

Number of thymus cells transferred ($\times 10^6$)	Without column		Glass bead column		Poly-L-lysine-coated glass bead column	
	DNP-TGL$_I$[c] (acidic)	DNP-TGL$_{II}$ (basic)	DNP-TGL$_I$ (acidic)	DNP-TGL$_{II}$ (basic)	DNP-TGL$_I$ (acidic)	DNP-TGL$_{II}$ (basic)
A. After transfer of thymus cells and 20×10^6 unfractionated bone marrow cells						
15	43	41	3	41	37	13
30	40	43	27	40	47	16
45	67	60	18	60	60	30
60	78	81	35	91	70	33
B. After transfer of bone marrow cells and 1×10^8 unfractionated thymus cells						
1	39	40	—	—	35	34
5	49	52	51	50	64	58
10	47	40	53	53	—	—
15	57	46	56	47	—	—

[a] (BALB/c × C57 Bl/6)F$_1$.

[b] From Karniely et al. (1973), tested by passive hemagglutination with sheep erythrocytes coated with DNP-bovine serum albumin.

[c] TGL = copolymer of tyrosine, glutamic acid, and lysine.

combining site proper (Licht *et al.*, 1971), and the thymus cell is considered a "helper" cell in the cooperation phenomenon (Mitchison, 1971).

IV. ARE SLOWLY METABOLIZED IMMUNOGENS THYMUS INDEPENDENT?

For most immunogens the above-mentioned cell cooperation seems necessary, and no antibodies are formed—at least in the mouse—in the absence of the thymus. Nevertheless, several immunogens have been recently described which are thymus-independent. These include polymerized flagellin (Feldmann and Basten, 1971), pneumococcal polysaccharide (Howard, 1971), *E. coli* lipopolysaccharide and polyvinylpyrrolidone (Andersson and Blomgren, 1971). Möller (1970a) has suggested that the common characteristic of all these thymus-independent antigens is that they possess repeating antigenic determinants. This may be a necessary, but not sufficient reason for their thymus independence, as several synthetic polypeptide antigens, all possessing repeating antigenic determinants, have been shown to need both T and B cells for an efficient immune response in mice. The thymus-dependent synthetic antigens include multi-copoly(LPhe, LGlu)-polyLPro—polyLLys (abbreviated as (Phe, G)-Pro—L; Mozes and Shearer, 1971), multi-copoly(LPhe, LGlu)-polyDLAla—polyLLys (abbreviated as (Phe, G)-A—L; Shearer *et al.*, 1972b), and multi-copoly(LTyr, LGlu)-polyDLAla—polyLLys (abbreviated as (T, G)—A—L; Lichtenberg *et al.*, 1972). It seemed possible that, in addition to repeating antigenic determinants, slow metabolism might be a reason for efficient responses in mice to some antigens in the absence of thymus cells.

To check this hypothesis, we made use of the known fact that immunogens composed of D-amino acids are metabolized slowly and incompletely (Gill, 1971). Moreover, in the case of the multichain polymers of the formula multi-copoly(Tyr, Glu)-polyPro—polyLys (abbreviated as (T, G)-Pro—L), four substances were prepared differing in the optical activity of their component amino acids (Jaton and Sela, 1968). The polymer is composed of two moieties: the *outside* determinants—peptides of tyrosine and glutamic acid; and the *inside* area—a multichain polyproline, i.e., polyproline side chains attached to a polylysine backbone. Thus, the following four enantiomorphs of (T, G)-Pro—L were obtained: (a) all L; (b) all D; (c) L outside and D inside; and (d) D outside and L inside. It is of interest that the polymer which is D outside and L inside (but more than 90% of the amino acids are of the L-configuration) behaved similarly to the all D polymer, both in its immunogenicity in rabbits being expressed only at very small doses (Jaton and Sela, 1968), and in its slow metabolism (Medlin et al., 1970). This is due to the lack of endopeptidases capable of splitting peptide bonds between two L-proline residues. As every poly-L-proline chain in multi-copoly(DTyr, DGlu)-polyLPro—polyLLys is linked to an ϵ-amino group of lysine on one end and to a peptide composed of D-amino acids on the other end, no significant digestion of this polymer can occur within the animal body, similarly to copolymers composed exclusively of D-amino acids.

The four different enantiomorphs of (T, G)-Pro—L were tested for their efficiency in provoking an immune response in irradiated mice into which various combinations of cells were transferred (Mozes et al., 1972a; Sela et al., 1972). As seen in Table III, the all L polymer was found to be thymus dependent. The other three polymers were thymus independent. If thymus-independence is related to slow metabolism of the antigen, this would be an adequate explana-

TABLE III

CELL COOPERATION AS A FUNCTION OF THE OPTICAL CONFIGURATION OF THE AMINO ACIDS COMPOSING THE IMMUNOGEN MULTI-COPOLY(TYR, GLU)-POLYPRO—POLYLYS[a]

Immunogen	10^8 Thymocytes	2×10^7 Marrow cells	10^8 Thymocytes and 2×10^7 marrow cells
L(Tyr, Glu)-LPro—LLys	0	8	100
L(Tyr, Glu)-DPro—DLys	ND[b]	73	56
D(Tyr, Glu)-LPro—LLys	0	70	64
D(Tyr, Glu)-DPro—DLys	0	63	59

[a] Percentage of syngeneic irradiated SJL/J mice producing antibodies (passive hemagglutination) after cell transfer.

[b] Not done.

tion for the all D polymer and for the polymer which is D outside and
L inside. The polymer which is L outside and D inside is expected
to be easily digested at least in its outside L moiety. The reason for
its thymus independence is that this particular polymer provokes in
SJL/J mice mainly an antipolyprolyl response and no anti(Tyr, Glu),
and thus the relevant determinants are composed of D-proline. To
verify this explanation we have investigated another polymer built
of L-amino acids on the *outside* and D-amino acids *inside*. This time we
used multi-copoly(LPhe, LGlu)-polyDPro—polyDLys (abbreviated as
(Phe, G)-DPro—DL) in DBA/1 strain of mice which are good
responders to both moieties of this immunogen. It is of interest
that whereas mice of the DBA/1 strain are good responders to the
copoly(LPhe, LGlu) moiety and poor responders to the polyLPro-
polyLLys moiety (Mozes *et al.*, 1969b), when immunized with the
all L polymer, they respond well to both moieties when immunized
with the polymer which is L outside and D inside (Mozes *et al.*,
1972b). As seen in Table IV, in this case the anti-poly-DPro response
is thymus independent, whereas the anti-(LPhe, LGlu) response was
found to be thymus dependent. It may be concluded, therefore, that
there is a direct correlation between metabolizability and thymus-

TABLE IV

CELL COOPERATION AS A FUNCTION OF THE OPTICAL CONFIGURATION OF THE ANTIGENIC
DETERMINANTS WITHIN THE IMMUNOGEN MULTI-COPOLY(LPHE, LGLU)-POLYDPRO—
POLYDLYS[a]

Antigen used for assay	10^8 Thymocytes	2×10^7 Marrow cells	10^8 Thymocytes and 2×10^7 marrow cells
L(Phe, Glu)-DLAla—LLys (for (Phe, Glu) specificity)	20	20	82
D(Tyr, Glu)-DProD—Lys (for Pro–Lys specificity)	10	60	67

[a] Percentage of syngeneic irradiated DBA/1 mice producing antibodies (passive
hemagglutination) after cell transfer.

dependence for the response towards these polymers in mice. More-over, this correlation seems to be valid at the level of unique immuno-potent determinants. It is conceivable that the role of thymus cells is mainly in helping the concentration and persistance of antigen, properties which are characteristic anyhow of nonmetabolizable antigens.

V. GENETIC CONTROL OF IMMUNE RESPONSE

The last topic I would like to discuss in this lecture is one in which the antigen design has been of paramount importance, and I am referring to the genetic control of immune response (McDevitt and Benacerraf, 1969; Shearer *et al.*, 1972a; Benacerraf and McDevitt, 1972). The immune state of an individual is not itself an inherited characteristic. Nevertheless, the ability of an animal to elicit an immune response to a specific immunogen is subject to genetically determined factors. Results of investigations reported during the last decade have indicated that the immune response potentials of several rodent species to natural and synthetic immunogens are under genetic regulation. Significant progress in elucidating the mechanisms responsible for generating genetic variations in the immune system has been made using immunogens possessing a restricted number of antigenic determinants. Thus, immunological studies using synthetic polypiptides, and haptens coupled to synthetic polypeptides, have opened the way for molecular and cellular studies of genetic control of immunological responsiveness. A single dominant autosomal gene determines whether or not guinea pigs can form antibodies to hapten-poly-L-lysine conjugates. The ability to respond does not depend in this case on the nature of the hapten but on the nature of the polymeric backbone.

Evidence for determinant-specific genetic control of antibody response in inbred strains of mice has been obtained with synthetic multichain polypeptide antigens in which short peptides containing glutamic acid and tyrosine, histidine, or phenylalanine were attached to the amino acid termini of multichain poly-DL-alanine (McDevitt and Sela, 1965, 1967). For example, C57 black mice are good producers of antibodies against the tyrosine-containing polymer and they respond poorly to the histidine-containing polymer;

the situation is completely reversed in CBA mice. In short, the genetic factors can discriminate clearly between tyrosine, histidine, and phenylalanine in the determinant. The genetic differences are dominant, unigenic, quantitative, and determinant specific.

The ability of mice to respond to the above antigens is a genetic trait which can be transferred with "responder" spleen cells, and which is closely associated with the major histocompatibility (H-2) locus in mouse linkage group IX. All strains of the same H-2 type exhibit the same pattern of immune response toward the above-mentioned three multichain antigens independently of the remainder of a given strain's genetic background (McDevitt and Chinitz, 1969; Benacerraf and McDevitt, 1972). When multichain polymers were built in which polyproline chains replaced the poly-DL-alanine side chains (Jaton and Sela, 1968), and when their immunogenicity in inbred strains of mice was tested, the response was different (and not linked to the H-2 locus), even though the same short sequences of tyrosine or phenylalanine and glutamic acid were attached to the polypeptide side chains in both series (Mozes et al., 1969a,b).

Different inbred strains of mice may produce against the same protein similar amounts of antibodies, but this may be due to the complexity of the multideterminant antigen, so that the specificity of the antibodies formed may differ. For example, two different mouse strains (DBA/1 and SJL) immunized with the same antigen, poly(Phe, Glu)-polyPro—polyLys, responded equally well but with the production of antisera of markedly different specificity. Antibodies formed in the DBA/1 strain cross-reacted well with copoly-(Phe, Glu)-polyDLAla—polyLys and only weakly with copoly(Tyr, Glu)-polyPro—polyLys. The opposite was true for the antibodies produced in the SJL strain (Mozes et al., 1969b). Thus, either the specificity of the antibodies produced or the recognition of antigenic determinants is under direct genetic control.

Direct evidence for genetic control at the level of unique antigenic determinants of native proteins came from a recent study on the "loop" peptide of lysozyme mentioned in this lecture previously. Although most inbred mice responded well to hen egg-white lysozyme, strains were found which did not respond to the "loop" region of this protein. This was true independently of whether the synthetic conjugate of loop with multichain poly-DL-alanine was used for immunization or whether lysozyme itself was the immunogen (Mozes *et al.*, 1971).

In order to determine whether the genetic control of immune response can be correlated with the number of antigen-sensitive precursor cells, spleen cell suspensions from normal and immunized SJL and DBA/1 donor mice were transplanted into lethally X-irradiated syngeneic recipients (incapable of immune response) along with the synthetic antigen (T, G)-Pro—L (Mozes *et al.*, 1970). By transplanting graded and limiting numbers of spleen cells, inocula were found which contained one or a few antigen-sensitive precursors reactive with the immunogen. Thus, it was found that spleen cell suspensions from immunized SJL donors contain about 25 times as many detectable precursors as suspensions from immunized DBA/1 donors (Fig. 9). In cell suspensions from normal spleens about 4 times more immunocompetent progenitors were detected in the SJL than in the DBA/1 strain. These results indicated that the genetic control of immunity to the synthetic polypeptide antigen investigated is directly correlated to the relative number of precursor cells reactive with the immunogen in high and low responder strains. Similar results were obtained using (Phe, G)-Pro—L as the immunogen (Shearer *et al.*, 1971). In this case it was possible to investigate two different specificities within the same strain, and to draw the

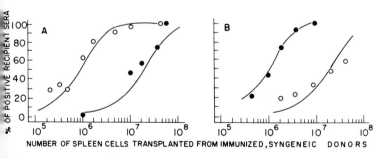

FIG. 9. Percentage of positive responses detected in sera of SJL (○) and DBA/1 (●) syngeneic recipients after irradiation and injection of graded numbers of spleen cells from immunized mouse donors and (A) (Phe, G)-A—L; or (B) (T, G)-Pro—L. From Mozes *et al.* (1970) and Shearer *et al.* (1972b), by permission of The Rockefeller University Press, New York.

conclusion that the phenotypic expression of the genetic control for immune responsiveness to different immunopotent regions is directly correlated with the number of immunocompetent response units detected in two inbred mouse strains (SJL and DBA/1).

Since expression of the genetic control of immune response has been demonstrated at the cellular level, it is important to establish which functional populations of immunocompetent cells exhibit the defect. Cooperation between thymocytes and bone marrow cells is needed for an efficient response to (Phe, G)-Pro—L (Mozes and Shearer, 1971). By limiting dilution experiments in which a non-limiting number of thymocytes was mixed with several limiting inocula of marrow cells and transferred into syngeneic, irradiated recipients, it was found that the genetic defect of the immune response to (Phe, G) in SJL mice and to Pro–L in the DBA/1 strain could be accounted for by differences in the relative number of stimulated immunocompetent cells found in the bone marrow of these two mouse strains. In contrast, experiments involving the transfer of graded numbers of thymocytes with an excess of marrow cells indicated that the genetic control of antibody responses to (Phe, G)-Pro—L in SJL and DBA/1 mice cannot be attributed to a deficiency in the relative numbers of available thymocytes. Similar results, suggesting that the genetic control is reflected in bone marrow cells, but not in thymus cells, were obtained also for (T, G)-Pro—L (Shearer *et al.*, 1972b), and are illustrated in Fig. 10.

Using the same techniques, involving transfer into irradiated recipients of graded inocula of cells of one type from syngeneic donors, while giving an excess of cells of the other type (thymus *versus* bone marrow), we found that in the case of (Phe, G)-A—L in strain SJL the genetic defect is expressed in cells derived both from thymus and bone marrow, as illustrated in Fig. 10 (Shearer *et al.*, 1972). The antigen (T, G)-A—L behaves in strain SJL just like (Phe, G)-A—L (Lichtenberg *et al.*, 1972). We see, thus, that the genetic defect is similar for antigens based on multichain poly-proline and those based on multichain polyalanine at the level of spleen cell (Fig. 9) and bone marrow cell (Fig. 10), but not at the level of thymocyte (Fig. 10). Thus, a major difference in the nature of the genetic control of immune response seems due to the details of chemical nature of the whole immunogenic macromolecule.

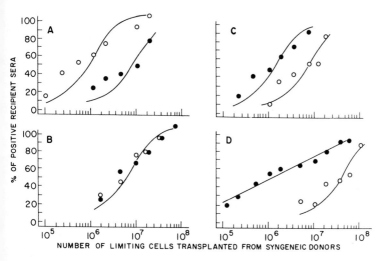

Fig. 10.   Percentage of positive responses detected in sera of SJL (○) and DBA/1 (●) syngeneic recipients after irradiation and injection of: (A) 10^8 thymocytes, graded numbers of marrow cells and (T, G)-Pro—L; (B) 2×10^7 marrow cells, graded numbers of thymocytes and (T, G)-Pro—L; (C) 10^8 thymocytes, graded numbers of marrow cells and (Phe, G)-A—L; and (D) 2×10^7 marrow cells, graded numbers of thymocytes and (Phe, G)-A—L. From Shearer *et al.* (1972b), by permission of The Rockefeller University Press, New York.

Several other differences are listed in Table V. The poor response toward antigens based on polyproline can be corrected with the polyadenylic–polyuridylic acid double strand and with syngeneic peritoneal exudate cells, whereas neither of these affects at all the poor response toward antigens based on polyalanine. Table V summarizes the emerging patterns of genetic control of immune responsiveness in SJL and DBA/1 mice to synthetic polypeptides built on multichain poly-L-proline and poly-DL-alanine.

While the above data show clearly the importance of the chemical structure in the detailed nature of the genetic control of immune response, experiments summarized in Table VI stress the importance of the mouse strain in the role assigned to various cell types in the genetic control. The same (T, G)-A—L antigen, for which a clear genetic defect has been observed in the thymus cells and in the bone marrow cells, when the analysis was carried out in the poor responder SJL/J mouse strain, does not exhibit any genetic effect in thymocytes when tested in the poor responder C3H/HeJ strain. It is of interest in this connection that the SJL/J strain is a poor responder toward any determinant attached to multichain poly-DL-alanine (the determinants tested until now are (Phe, G), (T, G) and lysozyme loop), whereas the strain C3H/HeJ is a poor responder toward (T, G)-A—L but not toward (Phe, G)-A—L. It seems thus that the T cell becomes of crucial importance as far as the genetic defect is concerned in those cases where the defect is at the "carrier" level.

On the basis of the limited information available until now I venture to hypothesize that the genetic defect in immune response

TABLE V

EMERGING PATTERNS OF GENETIC CONTROL OF IMMUNE RESPONSIVENESS IN SJL AND DBA/1 MICE TO SYNTHETIC POLYPEPTIDES BUILT ON MULTICHAIN POLY-L-PROLINE OR ON MULTICHAIN POLY-DL-ALANINE [a]

Immunogen studied: Response specific for:	(T, G)-Pro—L Pro–L	(Phe, G)-Pro—L Pro–L (Phe, G)	(Phe, G)-A—L (Phe, G)
Genetic characterization of response			
Low responder strain	DBA/1	DBA/1 SJL	SJL
High responder strain	SJL	SJL DBA/1	DBA/1
Linked to *H-2*	No	No Yes	Yes
Designation of gene	*Ir-3*	*Ir-3* *Ir-1*	*Ir-1*
Low responders enhanced by			
Poly(A)–poly(U) treatment	Yes	Yes No	No
Syngeneic peritoneal cells	Yes	Yes No	No
Methylated bovine serum albumin	Yes	Yes Yes	Yes
Ratio of precursor cells in high to low responder donors			
Spleen-secondary response	24:1	7:1 12:1	18:1
Spleen-primary response	4:1	11:1 3:1	7:1
Marrow-primary response (excess thymus)	8:1	5:1 5:1	5:1
Thymus-primary response (excess marrow)	1:1	1:1 1:1	(12–40):1

[a] From Shearer *et al.* (1972b).

TABLE VI

Role of Thymus Cells in the Response to Copoly(Tyr, Glu)-polyDLAla—polyLys as a Function of the Genetic Constitution of the Mouse Strain

Number of cells transplanted		Percentage of responder mice		
Thymus ($\times 10^6$)	Marrow ($\times 10^6$)	C57BL/6 (high)	C3H/HeJ (low)	SJL/J (low)
100	2	50	22	36
100	4	93	42	27
100	8	100	43	45
2.5	20	60	56	14
5	20	62	67	0
10	20	67	64	15
20	20	86	—	14

will reflect itself mainly in the T cells in those situations in which the poor response is a *carrier* effect, as is the case for polylysine in strain 13 guinea pigs and multichain polyalanine in SJL/J mice. On the other hand, in those situations in which the genetic defect is strictly at the *determinant* level, it will reflect itself mainly in the B cells.

VI. Concluding Remarks

I have tried to illustrate in this lecture the usefulness of precisely designed antigens for elucidation of both molecular and cellular aspects of immune response. I gave examples demonstrating the role of the steric conformation of the antigen in the definition of antibody specificity. These studies lead to the inevitable conclusion that an antigenic determinant is recognized at the biosynthetic site while the immunogenic macromolecule is still intact. Strong support for this view comes also from investigations, mentioned here, on the inverse relationship between the net electrical charge of antigens and that of antibodies elicited.

The successful synthesis of molecules capable of provoking the formation of antibodies that can react with unique antigenic conformation-dependent determinants on native proteins may potentially lead to synthetic vaccines of the future. Any developments in this direction will have to take into account both chemical and genetical parameters, especially in view of the apparent close genetic link in several species between good immune response to certain antigens and the major histocompatibility locus.

The relative simplicity of the synthetic molecules facilitates the interpretation of the results obtained with them, and sometimes permits the detection of effects, such as genetic variations in immune response, which are not easily observable with complex natural antigens. A detailed analysis of the genetic control of the immune response at cellular level permitted a tentative assignment of various roles to the different cell types.

Both cells derived from the thymus and from the bone marrow are needed for an efficient immune response in mice toward the synthetic polypeptide antigens which we have investigated in most detail. Recent studies have led us to conclude that when synthetic antigens are designed in such a way that they become very slowly metabolizable, they become thymus independent. These studies, as well as those showing the role of thymocytes in the net charge correlation and in the genetic control, stress again the role of the *carrier* moiety in determining the structure and biosynthesis of antibodies (Sela, 1967). Studies on antigenic competition (Schechter, 1968) and on immunological tolerance (Austin and Nossal, 1966; Rajewsky *et al.*, 1967; Bauminger and Sela, 1969) also corroborate this conclusion, which agrees well with the current hypothesis of cell cooperation (Claman *et al.*, 1966; Mitchell and Miller, 1968; Rajewsky *et al.*, 1969; Mitchison, 1971).

REFERENCES

Andersson, B., and Blomgren, H. (1971). *Cell. Immunol.* **2,** 411.
Anfinsen, C. B. (1967). *Harvey Lect.* **61,** 95.
Arnon, R., and Maron, E. (1970). *J. Mol. Biol.* **51,** 703.
Arnon, R., and Maron, E. (1971). *J. Mol. Biol.* **60,** 225.
Arnon, R., and Sela, M. (1969). *Proc. Nat. Acad. Sci. U.S.* **62,** 163.
Arnon, R., Maron, E., Sela, M., and Anfinsen, C. B. (1971). *Proc. Nat. Acad. Sci. U.S.* **68,** 1450.
Austin, C. M., and Nossal, G. J. V. (1966). *Aust. J. Exp. Biol. Med. Sci.* **44,** 341.

Bauminger, S., and Sela, M. (1969). *Isr. J. Med. Sci.* **5,** 177.

Benacerraf, B. (1973). *Harvey Lect.* **67,**

Benacerraf, B., and McDevitt, H. O. (1972). *Science* **175,** 273.

Benacerraf, B., Nussenzweig, V., Maurer, P. H., and Stylos, W. (1969). *Isr. J. Med. Sci.* **5,** 171.

Blake, C. C. F., Koenig, D. F., Mair, G. A., North, A. C. T., Phillips, D. C., and Sarma, V. R. (1965). *Nature (London)* **206,** 757.

Borek, F., Kurtz, J., and Sela, M. (1969). *Biochim. Biophys. Acta* **188,** 314.

Brew, K., Vanaman, T. C., and Hill, R. L. (1967). *J. Biol. Chem.* **242,** 3747.

Brown, R. K. (1963). *Ann. N.Y. Acad. Sci.* **103,** 754.

Browne, W. J., North, A. C. T., Philips, D. C., Brew, K., Vanaman, T. C., and Hill, R. L. (1969). *J. Mol. Biol.* **42,** 65.

Canfield, R. E. (1963). *J. Biol. Chem.* **238,** 2698.

Cinader, B., Suzuki, T., and Pelichova, H. (1971). *J. Immunol.* **106,** 1381.

Claman, H. N., Chaperon, E. A., and Triplett, R. F. (1966). *J. Immunol.* **97,** 828.

Clerici, E., Schechter, I., and Sela, M. (1970). *Immunology* **19,** 267.

Conway-Jacobs, A., Schechter, B., and Sela, M. (1970). *Biochemistry* **9,** 4870.

Crumpton, M. J. (1966). *Biochem. J.* **100,** 223.

Crumpton, M. J., and Small, P. A., Jr. (1967). *J. Mol. Biol.* **26,** 143.

Feinstein, R. N., Jaroslow, B. N., Howard, J. B., and Faulhaber, J. T. (1971). *J. Immunol.* **106,** 1316.

Feldmann, M., and Basten, A. (1971). *J. Exp. Med.* **134,** 103.

Freedman, M. H., and Sela, M. (1966a). *J. Biol. Chem.* **241,** 2383.

Freedman, M. H., and Sela, M. (1966b). *J. Biol. Chem.* **241,** 5225.

Gill, T. J., III (1971). *Curr. Top. Microbiol. Immunol.* **54,** 19.

Haber, E. (1964). *Proc. Nat. Acad. Sci. U.S.* **52,** 1099.

Howard, J. (1971). Quoted in Andersson and Blomgren (1971).

Jaton, J.-C., and Sela, M. (1968). *J. Biol. Chem.* **243,** 5616.

Jollès, J., Jauregui-Adell, J., Bernier, I., and Jollès, P. (1963). *Biochim. Biophys. Acta* **78,** 668.

Karniely, Y., Mozes, E., Shearer, G. M., and Sela, M. (1972). *Isr. J. Med. Sci.* **8,** 642.

Karniely, Y., Shearer, G. M., Mozes, E., and Sela, M. (1973). *J. Exp. Med.* **137,** 183.

Liberti, P. A., Maurer, P. H., and Clark, L. G. (1971). *Biochemistry* **10,** 1632.

Licht, A., Schechter, B., and Sela, M. (1971). *Eur. J. Immunol.* **1,** 351.

Lichtenberg, L., Shearer, G. M., Mozes, E., and Sela, M. (1972). *Isr. J. Med. Sci.* **8,** 649.

McDevitt, H. O., and Benacerraf, B. (1969). *Advan. Immunol.* **11,** 31.

McDevitt, H. O., and Chinitz, A. (1969). *Science* **163,** 1207.

McDevitt, H. O., and Sela, M. (1965). *J. Exp. Med.* **122,** 517.

McDevitt, H. O., and Sela, M. (1967). *J. Exp. Med.* **126,** 969.

Maoz, A., Fuchs, S., and Sela, M. (1972). *Isr. J. Med. Sci.* **8,** 657.

Maron, E., Shiozawa, C., Arnon, R., and Sela, M. (1971). *Biochemistry* **10,** 763.

Medlin, J., Humphrey, J. H., and Sela, M. (1970). *Folia Biol. (Prague)* **16,** 156.

Merrifield, R. B. (1965). *Science* **150,** 178.

Mitchison, N. A. (1971). *Eur. J. Immunol.* **1,** 18.

Mitchell, G. F., and Miller, J. F. A. P. (1968). *J. Exp. Med.* **128,** 821.

Möller, G. (1970a). *In* "Immune Surveillance" (R. T. Smith and M. Landy, eds.), p. 112. Academic Press, New York.

Möller, G. (1970b). *Cell. Immunol.* **1,** 573.

Mozes, E., and Shearer, G. M. (1971). *J. Exp. Med.* **134,** 141.

Mozes, E., McDevitt, H. O., Jaton, J.-C., and Sela, M. (1969a). *J. Exp. Med.* **130,** 493.

Mozes, E., McDevitt, H. O., Jaton, J.-C., and Sela, M. (1969b). *J. Exp. Med.* **130,** 1263.

Mozes, E., Shearer, G. M., and Sela, M. (1970). *J. Exp. Med.* **132,** 613.

Mozes, E., Maron, E., Arnon, R., and Sela, M. (1971). *J. Immunol.* **106,** 862.

Mozes, E., Shearer, G. M., and Sela, M. (1972a). *Isr. J. Med. Sci.* **8,** 647.

Mozes, E., McDevitt, H. O., and Sela, M. (1972b). *Eur. J. Immunol.* in press.

Pecht, I., Maron, E., Arnon, R., and Sela, M. (1971). *Eur. J. Biochem.* **19,** 368.

Rajewsky, K., Rottlander, E., Pettre, E., and Muller, B. (1967). *J. Exp. Med.* **126,** 581.

Rajewsky, K., Schirrmacher, V., Nase, S., and Jerne, N. K. (1969). *J. Exp. Med.* **129,** 1131.

Rotman, M. B., and Celada, F. (1968). *Proc. Nat. Acad. Sci. U.S.* **60,** 660.

Rüde, E., Mozes, E., and Sela, M. (1968). *Biochemistry* **7,** 2971.

Schechter, B., Schechter, I., and Sela, M. (1970). *J. Biol. Chem.* **245,** 1438.

Schechter, B., Schechter, I., Ramachandran, J., Conway-Jacobs, A., and Sela, M. (1971a). *Eur. J. Biochem.* **20,** 301.

Schechter, B., Schechter, I., Ramachandran, J., Conway-Jacobs, A., Sela, M., Benjamini, E., and Shimizu, M. (1971b). *Eur. J. Biochem.* **20,** 309.

Schechter, B., Conway-Jacobs, A., and Sela, M. (1971c). *Eur. J. Biochem.* **20,** 321.

Schechter, I. (1968). *J. Exp. Med.* **127,** 237.

Sela, M. (1966). *Advan. Immunol.* **5,** 29.

Sela, M. (1967). *In* "Nobel Symposium III on Gamma Globulins" (J. Killander, ed.), p. 455. Almqvist & Wiksell, Stockholm.

Sela, M. (1969). *Science* **166,** 1365.

Sela, M. (1971). *Ann. N.Y. Acad. Sci.* **190,** 181.

Sela, M., and Mozes, E. (1966). *Proc. Nat. Acad. Sci. U.S.* **55,** 445.

Sela, M., Katchalski, E., and Gehatia, M. (1956). *J. Amer. Chem. Soc.* **78,** 746.

Sela, M., White, F. H., and Anfinsen, C. B. (1957). *Science* **125,** 691.

Sela, M., Fuchs, S., and Arnon, R. (1962). *Biochem. J.* **85,** 223.

Sela, M., Schechter, B., Schechter, I., and Borek, F. (1967). *Cold Spring Harbor Symp. Quant. Biol.* **32,** 537.

Sela, M., Mozes, E., Shearer, G. M., and Karniely, Y. (1970). *Proc. Nat. Acad. Sci. U.S.* **67,** 1288.

Sela, M., Mozes, E., and Shearer, G. M. (1972). *Proc. Nat. Acad. Sci. U.S.* **69,** 269b.

Shearer, G. M., Mozes, E., and Sela, M. (1971). *J. Exp. Med.* **133,** 216.

Shearer, G. M., Mozes, E., and Sela, M. (1972a). "Progress in Immunology" (B. Amos, ed.), p. 509. Academic Press, New York.

Shearer, G. M., Mozes, E., and Sela, M. (1972b). *J. Exp. Med.* **135,** 1009.

Teicher, E., Maron, E., and Arnon, R. (1972). *Isr. J. Med. Sci.* **8,** 651.

Whitney, P. L., and Tanford, C. (1965). *Proc. Nat. Acad. Sci. U.S.* **53,** 524.

SUPPRESSION: A SUBVERSION OF GENETIC DECODING*

PAUL BERG

Department of Biochemistry, Stanford University Medical Center, Stanford, California

I. INTRODUCTION

IN deciphering the genetic message, transfer RNA (tRNA) mediates the recognition of each triplet codon by the appropriate amino acid: In essence, tRNA bridges the "information gap" between nucleotide and amino acid structures. It performs this adapter function in two stages: First, specific enzymes, amino acyl tRNA synthetases, esterify each amino acid to a cognate set of tRNA molecules; next, as each message codon appears in register at the ribosome, the matching amino acyl tRNA enters the "site" (or state) for polymerization to the growing polypeptide chain. Understandably the fidelity of translation, and therefore the quality of the proteins made, relies on the precision and specificity of these two reactions. [For a more extensive coverage of the discrete steps in protein synthesis, see the *Cold Spring Harbor Symposium on Quantitative Biology*, Vol. 34 (1969), particularly Lengyel's excellent summary; also a more recent review article by Lucas-Lennard and Lipmann (1971).]

What chemical and structural features of tRNA enable them to perform their task with such exquisite specificity? Specifically, what prevents the wrong amino acid from becoming esterified to a tRNA, or a particular tRNA from pairing with an incorrect triplet? Initially, my colleagues and I tried to answer these questions by examining the consequences of structural changes in tRNA on amino acyl tRNA synthetase and codon recognition. More recently we have directed our attention at modifications caused by mutation, but specifically, mutational changes which alter the translational

---

* Lecture delivered March 16, 1972.

specificity of the tRNA and thereby generate proteins with different amino acid sequences.

One class of such mutations, "suppressor" mutations, can be readily detected because they reverse the phenotypic manifestation of certain *missense* and *nonsense* mutations in a variety of structural genes for proteins. [In a *missense* mutation the base change produces a codon which can still be translated into one of the nineteen other amino acids. *Nonsense* mutations generate codons that cannot be translated as amino acids; instead, at a nonsense codon, premature termination of polypeptide chain growth and release of the incomplete polypeptide chain occurs (Garen, 1968).] As you will see, suppressor mutations are useful because the structural alteration they cause in tRNAs cannot readily be achieved by chemical means; more important, perhaps, is that such mutations can be selected because the mistranslation they cause may restore a defective function (e.g., the synthesis of an active rather than inactive enzyme).

My aim is to summarize two investigations of the mechanism of suppression, both of which yield interesting insight into structure–function relations of tRNAs. The first, concerning missense suppression, was initiated at Stanford in collaboration with Charles Yanofsky, John Carbon, and Peter Pouwels and later was joined by Charles Hill, Par Reid, and John Foulds; but the more recent and interesting findings of missense suppression come from the efforts of Carbon and his colleagues at the University of California, Santa Barbara, and from Hill's laboratory at Pennsylvania State's Hershey Medical Center. The second study, analyzing a novel example of nonsense suppression, was begun by one of my students, Larry Soll, and continued by long distance collaboration between Soll at Harvard and William Folk, Moshe Yaniv, and me at Stanford. For my part, knowing and working with these talented individuals has been a rewarding experience and genuine pleasure.

II. Missense Suppressors

The possibility that mutationally altered tRNA molecules could mistranslate certain codons and thereby correct or suppress a missense mutation was first suggested by Yanofsky and his colleagues (Yanofsky and St. Lawrence, 1960; Yanofsky *et al.*, 1961; Brody and

Yanofsky, 1963). Modified tRNAs able to translate chain termination codons as amino acids were similarly suggested as the explanation for nonsense suppression (Benzer and Champe, 1962; Garen and Siddiqi, 1962). But how could this theory be tested experimentally? During a conversation following one of our weekly tennis matches, Yanofsky and I devised an *in vitro* approach to studying the mechanism of missense suppression. Unbeknownst to us, Capecchi and Gussin (1965) and Engelhardt *et al.* (1965) were proceeding along somewhat similar lines on the problem of nonsense suppression.

Our approach utilized Yanofsky's extensive collection of tryptophan synthetase mutants and relied on an *in vitro* system to translate synthetic polynucleotides of defined sequence into specific polypeptides. Figure 1 summarizes the amino acid substitutions at sites specifying different glycine residues in the tryptophan synthetase α-protein: The *A36* mutation causes replacement of glycine by arginine at position 211, while *A58* and *A78* mutations result in replacement of glycine at position 234 by aspartic acid and cysteine, respectively (Yanofsky *et al.*, 1969). An extensive analysis of amino acid replacements at these sites in different mutant tryptophan synthetase α-proteins (Yanofsky *et al.*, 1969) permitted the assignment of GGA as the wild-type codon at position 211 and GG U/C

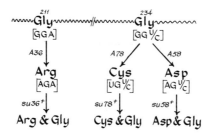

FIG. 1.   Consequences of missense mutational changes and suppressor mutations affecting tryptophan synthetase α-protein. *A36* is a missense mutation causing substitution of glycine at position 211 in the polypeptide chain; *A78* and *A58* cause substitutions of cysteine and aspartic acid for glycine at position 234. The triplets indicated in brackets are the most likely ones coding for the amino acids shown at the two positions. The *su36*[+] mutation permits the synthesis of both wild-type protein and the *A36* mutant protein (Brody and Yanofsky, 1963); the same is thought to be true for *su78*[+] and *su58*[+] though the synthesis of wild-type enzyme has not been established by sequence analysis.

to position 234; accordingly, the mutant codon in A36 is most likely AGA while UG U/C and GA U/C must be the mutant codons of A78 and A58, respectively.

One of the modes of reversion for each of these mutants is by a second, extragenic, mutation; these extragenic, or suppressor mutations, apparently cause mistranslation of the mutant codon so as to yield some polypeptide chains with the wild-type amino acid in place of the mutant amino acid. For example, *su36+*, the mutation which suppresses *A36*, causes the AGA codon to be occasionally translated as glycine instead of arginine (Brody and Yanofsky, 1963). Very likely *su78+* and *su58+* cause the cysteine and aspartic acid codons, respectively, to be occasionally mistranslated as glycine (Berger and Yanofsky, 1967). Of interest is the fact that *su36+* does not mistranslate the mutant codons of *A78* or *A58* nor does *su78+* cause the insertion of glycine in the *A36* mutant; that is, each suppressor causes the mistranslation of only a specific codon (Helinski and Yanofsky, 1966).

Based on this analysis, we surmised that the mistranslation caused by *su36+* could be detected *in vitro* with a synthetic messenger containing the AGA triplet (Fig. 2). Khorana's laboratory (Nishimura *et al.*, 1965) had already shown that the alternating copolymer rAG directed the synthesis of an alternating copolypeptide, arginine–glutamate. Would a cell-free protein synthesizing extract from *su36+* cells catalyze the occasional substitution of glycine for arginine with a poly rAG template? And if so, was it the ribosomes, soluble proteins or tRNA from *su36+* extracts that was essential for the misreading?

The answer was quite clear; even with all of the protein synthesizing ingredients from normal cells (*su36−*), the addition of

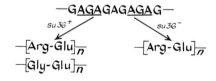

FIG. 2. Potential polypeptides which could be synthesized under the direction of an RNA containing alternating adenine and guanine bases when it is translated normally (*su36−*) or mistakenly (*su36+*).

purified $su36^+$ tRNA, but not tRNA from $su36^-$ or from $su58^+$ and $su78^+$ cells, caused the occasional insertion of glycine in place of arginine in the newly formed copolypeptide (Carbon et al., 1966a, b). Gupta and Khorana (1966), at the same time, showed that tRNA from $su78^+$ strains promoted the in vitro incorporation of glycine in place of cysteine in response to the UGU codon contained in the alternating copolynucleotide poly rUG (which normally codes for a cysteine-valine copolypeptide); tRNA from $su36^+$ or $su58^+$ did not mistranslate UGU as glycine. These two experiments established that suppression of missense mutations could be explained by the occurrence of mutationally altered tRNA molecules which can "misread" a particular codon.

In later studies (Hill et al., 1970) another suppressor of the $A36$ missense mutation was discovered; tRNA isolated from this new suppressor strain also misread the AGA codon as glycine in the in vitro assay mentioned above. But the mutation responsible for this altered tRNA species differs in its genetic location on the Escherichia coli chromosome from that of the Yanofsky suppressor. To distinguish the two suppressors, the original suppressor mutation has been designated $glyTsu36^+$ and the new one, $glyUsu36^+$.

Before going on to Carbon and Hill's analysis of the molecular changes caused by these suppressor mutations, I must digress briefly to introduce another point. If a suppressor mutation creates a tRNA with a new decoding specificity, one may wonder how the cell continues to translate the codon originally decoded by the wild-type tRNA. If there is more than one tRNA species capable of translating a given codon, loss of one of them would very likely be innocuous (provided it does not have some other special function). But if a codon is translated by a unique tRNA species, coded for by only one gene copy per cell, it is quite likely that the loss of that tRNA will be deleterious if not lethal.

With $glyTsu36^+$ this is not a moot point. To our surprise, the Yanofsky strains carrying $glyTsu36^+$ were found after genetic analysis to be heteroploid for the suppressor locus; both the $glyTsu36^+$ mutation and its $su36^-$ allele were represented within a chromosomal tandem duplication (Hill et al., 1969). Analogous, but haploid, $glyTsu36^+$ strains were eventually isolated, but most of these grew poorly and were unable to carry out normal cell division on complex

media (Hill *et al.*, 1969). These defects resulted not from an effect
of the suppressor, but rather from the absence of the corresponding
glyTsu36⁻ gene and its product from the cell. By introducing the
glyTsu36⁻ allele into haploid *glyTsu36⁺* strains, we could generate
glyTsu36⁺/glyTsu36⁻ heteroploids that grew and behaved indis-
tinguishably from the Yanofsky *su36⁺* strains (Hill *et al.*, 1969).

It seems that the UV mutagenesis used by Yanofsky to generate
su36⁺ mutations strongly favors the production of heteroploid
suppressors (99%); spontaneous and chemical induction markedly
increases the frequency of the haploid *glyTsu36⁺* and *glyUsu36⁺*
suppressors (Hill *et al.*, 1970). In some as yet unknown way, UV
light stimulates the frequency of duplication of this region of the
chromosome. Although the *glyTsu36⁺* mutation, in the absence of
the wild-type allele *glyTsu36⁻*, is deleterious for the cell, the
glyUsu36⁺ mutation is innocuous (Hill *et al.*, 1970). These experiments indicate that the product of the *glyT* gene is indispensable for
the cell whereas the *glyU* gene product is unessential. Although the
explanation for this is quite straightforward and predicted by the
arguments made above, the observations alerted and warned us to
the potential harmful consequences of suppressor mutations and was
to serve us in another phase of our work.

Now to Carbon and Hill's analysis (Hill *et al.*, 1970) of the tRNAs
that are affected by the different suppressor mutations. Gradient
chromatography on BD-cellulose columns displayed three distinct,
resolvable tRNA^{Gly} species: two minor components each comprising
about 20% of the total tRNA^{Gly} and one major species accounting
for the remaining 60% (Fig. 3). Using the binding of gly-tRNA to
triplet–ribosome complexes as an assay, tRNA$_I^{Gly}$ was bound to
GGG, tRNA$_{II}^{Gly}$ to GGA and GGG and tRNA$_{III}^{Gly}$ to GGU and
GGC (Carbon *et al.*, 1970). Thus, these three tRNAs can decode the
entire set of four glycine codons. By constructing the appropriate
merodiploids, i.e., strains carrying episomes duplicating different
segments of the chromosome, it could be established (Hill *et al.*,
1970; Carbon and Squires, 1971) that the *glyU* locus is the structural
gene for tRNA$_I^{Gly}$, *glyT* codes for tRNA$_{II}^{Gly}$, and another gene
which I shall mention later, *glyV*, determines the structure of
tRNA$_{III}^{Gly}$. As you will soon see there may be multiple copies of
the *glyV* gene located near each other.

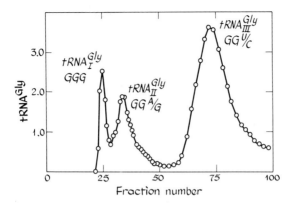

FIG. 3.   Elution profile of tRNA^{Gly} species on BD-cellulose column chromatography. The triplets shown in association with each peak indicate their decoding specificity as measured by binding to ribosome–triplet complexes (Carbon *et al.*, 1970).

The genetic locations on the circular map of *E. coli* for each of these genes is now known (Hill *et al.*, 1970; Carbon and Squires, 1971) (Fig. 4). A significant point is that the three tRNA structural genes are separate and not clustered. This may turn out to be a common feature of tRNA structural genes in contrast to the clustering of related protein structural genes.

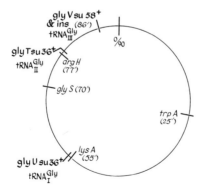

FIG. 4.   Genetic map location of structural genes for tRNA^{Gly} species; *glyU* codes for tRNA$_I^{Gly}$, *glyT* for tRNA$_{II}^{Gly}$ and *glyV* for tRNA$_{III}^{Gly}$; *glyS* is the structural gene for glycyl-tRNA synthetase.

Which tRNA is altered to yield each suppressor tRNA? And what
is the structural change which permits that modified tRNA to
translate a new codon? The first question was answered by comparing
the BD-cellulose chromatographic profiles of the tRNA^{Gly} species
from bacterial strains carrying each of the suppressor mutations with
tRNA^{Gly} from the wild-type counterparts (Hill *et al.*, 1970). Cochromatography of gly-tRNA from a *glyTsu36*$^{+}$ strain with that of
wild-type strains showed that tRNA$^{Gly}_{II}$, the tRNA which decodes
GG A/G is absent from the suppressor profile (Fig. 5a). The same

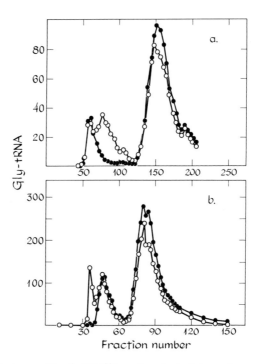

Fig. 5. Elution profile of tRNA^{Gly} species obtained by cochromatography on
BD-cellulose of radioactively labeled glycyl-tRNAs. In panel a, ^{3}H- or ^{14}C-labeled
glycyl-tRNAs from *glyTsu36*$^{-}$ (Wildtype) O——O and *glyTsu36*$^{+}$ (haploid) ●——●
were cochromatographed; panel b contains the profile for labeled glycyl-tRNAs from
glyUsu36^{-} (wild type) (O——O) and *glyUsu36*$^{+}$ (●——●). Reproduced from Hill
et al. (1970), by permission of Academic Press, New York.

kind of analysis with gly-tRNA from $glyUsu36^+$ strains (Fig. 5b) demonstrated that the GGG translating species, $tRNA_I^{Gly}$, is missing from the $su36^+$ strains. Actually, neither one is really missing; the modified $tRNA^{Gly}$ molecules, which mistranslate the AGA codon, are extremely poor glycine acceptors compared to the wild-type species, and unless a very high level of glycyl-tRNA synthetase is used for charging, glycine is not esterified to the suppressor tRNAs (Carbon and Curry, 1968; Squires and Carbon, 1971).

So, it seems that a $tRNA^{Gly}$, able to pair with GGG, can be mutationally altered to translate the arginine codon AGA; another $tRNA^{Gly}$ species, specific for GG A/G codons, can also be changed so that it can translate the AGA triplet. In both cases the structural change markedly reduces the capacity to react with the homologous glycyl-tRNA synthetase by several orders of magnitude.

The nature and location of the specific base change in each tRNA which confers it with a new specificity is not yet known. One might speculate that the $tRNA_{II}^{Gly}$ species, whose anticodon normally translates GGA, undergoes a change in one of the bases of the anticodon to permit AGA translation; it is more difficult to predict how $tRNA_I^{Gly}$, which is specific for GGG translation, is modified to permit AGA decoding. But as you shall see later, speculations, though plausible, are hazardous.

I have already pointed out that the $glyTsu36^+$ mutation, in the absence of the normal allele, is deleterious but that the $glyUsu36^+$ mutation is harmless. Both observations can be understood from the decoding specificity of the $tRNA^{Gly}$ species (see Fig. 3). A cell depleted of $tRNA_I^{Gly}$ can still translate the codon GGG; but loss of $tRNA_{II}^{Gly}$ leaves the cell without an obvious way to translate its GGA codons. It remains to be seen how the cell manages at all when it lacks the wild-type copy of $tRNA_{II}^{Gly}$.

Cells which carry the $glyTsu36^+$ mutation and therefore lack a $tRNA^{Gly}$ for translating GGA do not survive when plated on enriched media, such as tryptone; but tryptone-resistant survivors can be recovered at low frequency (Hill *et al.*, 1969). One class of these, referred to as *ins* mutants, are cells which have reacquired the capacity for translating GGA (Carbon *et al.*, 1970). The *ins* mutation is not due to regeneration of the wild-type glyT gene (since the cells remain *su36*⁺); moreover, the *ins* mutation maps in the *glyV* locus, the structural gene for tRNA$_{III}^{Gly}$ (Squires and Carbon, 1971).

Analysis of the chromatographic profile of the tRNA^{Gly} species from a strain carrying the *ins* mutation (Fig. 6) reveals a new glycine-accepting tRNA with decoding properties for GGA (Carbon *et al.*, 1970). This appears to arise at the expense of a portion of the tRNA$_{III}^{Gly}$. Since the tRNA$_{III}^{Gly}$ is the only component of the third peak and only about a third of tRNA$_{III}^{Gly}$ is converted to the new species, there very likely is more than one structural gene for tRNA$_{III}^{Gly}$.

Carbon and his colleagues have solved the base sequence of the tRNA$_{III}^{Gly}$ and tRNA$_{ins}^{Gly}$ (Squires and Carbon, 1971). In this case the change is the expected one (Fig. 7): a G to U base substitution in the anticodon sequence, thereby permitting translation of GG A/G instead of GG U/C. In effect, by converting one tRNA^{Gly} species into another, the cell has restored its ability to translate what had become a nontranslatable triplet.

Although the study of the *su58*⁺ and *su78*⁺ suppressors has not yet proceeded as far as the ones I have described, it seems that both

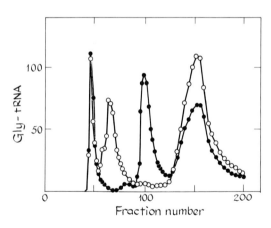

Fɪɢ. 6. Elution profile of tRNA^{Gly} species obtained by cochromatography on BD-cellulose of tRNA from *glyTsu36*⁻ (wild type) (O——O) and *glyTsu36*⁺ *ins* (●——●). Reproduced from Carbon *et al.* (1970), by permission of Academic Press, New York.

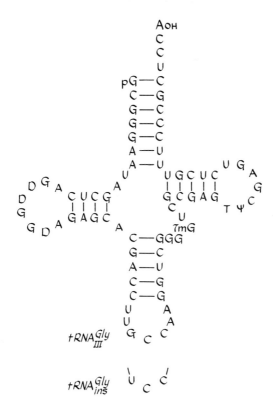

FIG. 7. Nucleotide sequence of tRNA$_{\text{III}}^{\text{Gly}}$ and the change in the anticodon sequence of that tRNA^{Gly} species caused by the *ins* mutation.

affect tRNA$_{\text{III}}^{\text{Gly}}$. The $su58^+$ mutation maps in the $glyV$ gene, the structural gene for tRNA$_{\text{III}}^{\text{Gly}}$ (Squires and Carbon, 1971). But the $su78^+$ mutation does not, suggesting a different mechanism of alteration of tRNA$_{\text{III}}^{\text{Gly}}$ (Carbon, private communication).

The information which I have reviewed concerning the mutationally altered tRNA^{Gly} isoacceptors is summarized in Fig. 8: (a) Mutation in $glyU$, the structural gene coding for a tRNA^{Gly} which normally translates GGG, can change that tRNA to one which translates AGA instead. (b) $GlyT$, which codes for a tRNA^{Gly} able to translate GG A/G can, by mutation, yield a tRNA that

Mutations	tRNA Alteration	Reactivity with gly-tRNA synthetase
GlyUsu36$^+$	tRNA$_{GGG}^{Gly}$ → tRNA$_{AGA}^{Gly}$	10^{-4} Lower
GlyTsu36$^+$	tRNA$_{GGA/G}^{Gly}$ → tRNA$_{AGA}^{Gly}$	10^{-4} Lower
GlyVsu58$^+$	tRNA$_{GGU/C}^{Gly}$ → tRNA$_{GAU/C}^{Gly}$	Markedly lower
GlyVins	tRNA$_{GGU/C}^{Gly}$ → tRNA$_{GGA/G}^{Gly}$	Unchanged
Su78$^+$	tRNA$_{GGU/C}^{Gly}$ → tRNA$_{UGU/C}^{Gly}$	10^{-3} Lower

Fig. 8. Summary of known mutations affecting the structure and function of tRNA^{Gly} species in *Escherichia coli*. In the first column are listed the different mutations discussed in the text. The second column indicates the functional change affected by the mutation: For example, the *glyUsu36$^+$* mutation alters the structure of a tRNA$_{GGG}^{Gly}$ so that it can translate the AGA codon; the *glyVsu36$^+$* causes a change in a tRNA$_{GG\ U/C}^{Gly}$ species enabling it to translate GA U/C. All the mutations shown, except *su78$^+$*, occur within the structural gene for the tRNA^{Gly} species shown to the left of the arrow; the *su78$^+$* mutation only indirectly affects the tRNA^{Gly} species. Except for the *glyV ins* mutation, the actual structural change is not yet known.

decodes AGA (and very likely AGG). (c) *GlyV*, which determines the structure of a tRNA specific for the codons GG U/C, can undergo two types of mutational change; the *su58$^+$* alteration, which permits translation of the aspartic acid codons, AG U/C, as glycine and the other, *ins*, which permits tRNA$_{III}^{Gly}$ to translate a different glycine codon pair, GG A/G. (d) The *su78$^+$* mutation appears to cause an alteration in tRNA$_{III}^{Gly}$ enabling it to decode the cysteine codon UGU (Carbon, private communication). But because the *su78$^+$* mutation does not map in *glyV*, the structural gene for tRNA$_{III}^{Gly}$, the mutation may cause a low frequency error in the modification of one of the bases of tRNA$_{III}^{Gly}$, thereby altering its translational specificity. This interpretation follows from Carbon's finding that although the *su78$^+$* suppressor tRNA species is derived from tRNA$_{III}^{Gly}$, there is no appreciable decrease in the wild-type tRNA$_{III}^{Gly}$ species in *su78$^+$* strains (Carbon, private communication). (e) The mutational changes affecting the translational specificity of tRNA$_I^{Gly}$ and tRNA$_{II}^{Gly}$ markedly alter their ability to react with the glycyl-tRNA synthetase in the charging reaction.

The precise chemical change in the three missense suppressor tRNAs still needs to be established. One would like to know what structural change enables them to translate different codons and why those changes profoundly affect the ability of the altered tRNA to react with the glycyl-tRNA synthetase. One interesting correlation we may note is as follows. Those modified tRNAs in which the change in translational specificity is directed to the first or second base of the codon (as is true for the tRNAs derived from the $glyUsu36^+$, $glyTsu36^+$, $su58^+$, and $su78^+$ mutations) have several orders of magnitude reduced activity for charging with the glycyl-tRNA synthetase; when the mutation affects translation of the third base of the codon (as with $tRNA_{ins}^{Gly}$) there is no detectable effect on the reactivity with the enzyme. Conceivably the anticodon bases which pair with the first two bases of certain codons play a role in the recognition with the activating enzyme. But clearly further studies with other altered tRNAs needs to be done to explore this possibility. Consistant with this view is the report that a change in the anticodon of $tRNA^{Tyr}$ from one which normally translates the UA U/C codons to one which translates UAG causes no alteration in the reactivity of the tRNA with tyrosyl-tRNA synthetase (Goodman et al., 1968). However, the $tRNA^{Leu}$ species, which normally decodes UUG and can be altered by mutation to produce a UAG suppressor (Gopinathan and Garen, 1970), still reacts normally with the leucyl-tRNA synthetase (Hayashi and Söll, 1971). Perhaps because leucyl-tRNA synthetase does not distinguish among its own five tRNAs, which must translate codons differing in the first position (Myers et al., 1971), that enzyme may be insensitive to the base in position one.

III. A NONSENSE SUPPRESSOR

Suppression of nonsense codons occurs by translation of chain termination signals as amino acids (see Garen, 1968; Gorini, 1970). Although mutationally altered ribosomes and tRNAs can mediate the misreading, my discussion will be confined to suppression caused by modified tRNAs.

The genetic map location, as well as the amino acids that are inserted by the widely studied nonsense suppressors (Fig. 9) has been

Suppressor	Amino Acid Inserted	Suppressed Codon
su1	Serine	UAG
su2	Glutamine	UAG
su3	Tyrosine	UAG
su4	Tyrosine	UAA ; UAG
su5	Lysine	UAA ; UAG
su6	Leucine	UAG
su7	Glutamine	UAG
su8	?	UAA ; UAG
su$_{UGA}$	Tryptophan	UGA

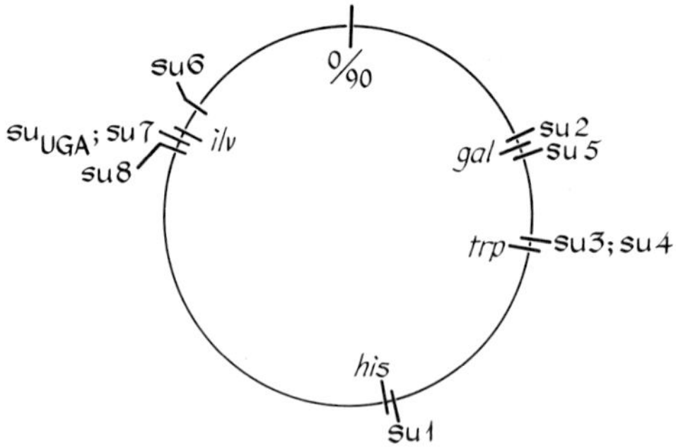

FIG. 9. Characteristics and genetic map location of a representative group of nonsense suppressor mutations in *Escherichia coli*.

well documented by many investigators (see Gorini, 1970). There are three classes of nonsense suppressors, each being specific for the codons they misread: those that respond to UAG alone, so-called amber suppressors; those that translate both UAG and UAA, the ochre suppressors; and suppressors that translate only UGA. Each suppressor mutation causes the insertion of the indicated amino acid in response to the codon shown (Fig. 9). Note that *su2*[+] and *su7*[+], both of which cause the insertion of glutamine for UAG, are located at opposite sides of the chromosome; I will refer later to the apparent congruent locations of *su7* and *su*$_{UGA}$.

Although each of the suppressors shown in Fig. 9 has been attributed to an altered tRNA molecule, for only two has the specific structural change caused by the mutation been confirmed by a sequence comparison of the suppressor and wild-type species of tRNA. The MRC-Cambridge group proved that $su3^+$ is a tRNA^{Tyr} with a single change, a G to C substitution in the anticodon, which permits translation of UAG instead of UA U/C (Goodman *et al.*, 1968). Because, at one time, it seemed reasonable to suppose that the other nonsense suppressor tRNAs would also result from altered anticodon sequences, enabling them to base-pair with UAG, Hirsh's analysis of su_{UGA} (Sambrook *et al.*, 1967) produced a surprise. Hirsh (1970, 1971) found that an altered tRNA^{Trp} is the UGA suppressor; but, instead of a changed sequence in the anticodon there is a substitution of A for G at position 24 (Fig. 10). This emphasizes how

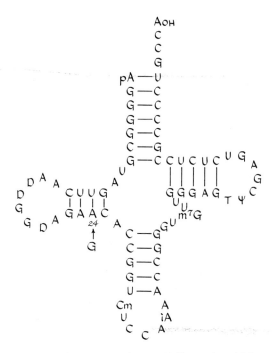

Fig. 10. The nucleotide sequence of the tRNA^{Trp} species which suppresses the UGA codon by translating it as tryptophan; the wild-type tRNA^{Trp} contains G at position 24.

perilous it is to speculate on the nature of the mutational change
which causes the mistranslation.

As I mentioned earlier, certain suppressor mutations which affect
tRNA structure can have deleterious consequences. Since one of the
objectives in studying suppression was to generate a variety of mutationally altered tRNAs for structure–function investigations,
changes which are lethal, and therefore not detectable, would
clearly restrict the usefulness of this approach. Accordingly, Soll
and I devised a protocol which would enable us to isolate lethal
nonsense suppressor mutations.

Although a particular structural change in a tRNA might allow
it to translate a nonsense codon (assuming the change does not also
prevent its aminoacylation), that change would never be detected
if the original function performed by the tRNA was indispensable.
But such mutations should be recoverable in cells carrying more than
copy of the affected gene: If a cell retains at least one wild-type
copy of the gene for an essential tRNA, it can accommodate an
otherwise lethal suppressor mutation in another copy of that gene.
Our strategy, therefore, was to isolate nonsense suppressor mutations
in a strain which contained an additional chromosomal segment;
for example, the episome F′14, which duplicates about 5% of the
bacterial chromosome in the region of the *ilv* genes (see Fig. 9).
Any suppressors arising in the duplicated region of the genome could
then be tested to determine whether they were lethal in cells without
the genetic duplication.

To do this, cells containing the F′14 episome and two UAG
mutations in structural genes for histidine and tryptophan biosynthetic enzymes were used (Soll and Berg, 1969b). In such a strain,
reversion to amino acid independence by a single step occurs most
frequently by suppressor mutations. Soll and I found that a sizable
proportion of the suppressor mutations that were detected occurred
within the episome segment. These were of two types: *su7*+, which
suppressed UAG codons only, and *su8*+, which suppressed UAG
and UAA. The UAG suppressor could be located very close to the
ilv gene cluster (74 minutes) on the genetic map of the *E. coli* chromosome (Fig. 9).

It was significant that *these two* suppressor mutations did not
arise in cells lacking the F′14 episome (although the usual suppres-

sors were found); moreover, attempts to transduce the suppressor gene from the F'14 merodiploid to its haploid progenitor were unsuccessful (except where gene duplications to produce $su7^+/su7^-$ heteroploids arose in the course of the P1-mediated transduction) (Soll and Berg, 1969b; Soll, 1971). By these criteria and from other data, it seemed likely that these suppressors were the type of recessive lethal mutation we were looking for.

Suppressor $su7^+$ causes insertion of glutamine at the UAG codon; Soll and I found that a tryptophan synthetase α-protein mutant, having a UAG triplet instead of GAG at the 48th codon, synthesized a complete protein with glutamine at position 48 when the cells carried $su7^+$ (Soll and Berg, 1969a). The efficiency with which UAG is translated as glutamine, relative to chain termination, is high, 75%. As is the case with other ochre suppressors, $su8^+$ has a much lower suppression efficiency, about 4% (Soll and Berg, 1969b). The suppression efficiency of the other glutamine-inserting UAG suppressor, $su2^+$, is of the order of 10–20%, depending upon the particular UAG mutation (Soll, 1971).

Suppression mediated by $su7^+$ could be shown to be caused by tRNA by *in vitro* experiments using as messenger the phage R17 RNA containing a UAG codon (Cordes and Primakoff, unpublished results). Fractionation of tRNA from normal cells $(su7^-)$ on DEAE-Sephadex yields only two peaks of tRNA^{Gln} activity whether the fractions are assayed with *low* or *high* levels of glutaminyl tRNA synthetase (Fig. 11). The same two peaks of tRNA^{Gln} are seen when the tRNA from cells containing the $su7^+$ and $su7^+$ alleles is chromatographed and the fractions are assayed with low amounts of glutaminyl-tRNA synthetase (Fig. 11). But if, in the latter case the column fractions are assayed with high levels of glutaminyl-tRNA synthetase, three peaks of glutamine acceptor are seen (Fig. 11); the tRNA in the first peak, which is unique to $su7^+$ cells, is evidently only very poorly charged with glutamine.

When the three species of tRNA^{Gln} isolated by chromatography were tested for their decoding specificity by ribosome binding in response to different codons, the material in the first peak paired with UAG whereas that from the second and third peaks pair best with the two known codons for glutamine, CAA and CAG, respectively (Fig. 12). Thus, in strains containing $su7^+$, there is a new

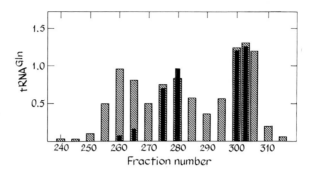

Fig. 11. The elution profile of glutamine-acceptor tRNAs obtained by DEAE-Sephadex chromatography of tRNA isolated from an *Escherichia coli* strain containing both the *su7+* and *su7−* alleles. The hatched bars represent the values obtained by assaying selected fractions with an excess of pure glutaminyl-tRNA synthetase (GlnRS) (3 μg); the filled bars show the values found when peak fractions of the first profile were assayed with lower levels of GlnRS (0.03 μg).

species of glutamine-accepting tRNA which can pair with UAG; presumably, this is the one that accounts for suppression of UAG *in vivo*. These cells also contain the usual two wild-type species of tRNA^{Gln}, one of which pairs with CAA and the other with CAG. The finding of discrete tRNA molecules with specificity for either CAA or CAG, but not both, was unexpected; according to the "Wobble" hypothesis (Crick, 1966) tRNA capable of pairing with

Triplet or Polymer	tRNA$^{Gln}_{su}$	tRNA$^{Gln}_{1}$	tRNA$^{Gln}_{2}$
	Gln-^{14}C bound, pmoles		
poly UA	0.07	0.06	0.07
poly AC	0.11	_0.51_	0.19
poly UAG	0.23	0.10	0.10
CAG	0.09	0.12	_0.80_
UAG	_0.60_	0.06	0.11

Fig. 12. Coding properties of the tRNA^{Gln} species shown in Fig. 11. Transfer RNA from the peak fractions, charged to their limit with ^{14}C-labeled glutamine (10 pmoles) was tested for its ability to bind to ribosomes (1 A_{260}) in the presence of either the indicated polymers (0.27 A_{260}) or triplets (0.19 A_{260}) by the method of Nirenberg and Leder (1964). The blank value with no added polymer or triplet has been subtracted.

CAA should also bind to CAG. The explanation for this "anomaly" will be evident in a moment.

Since it was reasonable to expect that the $su7^+$ tRNA was derived from one of the two normal tRNA^{Gln} species (assuming a single base change, tRNA$^{Gln}_{II}$, which pairs with CAG, was the most logical candidate), Folk and Yaniv set out to determine the base sequence of the two wild-type tRNA^{Gln} species. The two sequences turned out to be very similar (Folk and Yaniv, 1972) (Fig. 13). But they differ in a crucial way—in the anticodon sequence. The tRNA$^{Gln}_{II}$ species which translates CAG is classical; it contains an anticodon sequence complementary to CAG. The CAA translating tRNA^{Gln}, however, has a modified uridine in the anticodon; a uridine with a sulfur substituted for oxygen at position 2. Very likely, the 2-thiouridine

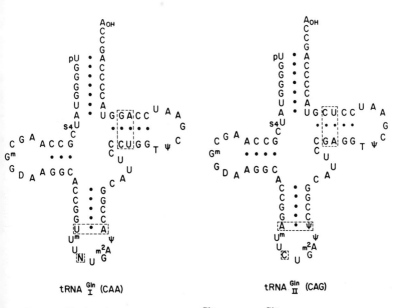

tRNA$^{Gln}_{I}$ (CAA)   tRNA$^{Gln}_{II}$ (CAG)

Fig. 13. Nucleotide sequences of tRNA$^{Gln}_{I}$ and tRNA$^{Gln}_{II}$ which translate CAA and CAG, respectively, written as cloverleaf structures. The unusual nucleosides are abbreviated: s4U, 4-thiouridine; G_m, 2′-o-methylguanosine; D, dihydrouridine; U_m, 2′-o-methyluridine; m²A, 2-methyl adenosine; ψ, pseudouridine; T, ribosylthymidine; N, an unknown base, probably a 2-thiouridine derivative. The base pairs enclosed in the dashed boxes differ in the two tRNAs.

derivative (the precise structure of the modified base in $tRNA_I^{Gln}$ is not yet known), while able to base-pair with A, probably cannot form a "Wobble" base pair with G. A similar finding has been made with other tRNAs that decode triplets differing only by A or G in the third position (Yoshida et al., 1970; Ohashi et al., 1970).

At this point it seemed that the structure of the su7 suppressor and the reason for its lethality was solved; it only remained for us to confirm that the sequence change was in the anticodon of the tRNA specific for CAG, enabling it to translate UAG. If this was the case, the lethality could be seen as due to lack of a tRNA to translate CAG as glutamine. Our attempts to confirm that hypothesis, however, were frustrated by an inability to isolate the suppressing $tRNA^{Gln}$ in sufficiently pure form for base sequence analysis.

Besides there were some disquieting facts which troubled us. First, there was $su2^+$, another UAG suppressor which inserts glutamine (see Garen, 1968; Gorini, 1970). If $su2^+$ generates an altered tRNA, that species would also be expected to arise from a tRNA translating CAG. Yet, $su2^+$ is not lethal; moreover, $su2^+$ and $su7^+$ map in different chromosomal locations. If there are two structural genes for a $tRNA^{Gln}$ decoding CAG, why should mutation in one be lethal? Even more paradoxical were the findings of Miller and Roth (1971). Using the related organism Salmonella typhimurium, they isolated what appeared to be the same recessive-lethal UAG suppressor on F'14 that Soll and I had. But they also reported the isolation of recessive lethal mutants which suppress UGA. Because the two suppressors were closely linked genetically and mutually exclusive, they suggested that both arose by different anticodon changes of a common tRNA structural gene. The paradox was, how could a tRNA able to translate UGA be derived from one designed to translate CAG?

At this point Soll's genetic skills enabled us to make another approach to solving the structure of the $su7^+$ tRNA. The MRC-Cambridge group had already shown how useful it was to have a tRNA structural gene incorporated into the $\phi80$ phage genome; infection by such a phage or induction of its lysogens increased dramatically the amount of that specific tRNA, presumably because of the multiple copies of the $su3^+$ gene (Smith et al., 1966). In a way which I cannot detail here, Soll constructed a $\phi80$ phage which carried the *su7* gene; it could carry that gene in the wild-type state, *su7⁻*, in the UAG-suppressor form, *su7⁺*, or in an ochre-suppressor form, *su7* ochre (Soll, to be published). With these strains in hand, Yaniv's observation that φ80 *su7* lysogens contained more than twice the normal level of tRNA^Trp, but nearly normal levels of tRNA^Gln, shifted our attention toward the possibility that the *su7* gene coded for tRNA^Trp instead of tRNA^Gln. But the proof that *su7⁺* was indeed a modified tRNA^Trp came from base sequence analysis of the tRNA produced after infection by the various phages.

Using Sanger and his colleagues' elegant procedures for analyzing the sequence of tRNAs (Sanger *et al.*, 1965; Brownlee and Sanger, 1967; Brownlee *et al.*, 1968, 1969), Yaniv undertook an analysis of the tRNAs produced by infection of *E. coli* cells with Soll's φ80 phages carrying the different forms of the *su7* gene. He found to our surprise, that the T1-RNase digest of the unfractionated ³²P-labeled tRNA recovered after infection, yielded a two-dimensional fingerprint which contained no readily detectable fragments characteristic of the tRNA^Gln; instead there was unmistakable evidence of an enrichment of oligonucleotides derived from tRNA^Trp (Fig. 14). Ordinarily tRNA^Trp comprises less than 1% of the total tRNA and its oligo-

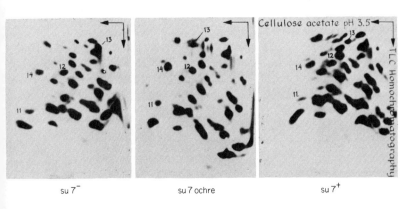

Fig. 14. Radioautogram of a two-dimensional fingerprint of the T1 RNase oligonucleotide fragments from ³²P-labeled tRNA isolated from *Escherichia coli* cells infected with φ80dsu7⁻, φ80dsu7 ochre, and φ80dsu7⁺. The numbers indicate the position of the oligonucleotides from tRNA^Trp: 11, Um⁷GUUG; 12, UCUCUCCG; 13, see Fig. 15; 14, UUCAADUG.

nucleotides would not be seen in a T1 digest of the total tRNA; yet the T1-RNase digest of the ^{32}P-labeled tRNA recovered after infection with ϕ80 su7$^-$ showed four spots characteristic of some of the larger oligonucleotides produced from tRNA^{Trp} (spots 11–14 on the left-hand panel of Fig. 14). The sequence of each of these did indeed correspond to one of the known T1-RNase generated segments of tRNA^{Trp} (see legend to Fig. 14). But spot 13 was the key one, for it contains the base sequence of the anticodon of tRNA^{Trp} (Fig. 15). When the fingerprints of the T1 RNase digest of tRNA isolated after infection with ϕ80dsu7ochre or ϕ80dsu7$^+$ were examined (Fig. 14), the position of spot 13 changed. Sequence analysis of the material from spot 13 in each of these digests showed that they contain the same oligonucleotide sequence but with one or two bases changed in what corresponds to the anticodon (Fig. 15). The anticodon sequence from the tRNA derived after ϕ80dsu7$^+$ infection quite clearly corresponds to what would be expected of a UAG suppressor and the one from the tRNA induced by ϕ80dsu7ochre could also explain translation of both UAA and UAG.

Although these findings were made with unfractionated ^{32}P-labeled tRNA from the phage infected cells, it remained to be established that it was the glutamine-accepting tRNA per se which was derived from tRNA^{Trp}. Yaniv partially purified the glutamine-acceptor ^{32}P-labeled tRNA from cells infected with ϕ80dsu7$^+$ phage (see Folk and Yaniv, 1972) and after T1 RNase digestion found that virtually all of the spots on the fingerprint corresponded to those produced by tRNA^{Trp}. So, a glutamine-accepting species of tRNA in $su7^+$ cells has the base sequence of what was a tryptophan-accepting tRNA.

Our present interpretation of the origin of the $su7^+$ and the other suppressor forms of that gene is summarized in Fig. 16 and as follows:

a. The structural gene which codes for tRNA^{Trp} is the locus of the $su7^+$ suppressor mutation (arrow 1). The mutation changes the middle C of the anticodon to a U enabling it to translate UAG but probably no longer UGG; the same change causes the tRNA to accept glutamine, albeit poorly. (We do not yet know whether the $su7^+$ tRNA also accepts tryptophan.)

b. The $su7^+$ change is lethal because the translation of UGG as tryptophan is either completely lost or limiting.

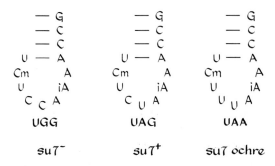

Fig. 15. Nucleotide sequence of the anticodon-containing oligonucleotides isolated from spot 13 in each of the fingerprints of Fig. 14.

c. The same structural gene can also give rise to a UGA suppressor by a mutational change which converts C to U in the first base of the anticodon (arrow 2). Although Soll accomplished this by mutation of φ80dsu7⁻ to φ80dsu_UGA (to be published), it might correspond to the same mutation observed by Miller and Roth (1971) in *Salmonella typhimurium*. But according to the "Wobble" hypothesis, this altered tRNA should be able to translate UGG and UGA. Why then is the mutation lethal? Conceivably the change impairs the ability to charge tryptophan so that even if it can pair

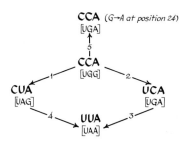

Fig. 16. Relationships between the anticodons of tRNA^Trp and those tRNAs derived from tRNA^Trp which can translate the codons UAG, UAA, and UGA. The change described by arrow 5 is the one described by Hirsh (1970, 1971); the changes indicated by arrows 1 and 4 are reported here; those indicated by arrows 2 and 3, though demonstrated genetically (Soll, unpublished data) have not yet been confirmed by structure proof.

with UGG it may be unable to perform the first act of its adapter role correctly (Soll, unpublished data).

d. Either the UAG suppressor ($su7^+$) or the UGA suppressor (su_{UGA}) form of the structural gene can be mutated to yield a UA A/G suppressor ($su7$ ochre) by changing the appropriate C to U in the anticodon (arrows 3 and 4). Nothing is known of the lethality of that change or of the acceptor specificity of that tRNA.

e. tRNA^Trp can also be changed in another way to permit it to translate UGA (arrow 5). Hirsh (1971) has shown this occurs by a base change outside the anticodon sequence; no alteration of amino acid acceptor specificity accompanies this change. As expected, this mutation is not lethal.

How does a tRNA^Trp become recognizable by glutaminyl-tRNA synthetase, and thereby a glutamine acceptor? Without knowing more about the structural basis for this recognition one can only guess. A comparison of the structures of tRNA^Trp and tRNA^Gln

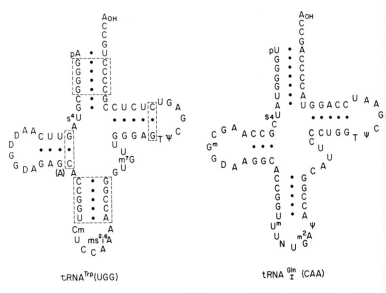

Fig. 17. Nucleotide sequence of tRNA$_I^{Gln}$ and tRNA^Trp. The dashed boxes in the tRNA^Trp sequence indicate those nucleotides that are identical to the corresponding nucleotides of tRNA$_I^{Gln}$.

reveals few similarities except in the anticodon and CCA stems (Fig. 17). It will be interesting to learn what role, if any, these regions play in the interaction of tRNA^{Gln} with glutaminyl-tRNA synthetase or of tRNA^{Trp} with tryptophanyl-tRNA synthetase.

REFERENCES

Benzer, S., and Champe, S. P. (1962). *Proc. Nat. Acad. Sci. U.S.* **47**, 1025; **48**, 1114.

Berger, H., and Yanofsky, C. (1967). *Science* **156**, 394.

Brody, S., and Yanofsky, C. (1963). *Proc. Nat. Acad. Sci. U.S.* **50**, 9.

Brownlee, G. G., and Sanger, F. (1965). *J. Mol. Biol.* **13**, 373.

Brownlee, G. G., and Sanger, F. (1969). *Europ. J. Biochem.* **11**, 395.

Brownlee, G. G., Sanger, F., and Barrell, B. G. (1968). *J. Mol. Biol.* **34**, 379.

Capecchi, M. R., and Gussin, G. N. (1965). *Science* **149**, 417.

Carbon, J., and Curry, J. B. (1968). *J. Mol. Biol.* **38**, 201.

Carbon, J., and Squires, C. (1971). *Cancer Res.* **31**, 663.

Carbon, J., Berg, P., and Yanofsky, C. (1966a). *Proc. Nat. Acad. Sci. U.S.* **56**, 764.

Carbon, J., Berg, P., and Yanofsky, C. (1966b). *Cold Spring Harbor Symp. Quant. Biol.* **31**, 487.

Carbon, J., Squires, C., and Hill, C. W. (1970). *J. Mol. Biol.* **52**, 571.

Crick, F. H. C. (1966). *J. Mol. Biol.* **19**, 548.

Engelhardt, D. L., Webster, R. E., Wilhelm, R. C., and Zinder, N. D. (1965). *Proc. Nat. Acad. Sci. U.S.* **54**, 1791.

Folk, W. R., and Yaniv, M. (1972). *Nature (London) New Biol.* **237**, 165.

Garen, A. (1968). *Science* **160**, 149.

Garen, A., and Siddiqi, O. (1962). *Proc. Nat. Acad. Sci. U.S.* **48**, 1121.

Goodman, H. M., Abelson, J., Landy, A., Brenner, S., and Smith, J. D. (1968). *Nature (London)* **217**, 1019.

Gopinathan, K. P., and Garen, A. (1970). *J. Mol. Biol.* **47**, 393.

Gorini, L. (1970). *Annu. Rev. Genet.* **4**, 107.

Gupta, M., and Khorana, H. G. (1966). *Proc. Nat. Acad. Sci. U.S.* **56**, 772.

Hayashi, H., and Söll, D. (1971). *J. Biol. Chem.* **246**, 4951.

Helinski, D. R., and Yanofsky, C. (1966). *In* "The Proteins" (H. Neurath, ed.), 2nd ed., Vol. 4, p. 1. Academic Press, New York.

Hill, C. W., Foulds, J., Soll, L., and Berg, P. (1969). *J. Mol. Biol.* **39**, 563.

Hill, C. W., Squires, C., and Carbon, J. (1970). *J. Mol. Biol.* **52**, 557.

Hirsh, D. (1970). *Nature (London)* **228**, 57.

Hirsh, D. (1971). *J. Mol. Biol.* **58**, 439.

Lengyel, P. (1969). *Cold Spring Harbor Symp. Quant. Biol.* **34**, 828.

Lucas-Lennard, J., and Lipmann, F. (1971). *Annu. Rev. Biochem.* **40**, 409.

Myers, G., Blank, H. U., and Söll, D. (1971). *J. Biol. Chem.* **246**, 4955.

Miller, C. G., and Roth, J. R. (1971). *J. Mol. Biol.* **59**, 63.

Nirenberg, M., and Leder, P. (1964). *Science* **145**, 1399.

Nishimura, S., Jones, D. S., and Khorana, H. G. (1965). *J. Mol. Biol.* **13**, 302.

Ohashi, Z., Saneyoshi, M., Harada, F., Hara, H., and Nishimura, S. (1970). *Biochem. Biophys. Res. Commun.* **40,** 866.

Sambrook, J. F., Fan, D. P., and Brenner, S. (1967). *Nature (London)* **214,** 452.

Sanger, F., Brownlee, G. G., and Barrell, B. G. (1965). *J. Mol. Biol.* **13,** 373.

Smith, J. D., Abelson, J. N., Clark, B. F. C., Goodman, H. M., and Brenner, S. (1966). *Cold Spring Harbor Symp. Quant. Biol.* **31,** 479.

Soll, L. (1971). Ph.D. Dissertation, Stanford University, Stanford, California.

Soll, L., and Berg, P. (1969a). *Nature (London)* **223,** 1340.

Soll, L., and Berg, P. (1969b). *Proc. Nat. Acad. Sci. U.S.* **63,** 392.

Squires, C., and Carbon, J. (1971). *Nature (London) New Biol.* **233,** 274.

Yanofsky, C., and St. Lawrence, P. (1960). *Annu. Rev. Microbiol.* **14,** 311.

Yanofsky, C., Helinski, D. R., and Maling, B. D. (1961). *Cold Spring Harbor Symp. Quant. Biol.* **26,** 11.

Yanofsky, C., Berger, H., and Brammar, W. J. (1969). *Proc. Int. Congr. Genet. 12th* Vol. 3, p. 155.

Yoshida, M., Takeishi, K., and Ukita, T. (1970). *Biochem. Biophys. Res. Commun.* **39,** 852.

CURRENT ENIGMAS IN CANCER RESEARCH*

LLOYD J. OLD AND EDWARD A. BOYSE

Division of Immunology, Sloan-Kettering Institute for Cancer Research, New York, New York

I. INTRODUCTION

IN choosing the topics for discussion, it was our intention to present some areas of current research that offer outstanding challenges to cancer biologists. The subjects to be discussed are diverse, but there is a thread which connects them, and that is the widely held contention that the cell surface holds many of the keys to cellular differentiation and morphogenesis, and to the aberrations of these processes which are characteristic of cancer.

Our own special interest in the cell surface began with the fundamental question facing immunologists with an interest in cancer more than a decade ago: Do malignant cells have specific antigens? The various demonstrations at that time showing that this is so, was a major advance in cancer biology, and underlies all modern aspirations to control cancer by immunological means; this is an area to be explored briefly at the end of this presentation. But it was obvious in those early days of defining tumor antigens, first by transplantation techniques *in vivo* and later serologically, that the significance of the antigenic changes in cancer, and their relation to the aberrant behavior of the cancer cell, must largely remain obscure until far more was known about the surface composition of *normal* cells.

Progress in relating the cell surface to normal and abnormal differentiation involves a fusion of immunology, genetics, and virology, and first we should deal with some of the questions it has been possible to approach with these powerful techniques.

II. IMMUNOGENETICS OF CELL SURFACES

The cell surface is a meeting ground of interest for various disciplines in biology. A number of precise methods are being applied

* Lecture delivered April 20, 1972.

in studying its properties; these include such techniques as electron spin resonance, X-ray defraction, and fluorescence probes, but none of these at the moment has the discriminating power of immunogenetics, which has the potential of resolving the cell surface into an assembly of products, each of which can be tracted to a particular gene. The antigenic properties of cell surfaces are of interest for several quite different reasons. (a) The transplantation biologist is concerned with the antigenic differences between individuals that decide the fate of transplanted tissues. (b) From the viewpoint of tumor virology, the presence or absence of a particular antigen may signify the presence or the absence of an oncogenic virus, with implications as to the etiology of that tumor. (c) In the context of cancer immunology generally, the fact of antigenicity is the starting point of attempts to explain the malignant phenotype in terms of cell surface changes, and of attempts to control cancer by immunological means. (d) And in the most general biological setting, the different spectra of antigens appearing on contrasted cell types, implying patterns of selective gene action geared to cellular differentiation, are of interest to all who are concerned with the role of the cell surface in embryogenesis and morphogenesis.

Immunogenetic investigations of the cell surface begin with the recognition of an antigen. In some instances this is known only from observations *in vivo*, namely from the rejection of grafted tissue. This gives rise to the term "transplantation antigen," which is borrowed by tumor immunologists for use also in reference to the regression of tumors in their original hosts or in genetically compatible recipients. Analysis of antigenic systems recognizable only in this way, however, is limited in comparison with the detailed analysis which is possible once an antigen can be recognized and identified serologically, i.e., by an antibody reaction *in vitro*. So it is not unexpected that most of what we know about cell surface immunogenetics has been ascertained by the use of serology.

For convenience, we can distinguish five categories of serologically demonstrable cell surface antigens. These are listed in Table I together with some examples in the mouse. In certain cases, notably alloantigens such as H-2, the specification of the antigens is straightforward and is traceable to cellular genes; in other instances coding for the antigen can be ascribed to viral genes, as is almost certainly

TABLE I

SEROLOGICALLY DEMONSTRABLE CELL SURFACE ANTIGENS

Categories recognized	Examples in the mouse
Alloantigens	H-2, θ, Ly-A, Ly-B,C, TL^a, G$_{IX}$^{a}, Sk, PC
"Species" antigens	MSLA, MBLA, MSPCA, H-Y
Surface immunoglobulins	κ μ
Virus-related antigens	GCSA, G$_{IX}$^{a}, GVe, FMR, ML
Tumor-specific antigens	Individually distinct antigens of chemically induced tumors, TL^a

^{a} Note that the categories need not be mutually exclusive—see text.

the case with leukemia virus envelope antigens, such as GVe (see below), that are found on the cell surface. There are other antigens, especially the individually distinct transplantation antigens of chemically induced tumors listed last in Table I, whose mode of specification is problematical, and whose origin may not be *directly* attributable to either viral or cellular genes (see Boyse and Old, 1970, and below). The five categories listed are arbitrary, and are not intended as anything more than a convenience. This is clear from the fact that TL and G$_{IX}$ antigens appear as alloantigens in some circumstances, and as tumor-specific or virus-related antigens under other circumstances.

Although other serological tests are available, and although many different cell types can be studied, most knowledge of surface antigens on nucleated cells comes from the use of cytotoxicity tests applied to thymic lymphocytes and leukemia cells derived from them. With this as a foundation, it has been possible more recently to begin the study of other cell populations that are more difficult to work with, including plasma cells, epidermal cells, and sperm (reviewed by Boyse *et al.*, 1971).

To start with, let us consider some basic questions about the cell surface which are approachable serologically:

1. *Do different cell types in an organism express different surface phenotypes?* Table II illustrates that this is indeed the case and justifies the conclusion that particular pathways of differentiation entail

TABLE II

Selective Gene Action Revealed by Distinctive Spectra of Surface Antigens Related to Particular Pathways of Differentiation[a]

Site	H-2	TL	θ	Ly-A Ly-B,C MSLA	PC	MBLA MSPCA	Ig	Sk	H-Y
Thymic lymphocyte	+	+	+	+	−	−	−	−	+
B lymphocyte/ plasma cell	+	−	−	−	+	+	+	−	
Epidermal cell	+	−	+	−	−	−	−	+	+
Sperm	+	−	−	−		−	−	−	+
Brain	+	−	+	−	+		−	+	+

[a] + Antigen expressed; − antigen not expressed.

characteristic surface compositions, just as they give rise to characteristic *functions* appropriate to the cell type. Some antigens are widely expressed and many others are more restricted. At one extreme are antigens like H-2, which are expressed probably on all cells, and at the other extreme are the TL antigens, which appear on only one normal cell type, the thymocyte. There are other antigens that have a limited tissue representation, but are not restricted to a single cell type; for example θ, which appears on thymic lymphocytes, brain, and epidermal cells. Antigens whose appearance on the cell surface is conditional on particular pathways of differentiation are appropriately termed "differentiation antigens" (Boyse and Old, 1969). The appearance of these antigens is regulated by the program of selective gene action which is in force for a given pathway of differentiation; Table II is a summary of what we know about the genetic programming of surface antigens for a few different cell types of the mouse.

2. The next question concerns *the chromosomal location of genes responsible for cell surface components*. The mouse is a favorable subject for genetic mapping because of the many chromosomal markers available, covering some 70% of its genome. There are at least two

good reasons for wanting to know where the genes are that code for cell surface components: First, to find out whether there is any significant grouping of genes specifying elements of the cell surface. Second, in cases where the presence of a cell surface antigen is related to a viral genome, to find out whether the coding gene is part of the chromosomal complement, as evidenced from its having definable linkage to known genomic markers.

Figure 1 shows some of the loci which specify cell surface components in the mouse and whose linkage groups are known. These are scattered throughout the genome, the only case of close linkage being that between *H-2* and *Tla* in linkage group IX. This linkage between *H-2* and *Tla* should be remembered in connection with the map of cell surface antigens (indicating where they are placed in the cell surface assembly in relation to one another), which is discussed in the following section.

3. *Do the various gene products that make up the cell surface have pre- ferential locations as part of a prescribed organization of surface elements? In short, is there a surface map?* This has been studied by a technique which indicates whether any two antigens on the cell surface are or are not situated in close proximity to one another. The principle is to determine what effect the attachment of antibody to one antigen has on the ability of the cells to combine with antibody of a second specificity. If the two antigens are sufficiently close, then previous attachment of the first antibody impedes uptake of the second anti- body, and this interference can be accurately measured. An extensive series of tests of this kind enabled us to contruct a rudimentary

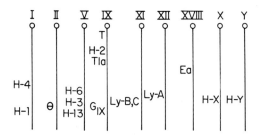

FIG. 1.   Chromosomal location of some genes specifying cell surface antigens of the mouse; see particularly Snell (1971) and Itakura *et al.* (1972).

"map" for the mouse thymocyte (Fig. 2) (Boyse *et al.*, 1968). This should not be taken as a literal representation of how the antigens are disposed; it represents only one arrangement that would fit the blocking data. The important point is not the detail of the map, but the fact that an orderly assembly of gene products at the cell surface is discernible.

It was obviously worthwhile to establish whether these topographical relations of the gene products on the cell surface could be related to the chromosomal sites of the genes, because (as noted above) *Tla* and *H-2* are closely linked genes, and their gene products, carrying TL and H-2 antigens, are situated close together on the cell surface. This is a tantalizing finding, but it has not so far been duplicated with any other pair of antigens that are known to be closely associated on the cell surface. Thus, no pattern relating genomic arrangements to cell surface location of gene products has yet emerged; but it may be that the present inventory of antigens is too small for this to be apparent.

We hope to be justified in regarding this as the beginning of a descriptive molecular anatomy for the cell surface, which may allow us to inquire into how surface molecular dispositions may be altered in malignancy, and how this may be related to the intrusion of new cell surface elements recognized as tumor antigens.

4. *What new surface components appear as a consequence of malignancy, and how does their appearance affect the existing display of surface constituents?* First, it must be emphasized that such new components, collectively termed tumor antigens, comprise a number of distinct categories (Table III). Antigens that are recognized primarily by their capacity to cause the rejection of tumors are known as tumor-specific transplantation antigens (TSTA) (see Klein, 1966). It appeared at one time that a distinction could be made between chemically induced tumors, each of which typically possesses a unique TSTA, and virus-induced tumors, which characteristically

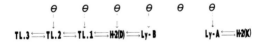

FIG. 2. Relative positions of eight alloantigens on the surface of mouse thymocytes: evidence for a surface "map."

TABLE III

SURFACE ANTIGENS OF SPECIAL RELEVANCE TO MALIGNANT CELLS

Category	Example
1. Individually distinct transplantation antigens	Chemically induced tumors
2. Viral envelope (Ve) antigens	Leukemias and solid tumors induced by oncogenic RNA viruses
3. Virus-specified (but nonvirion) antigens	Transplantation antigens of tumors induced by DNA oncogenic viruses
	Surface antigen (GCSA, G_{IX}) of leukemias induced by murine leukemia virus
4. Derepression antigens	TL antigens occurring on leukemias of mice not normally expressing them

share a TSTA which is common to all tumors produced by the same virus (Old and Boyse, 1964). It now seems likely that this distinction is relative rather than absolute, and that individually distinct TSTA may turn out to be characteristic of tumors generally, although this will frequently be overshadowed by the presence of cross-reacting antigens in virus-induced tumors (Old and Boyse, 1965).

The antigens demonstrable primarily by serological techniques are a diverse group. There are antigens that belong to the envelope of leukemia viruses and other viruses that bud from the cell surface. Other cell surface antigens, while not structural components of the virus, are either coded by the viral genome or under control by the viral genome.

The TL (thymus leukemia) antigens fall into a class of their own (Table IV), for they have features that indicate straightforward determination as alloantigens and yet their intimate association with leukemogenesis suggests coding by occult leukemia virus (Boyse and Old, 1969). TL antigens are specified by genes in linkage group IX near H-2, as we have seen. In normal mice their inheritance is Mendelian, like other alloantigens, and their expression is confined to thymocytes. Some mouse strains however, do not carry TL antigen on their thymocytes, and these are referred to as TL⁻ strains.

TABLE IV

TL (THYMUS-LEUKEMIA) SYSTEM OF ANTIGENS

TL antigens of normal mice	TL antigens of leukemic mice
1. Inheritance is Mendelian (*Tla* locus in linkage group IX) 2. Confined to thymocytes 3. Are alloantigens (mouse strains are either TL$^+$ or TL$^-$)	1. TL antigens may occur on leukemias of TL$^-$ mouse strains as well as TL$^+$ mouse strains 2. TL antigens occurring on TL$^+$ leukemias of TL$^-$ mouse strains are *leukemia-specific* (host is therefore capable of producing TL antibody)

The phenomenon that links the *Tla* locus with leukemogenesis is that when leukemias occur in such TL$^-$ strains the leukemia cells frequently *do* express TL antigens. This anomalous appearance of TL antigens on malignant cells arising from a progenitor cell on which they were not expressed, indicates derepression of *Tla* genes accompanying malignant transformation.

This brief description of the TL system is helpful also in illustrating how we can begin to inquire about the disposition of surface antigens on malignant cells. The particular question here relates to TL antigens appearing on leukemia cells of mice that do not normally express them: Do these aberrant TL antigens in leukemia cells occur in the same place they occupy on the surface of cells that normally express TL antigens (see above)? The answer from blocking tests appears to be "*yes*, they do." So the presence of TL antigen is anomalous on these leukemia cells, but its location on the cell surface is at least not grossly so.

5. *The next question to be considered regarding antigenic cell surface components is their representation on the cell surface as a whole.* We have already touched on the matter of molecular grouping revealed by antibody blocking. Ideally one would wish to visualize these cell surface arrays with labeled antibody, but this is at present beyond the scope of immunoelectronmicroscopy. In practice the principal use to which this valuable tool has been put is in ascertaining the representation of particular antigens over the cell surface as a whole. Immunoelectronmicroscopy refers to the labeling of antibody with

an electron-dense visual marker such as ferritin, to identify the location of the antigen visually. Originally the ferritin was covalently linked directly to the antibody (Singer, 1959). A more recent alternative (Hämmerling *et al.*, 1968) is to prepare a hybrid antibody by combining F(ab) fragments from antibodies of two specificities, one directed to the visual marker and the other to (a) a selected antigen (direct test) or to (b) immunoglobulin ("indirect" reagent for use with antibody to any antigen). This method of labeling increases precision, because each hybrid molecule combines with a single ferritin molecule, and it lends itself to the employment of different visually distinct markers. For this purpose, we have successfully used a small plant virus, Southern bean mosaic virus (SBMV). Figure 3 shows the clear distinction between the two

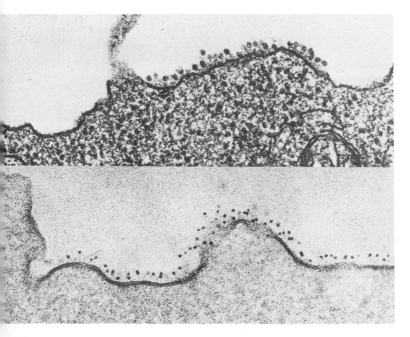

FIG. 3. Immunoelectron microscopy of cell surface antigens; comparison of Southern bean mosaic virus (above) and ferritin (below) as visually distinguishable markers. Hybrid antibody technique.

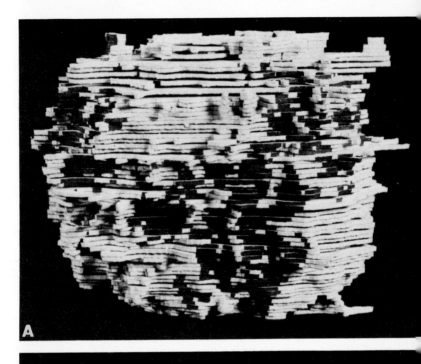

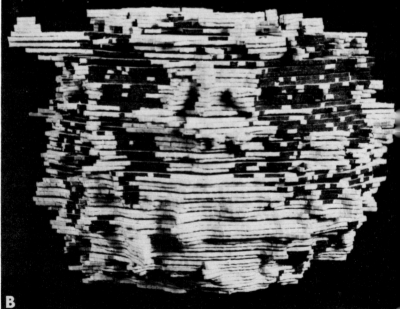

markers, which we hope will ultimately permit the visualization of two different antigens simultaneously on the same cell.

Figure 3 also shows a discontinuous representation of antigen over the cell surface. In our experience this has been characteristic of all cell surface components so far tested (Aoki *et al.*, 1969). This discontinuity is shown most clearly in reconstructions built up from single cells exposed to the labeling reagents and then serially sectioned. Figure 4 illustrates two views of a lymphocyte model constructed in this way and showing the patchy distribution of H-2 antigens on the cell surface (Stackpole *et al.*, 1971).

In looking at this irregular representation of surface antigens, one must bear in mind many indications that the surface phenotype is susceptible to adaptive changes. An indication that surface topography is not necessarily constant under all conditions comes from the work of Frye and Edidin (1970), who observed rapid admixture of at least some human and mouse surface components when human and mouse cells were hybridized. The question is: To what extent does the segregation of visual labeling into discrete areas reflect the natural distribution of the antigen on the cell, and to what extent may it be due to aggregation brought about by reaction of surface antigens with the antibodies used for labeling (Davis, 1972)? It is perhaps too early to attempt a definitive statement about this. The eventual solution of this problem of the native distribution of antigens is likely to come from modifications in technique, particularly in regard to inhibiting surface mobility, and from improved uses of antibody labeling in ways that preclude aggregation.

6. And so to the last of this series of questions about the cell surface: *Is the expression of any or all of these antigens a stable irreversible character of the cell, or is it amenable to quantitative or qualitative adaptive variation?* We ourselves first realized the importance of this while studying the TL system of antigens. When TL$^+$ leukemias occur in TL$^-$ mice, the antigen is leukemia-specific, and syngeneic mice can by appropriate immunization be made to produce high titers of cytotoxic TL antibody. However, when such immunized mice are

FIG. 4. Distribution of H-2 antigen on the lymphocyte surface according to the hybrid-antibody labeling method. Two views of a model based on serial sections of a single lymphocyte.

challenged with TL⁺ leukemias originating in the same inbred strain there is in fact little or no resistance, which is contrary to what is expected on the supposition that TL, being a readily demonstrable cell surface antigen should also be an effective transplantation antigen. The reason for this lack of resistance was found to be an apparently complete disappearance of TL antigen, which persists as long as the cells remain in the immune environment, and can in fact be brought about by exposure of TL⁺ cells to TL antibody *in vitro* (Old *et al.*, 1968). Both *in vivo* and *in vitro*, the negative phenotype persists only as long as antibody is present, the TL⁺ phenotype recurring when antibody is removed. This shift between the positive and negative phenotype is called antigenic modulation, and it can be inhibited by exposure to certain metabolic inhibitors or by lowering the temperature. At first antigenic modulation appeared to be confined to the TL system of antigens, but it now seems that other surface antigens can show antigenic modulation or something akin to it. These other possible examples of surface antigenic modulation involve antigens of two other lymphoid malignancies: Burkitt's lymphoma in man (Smith *et al.*, 1968) and leukemias induced by Gross leukemia virus in the mouse (Aoki and Johnson, 1972), which raises the ominous possibility that antigenic modulation is an effective escape mechanism for malignant cells under attack from immunological responses.

Phenotypic deletion of antigen, exemplified by modulation of TL, is not confined to malignant cells nor to antigens related particularly to malignancy. Thus TL antigens on normal thymocytes are subject to modulation by TL antibody (Boyse *et al.*, 1967). Again, the immunoglobulins which lymphocytes carry incorporated in their surfaces undergo modulation when the lymphocyte is exposed to anti-immunoglobulin antibody (Takahashi, 1971). The process has been visualized with fluorescein-labeled anti-immunoglobulin, which shows that the cell surface immunoglobulin is first rounded up into patches, and that these then move to one pole of the lymphocyte to form a cap, which is eventually pinocytosed (reviewed by Raff, 1971).

Can the induction of aggregates, and subsequent capping, occur with other cell surface antigens? Is either of these processes essential for antigenic modulation? These are certainly crucial questions which can be resolved with present techniques. Just as the topography of surface antigens has introduced us to the microanatomy of the cell surface, so observations of their mobility is an introduction to another aspect of what might be thought of as the physiology of the cell surface.

These induced surface phenomena, in addition to their relevance to tumor immunology, may signify general physiological processes of wider biological significance, concerned with eliciting responses from cells after attachment of specific molecules to surface receptors; in the case of surface immunoglobulin, the purpose of the response presumably has to do with immune reactivity. There is evidence that modulation can affect even H-2 histocompatibility antigens if an antiglobulin antibody is added to the H-2 antibody itself (Takahashi, 1971). But the very fact that H-2 is a strong transplantation antigen indicates that not all components of the cell surface are equally susceptible to antigenic modulation.

III. Immunogenetics of Leukemia Virus

The first part of this talk was directed to the genetic specification of cell surfaces, and we saw that it is not possible to separate this entirely from the subject of viruses and what they contribute to cell surface composition. In this section, viral oncogenesis will be considered more directly, particularly in relation to leukemia, with illustrations drawn from our own findings.

The original reason for concentrating on leukemia cells as an object of study, rather than on malignant cells of other types, was a technical one, namely, that serological analysis of surface antigens requires dispersed suspensions of viable cells; for this purpose leukemias are ideal (Gorer, 1956). It is for the same reason that vastly more is known about the surface structure of thymic lymphocytes than about any other nucleated normal cell type (Boyse and Old, 1969). Leukemias of the mouse are characteristically derived from thymic lymphocytes, so the availability of the malignant cell population (leukemia cells) together with the comparable normal population from which they arise presents unrivaled opportunities for studying the immunogenetics of the cell surface in relation to malignancy.

During the early serological study of leukemia cells a number of cell surface antigens came to light, most of which could be traced to the presence of leukemia virus. So the first task resolved itself into one of defining as closely as possible the spectrum of antigens present in leukemia virus itself and in cells which they infect and transform. Before reviewing this work and relating it to viral leukemogenesis, let us consider the following statements about viral oncogenesis.

There are two broad aspects of the relation of viruses to cancer research:

First, oncogenic viruses causing malignant transformation of cells under laboratory conditions, both *in vitro* and *in vivo*, provide excellent models for studying events that lead to cancer, regardless of whether or not the same viruses induce malignancy in nature. The small DNA viruses SV40 and polyoma, for example, which have contributed greatly to what might be called the molecular biology of oncogenesis, are in fact not known to be natural causes of cancer.

Second, there are now several impressive examples of natural cancers that are regularly associated with certain viruses, and possibly or probably are caused by them. The two groups of such viruses that are receiving most attention at the moment are the oncogenic RNA viruses, for which we have coined the term "oncornaviruses" (Nowinski *et al.*, 1970), and the DNA oncogenic viruses of the Herpes class.

In regard to the oncornaviruses, much of what was known earlier about chicken leukosis and sarcoma viruses is now being found to apply, even in detail to similar viruses of mammals, notably of the mouse and cat. Now that oncornaviruses are known to be indigenous in such widely diverse hosts as snakes and monkeys, it seems very likely that they will be found in all vertebrates, including man.

Herpesviruses were first suspected of involvement in natural oncogenesis when virus of this type was found in renal adenocarcinomas of the frog. Later a Herpesvirus was found to be associated with Marek's disease (neurolymphomatosis) of chicken. This disease, which is a serious menace to commercial flocks, is now preventable by immunization with a related Herpesvirus. Another Herpesvirus, from a primate source, has now been shown to cause leukemias and lymphomas on inoculation into monkeys. And in man himself a good case has been made out for the Epstein-Barr Herpesvirus as the cause of Burkitt's lymphoma (Klein, 1972).

Speaking of viral oncology generally, two important principles need to be emphasized. First, in tumors induced by both DNA and RNA viruses the viral genome persists. Its presence is obvious in the case of leukemias and sarcomas produced by oncornaviruses where complete infectious virus continues to be produced. In the case of tumors induced by DNA viruses, where infectious virus is characteristically not found, the persistence of the viral genome is betrayed by the presence of virus-coded products or by recovery of infectivity on hybridization of the transformed nonproducing cell with a so-called permissive cell. The lesson seems to be that probably in all cases the maintenance of the malignant phenotype depends on the continued presence of the viral genome.

The second principle is that there is generally and perhaps always an intimate association between the viral and cellular genomes. The discovery of reverse transcriptase has done away with the necessity to consider separate mechanisms for oncogenesis by the DNA and RNA tumor viruses. This, coupled with a variety of evidence that oncogenic viral genes occupy chromosomal sites, has gone a long way to substantiating the relevance of lysogeny in bacteria to the state of occult tumor virus genomes in cells that carry them. Evidence is now forthcoming that two hallmarks of lysogeny in bacteria, integration and inducibility, are also characteristic of oncogenic viruses. But valuable though the lysogeny model may be in explaining the inheritance and transmission of oncogenic viruses in normal cells, it does not itself offer an explanation of malignant transformation.

With this as a background, we can go on to consider, in relation to leukemia viruses of mammals, how immunogenetic methods help to clarify their relationship to the host organism.

Several characteristics distinguish the oncornaviruses as a group (Nowinski et al., 1970):

1. Oncogenic to some degree in their natural hosts (leukemia, sarcoma, mammary tumor)
2. Widespread in vertebrates
3. Noncytopathic

4. Maturation by budding from cell surface
5. Single-stranded 60–70 S RNA
6. Reverse transcriptase
7. Transmitted both vertically (parent to progeny via gametes) and horizontally (contagion)
8. Viral group-specific antigen (gs1) shared by leukemia-sarcoma viruses of each host species
9. Other group-specific antigen (gs3) shared by leukemia-sarcoma viruses of different mammalian host species
10. Specify virion envelope antigens, and nonvirion antigens, at the cell surface

Figure 5 shows successive stages in the budding of a murine leukemia virion from the cell surface. The earliest visible stage is a crescent immediately beneath the cell surface. As this extends to become the nucleocapsid, the overlying cell surface forms a bud, which eventually is pinched off, and the virion is released.

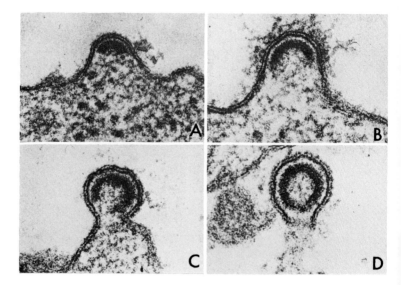

Fig. 5. Steps in the maturation of an MuLV virion at the cell surface.

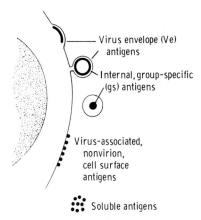

FIG. 6.   Antigens associated with murine leukemias and murine leukemia viruses.

Figure 6 indicates various antigens associated with infection. First there are the antigens of the virus itself, comprising envelope antigens and internal group-specific antigens. There are also antigens on the cell surface which are a consequence of viral infection but are not part of the virion. This explains how it is possible to prepare mouse antisera that are highly cytotoxic for cells carrying leukemia virus, but have little or no neutralizing capacity for the virus. Also, soluble antigens are released by infected cells and are found in extracellular fluids, including blood (Stück *et al.*, 1964; Aoki *et al.*, 1968); it has not been determined whether these are virion components, or exfoliated cell surface antigens, or both.

Envelope antigens of leukemia virus are demonstrable by the capacity of the relevant antisera to neutralize the virus. Immuno-electronmicroscopy also is a highly effective method for discriminating between these and other antigens (Aoki and Takahashi, 1972). Figure 7 shows a leukemia cell and virion after exposure to antibody to envelope antigen and labeling by the hybrid antibody method with SBMV as the visual marker. The small SBM virions, marking the site of antibody attachment are seen surrounding the relatively massive leukemia virion. There is no label at other sites.

Internal group-specific (gs) antigens of oncornaviruses were demonstrated first in avian leukemia-sarcoma viruses (Huebner *et al.*, 1964) and later in mouse leukemia viruses (Geering *et al.*,

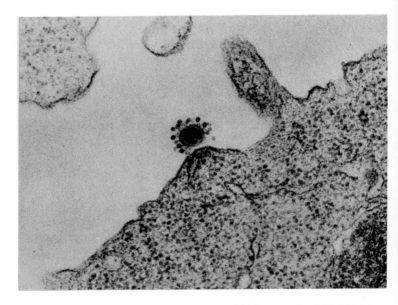

Fig. 7.   Electron micrograph of a leukemia cell and an associated MuLV virion. Viral envelope antigen has been visually labeled with SBMV (hybrid antibody method); there is no labeling of the cell surface.

1966; Huebner, 1967). Figure 8 shows that the antigen called gs1 (Gregoriades and Old, 1969), which is released from virions when the viral envelope is disrupted, is shared by all leukemia viruses of the mouse, but not by the mouse mammary tumor virus. It has now been shown for several mammalian hosts that the indigenous leukemia–sarcoma viruses of a particular species share a common gs antigen, homologous with gs1 antigen of the mouse, and that this is confined to that species (Schäfer et al., 1969; Hardy et al., 1969; Nowinski et al., 1971; Gilden and Oroszlan, 1972). Another group antigen, discovered by Geering et al. in 1970, is shared by all known mammalian leukemia–sarcoma viruses; this is called gs3 (or "interspec") (Schäfer et al., 1970; Oroszlan et al., 1971), and Fig. 9 illustrates that it is found in leukemia viruses of the mouse, cat, hamster, and rat, but not of the chicken.

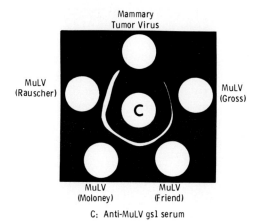

Fig. 8. Demonstration of a group-specific antigen (MuLV-gs1) common to murine leukemia viruses.

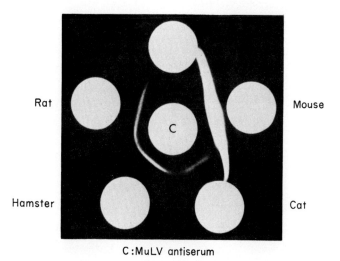

Fig. 9. Mammalian leukemia–sarcoma viruses share a common group-specific antigen, gs3 (also called "interspec") which avian leukemia–sarcoma viruses lack. The outer wells in this Ouchterlony plate contain ether-disrupted leukemia virus from the species named. The major band with MuLV is gs1 antigen, which is restricted to leukemia-sarcoma viruses from the mouse.

The existence of cell surface antigens specified directly or indirectly by the virus but not part of it was suspected on serological grounds (Klein and Klein, 1964; Pasternak, 1968; Steeves, 1968). Immuno-electron microscopy provides direct proof of this (Aoki *et al.*, 1970). Figure 10 shows labeling of one of the cell surface antigens specified by Gross leukemia virus, GCSA (Old *et al.*, 1965). (The method of locating antigen was again the hybrid antibody technique with Southern bean mosaic virus as the visual marker.) In contrast to Fig. 7, illustrating envelope antigens, it is in this case the cell surface only that is labeled, not the virion.

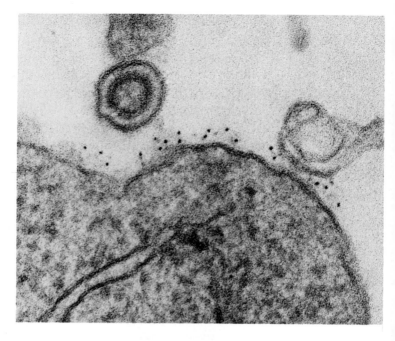

Fig. 10. Electron micrograph of a leukemia cell and budding virion exposed to mouse antiserum to the MuLV-related antigen GCSA. The cell surface is labeled, but the viral envelope is not (hybrid antibody method with ferritin as the visual marker); compare with Fig. 7.

TABLE V

GCSA AND G_{IX} SURFACE (NONVIRION) ANTIGENS OF MuLV-INFECTED CELLS

Features shared with differentiation alloantigens	Features not shared with differentiation alloantigens
1. Present in some mouse strains: absent in others (antigen-negative strains)	1. Antigen induced in rats and mice inoculated with MuLV
2. Present on some tissues: absent on others	2. *De novo* appearance of antigen in leukemias, solid tumors, or aging tissues, of antigen-negative mice
3. Half-quantity on cells of heterozygotes	3. Antigen-negative mice have no alternative antigen specified by an alternative allele
4. Segregation data: Mendelian (G_{IX})	4. G_{IX} system shows quantitative differences characteristic for different mouse strains (3:2:1:0)
	5. In GCSA system, progeny of $+ \times -$ matings may be $-$

The two most studied cell surface nonvirion antigens associated with MuLV are GCSA and G_{IX} (Old *et al.*, 1965; Stockert *et al.*, 1971). Had their association with MuLV not been evident from the outset, they might both have been accepted as conventional differentiation alloantigens. This is because they have some of the properties of differentiation alloantigens, being present in some mouse strains and absent in others, being present on some cell types but absent on others, showing half-expression on heterozygous cells, and in the case of G_{IX} antigen (GCSA has been so far less studied in this respect) showing Mendelian inheritance (Table V). Nevertheless the features listed on the right side of Table V clearly point to direct or indirect specification by leukemia virus, the major point being that these antigens can be induced in the rat or in mice of strains that normally do not express them, by inoculation of MuLV. So a mouse cell may be G_{IX}^+ either because it inherited the antigen as a Mendelian trait, or because the cell became productively infected with MuLV, as a result of either spontaneous induction or exogenous infection. There is a striking parallel here with the TL system of antigens, for TL antigens make their appearance in malignant cells of mice that are hereditarily negative for TL antigens. This strengthens earlier suspicions that the *Tla* locus may be an integrated viral genome (Boyse *et al.*, 1972).

It is characteristic of the TL and G_{IX} systems that alternative antigens, specified by alternative alleles, have not been identified. This is to be expected from the fact that the structural genes are to be found in all mice, and that it is *expression* vs. *nonexpression* which is inherited by normal mice as a Mendelian trait. Another peculiarity of the G_{IX} system is the existence of quantitative differences in the representation of antigen from strain to strain, whereby most mouse strains can be placed in one of four categories according to the relative amounts of G_{IX} antigen which they express on their thymocytes (3:2:1:0). Possibly this unusual feature may have its origin in different numbers of copies of MuLV in different strains.

Table VI is a list of the several MuLV (Gross: wild type) antigens now recognized, including 3 distinct envelope antigens, 3 gs antigens, the 2 nonvirion cell surface antigens discussed above, and the soluble antigens. And assuredly this is not a complete inventory of the products of the viral genome (e.g., it probably does not include reverse transcriptase).

Provided with these several antigenic markers, we can attempt to answer a number of questions concerning the relation between virus

TABLE VI

ANTIGENIC MARKERS OF WILD-TYPE MuLV

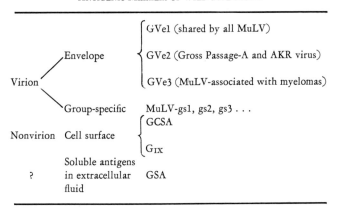

	Envelope	GVe1 (shared by all MuLV)
		GVe2 (Gross Passage-A and AKR virus)
Virion		GVe3 (MuLV-associated with myelomas)
	Group-specific	MuLV-gs1, gs2, gs3 . . .
		GCSA
Nonvirion	Cell surface	G_{IX}
?	Soluble antigens in extracellular fluid	GSA

TABLE VII

MuLV-Associated Antigens

	Antigen	Has antigen been found in virus-negative cells?	Expression in heterozygote	Linkage of specifying genes (tentative)
Nonvirion	G_{IX}	Yes	$\frac{1}{2}$ Closely	
	GCSA	No	0 or $\frac{1}{2}$[a] linked	
				Loosely linked
Virion	GVe	No		
	gs1	Yes	$\frac{1}{2}$[a] Closely	
	gs3	Yes	$\frac{1}{2}$[a] linked	

[a] Depends on which negative strain is used for the cross.

and cell. One of the most immediate tasks is to find out which of the genes responsible for specifying these antigens exhibit Mendelian inheritance, and to locate these in the cellular genome, as an approach to the question whether each gene is part of an integrated viral genome. In this context, Table VII is a sketch of the sort of information now being obtained.

The important points that have been established are that some of these antigens can be expressed independently of virus production, indicating that the genes responsible must be subject to independent control. In general, expression in heterozygotes is 50% of that in homozygotes, which is characteristic of antigens specified by cellular genes. (GCSA is exceptional in that there may be no demonstrable expression of this antigen in certain heterozygotes, so that in these circumstances the antigen is unusual in that its detectability is apparently recessive; a provisional interpretation is that expression of GCSA antigen depends on virus production, and that this is suppressed by genes of the GCSA-negative parent of the heterozygote.) Genetic analysis is still in its early stages, but segregation data suggest a close association or linkage between the nonvirion antigens G_{IX} and GCSA on the one hand, and between the envelope and internal gs virion antigens on the other. These two loci appear loosely associated or linked with one another in segregating populations. Linkage group IX is the likely site for this block of genes, because one of them, expressed independently (G_{IX}) has been clearly identified in that linkage group by segregation tests (Stockert *et al.*, 1971). A reason for caution in generalizing from this finding is that there are no grounds for assuming that integrated viral genes need reside at the same chromosomal site in different strains of mice; in fact we are now occupied with that question, namely, whether the linkage relation of MuLV-associated genes in strains with a high incidence of leukemia is or is not the same as in strains with a low incidence of leukemia.

To complete this brief sketch of the immunogenetics of the mammalian leukemia viruses, here are a few statements as to what the present goals are in this field, and what sort of facts ought to be established in the near future.

To begin with, there is a growing conviction in many quarters, and from a variety of evidence, that probably all mice carry MuLV genomes, and it is from considerations of this kind that the well-known "oncogene theory" of cancer originated (Huebner and Todaro, 1969). So it is not the presence or the absence of viral genes that accounts for the fact that some mice exhibit overt infection with leukemia virus and others do not; nor can malignancy be attributed simply to the presence of viral genomes. The emphasis is rather on factors that influence the expression of viral genes (Table VIII).

Malignant cells induced by chemical carcinogens or by radiation frequently produce MuLV and its associated antigens. This was one of the earliest pieces of evidence that leukemia virus genomes might

TABLE VIII

FACTORS THAT INFLUENCE SYNTHESIS OF MuLV
AND MuLV-RELATED ANTIGENS IN MOUSE CELLS

Exposure to physical and chemical carcinogens
Age of the mouse
Culture *in vitro*
Bromodeoxyuridine, mitomycin C
Genes: H-$2/Ir$
        NB ($= Fv$-1)
Pathway of cellular differentiation

---

be ubiquitous in mice, since this was seen to occur in tumors of mouse strains that showed no evidence of overt infection. Aging is clearly conducive to activation of latent leukemia virus; this was recognized by observing that mice of certain strains that show no evidence of infection when young convert to the virus-positive carrier state later in adult life (Nowinski *et al.*, 1968; Huebner, 1970). Embryo cells from mouse strains that commonly do not produce demonstrable MuLV may spontaneously produce virus and associated antigens after a period in tissue culture (Aaronson *et al.*, 1969). Exposure to (for example) bromodeoxyuridine can induce the production of virus in cloned lines of cultured cells that do not spontaneously release virus (Lowy *et al.*, 1971).

With regard to the intact organism, as distinct from individual cells, it is necessary to consider further the consequences of the initiation of productive infection in one or more cells, particularly in regard to the extent to which infection may become generalized. This is doubtless influenced by several genes; two of these will be discussed here because something is known of the way in which they may influence generalization of infection and hence may affect the number of cells at risk of leukemogenic transformation. The influence of *H-2* was first suspected from the observation that the three best-known strains of mice with a high incidence of leukemia are H-2^k, and that other H-2^k mice are highly sensitive to inoculated leukemia virus (Lilly *et al.*, 1964). This association between H-2 types and susceptibility to leukemogenesis has since been confirmed in numerous formal genetic tests (Lilly, 1970a). It is now known that an immune response (*Ir*) locus is situated in or near *H-2* (McDevitt and Benacerraf, 1969), so possibly it is this that controls susceptibility to leukemia by affecting immune responsiveness to the virus and viral antigens.

A second locus, *Fv-1* (see Lilly, 1970b) now thought to be identical with NB (Pincus *et al.*, 1971), is recognizable by effects *in vivo* and *in vitro*. *In vivo*, the locus governs *susceptibility* vs. *resistance* to certain leukemia viruses; *in vitro* it determines levels of susceptibility of mouse embryo cultures to infection by leukemia viruses classified as either N-tropic or B-tropic. The mechanism, it appears, does not involve a cell surface virus receptor, but more likely some later step in virus infection which depends upon the number of virus particles required to initiate productive infection in individual cells. So the influence of *Fv-1 in vivo* is probably on dissemination rather than on initiation of infection (Rowe and Hartley, 1972).

The influence of cellular differentiation on viral or virus-controlled characters is seen in the fact that G_{IX} antigen in normal mice is expressed only on thymic lymphocytes; probably therefore other viral or virus-controlled genes come under the influence of selective gene controls that regulate cellular differentiation.

So the conclusion that all mouse cells carry inherited MuLV genomes may imply that these are integrated in the cellular genome; this is supported by the Mendelian segregation of virion antigens and virus-associated cell surface antigens in mouse and chicken (see "RNA Viruses and Host Genome in Oncogenesis"). The fact that gs and other viral antigens can under appropriate conditions appear in mice that have not inherited the antigen as a Mendelian trait must indicate that it is not the structural genes which show Mendelian segregation, but genes governing their expression. Thus, until more direct evidence is forthcoming, there remains the possibility that the MuLV genome itself is episomal, and that only genes which control or are controlled by MuLV are chromosomal. Whether and when it may be technically feasible to make the critical demonstration that a given chromosome or linkage group contains DNA homologous with the complete viral RNA, it is not possible to predict.

It is obvious that neither viral integration, nor productive infection, is itself responsible for malignant transformation. So a vital question is: What is the gene product, if there is such a single gene product, which initiates and maintains the malignant state of the cell? A virological approach to this is to develop virus mutants which can distinguish transforming function from virus-producing function (Dulbecco, 1969). An immunological approach is to identify antigenic products specifically associated with malignancy. Perhaps the most promising cells for study in this connection are those that have been transformed by viruses and retain the virus genome but produce no demonstrable virus or virion antigen.

As an extension of the idea of searching for a gene product responsible for initiation and maintenance of malignancy, one may ask whether a particular *region* of the genome is involved in malignant transformation. The finding that genetic derepression of the *Tla* locus occurs in many mouse leukemias drew attention to linkage group IX in this connection, and now the finding of the G_{IX} locus on the same chromosome focuses attention once again on this chromosome as a center of interest for leukemic transformation in the mouse (Fig. 11). There are methods of exerting immunoselection pressures on leukemic cell populations to yield variant lines lacking one or other of the *H-2/Tla* segments of linkage group IX (Boyse *et al.*, 1970); these deletion variants are being used to determine whether the malignant phenotype of leukemia cells is dependent on retention of these particular genes. Cell hybridization offers another approach to relating particular chromosomes to the malignant state (Harris, 1970; Barski, 1972).

Finally, the question of how oncornaviruses are transmitted in nature is important not only for the light it may shed on the relation between virus and cell, but also because the facts are needed for an understanding of how infection may be controlled. To recapitulate, the probable ubiquity of the viral genome in mammalian cells, and the fidelity with which it is transmitted from generation to genera-

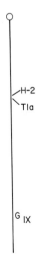

FIG. 11.   Linkage-group IX genes related to leukemia.

tion, accords with current views that it is in fact integrated and transmitted as part of the cellular genome. This mode of infection, which is what is usually implied in the terms "vertical transmission" or "transmission by gametes" (Gross, 1951) does not of course exclude horizontal transmission, i.e., passage of infection from one individual to another. Vertical and horizontal transmissions are in no way mutually exclusive; in fact the spread of infection from one individual to another is comparable to the spread of infection from cell to cell which is believed to follow the spontaneous initiation of productive infection in individual cells (see above). In chicken there is ample evidence of horizontal transmission of leukemia virus from bird to bird, carrying with it a heightened risk of leukemia (Rubin et al., 1962). In the mouse there is little evidence that horizontal transmission plays much part in the natural incidence of leukemia, and accordingly there might be a temptation to assume that horizontal transmission is a negligible factor in mammals generally. But recent work in the cat indicates the opposite.

The development of serological tests for the cat leukemia virus (Hardy et al., 1969; Sarma et al., 1970; Fink et al., 1971) has made it possible to study the epidemiology of this virus and its relationship to leukemia in the cat. Helped by past experience with similar serological methods applied to the chicken and mouse, the natural history of the cat leukemia virus is being elucidated rapidly (Table IX). In Hardy's series, virus was demonstrable in a high proportion of cats with leukemia and also particularly in many cases of infectious peritonitis. As the cat is a domestic animal, living in close association with man, it is noteworthy that the cat leukemia virus antigens so far identified have not been found in tumors and leukemias of man.

Study of the spread of the virus in cats became possible with the development of an immunofluorescence test on peripheral white cells (Hardy et al., in press). This identifies overtly infected cats. Hardy's (unpublished data) survey of 378 apparently normal cats from a variety of sources revealed that 44 were overtly infected with leukemia virus (Table X). All these virus-positive cats came from households in which another cat had previously been diagnosed as suffering from either leukemia or infectious peritonitis. In most

TABLE IX

Occurrence of FeLV in Tissues of Cats[a]

Case	Number of cases in which FeLV antigen was demonstrable
Cats with malignant disease	
Leukemia	114/142
Sarcoma	4/20
Mammary adenocarcinoma	0/22
Cats with nonmalignant conditions	
Infectious peritonitis	20/42
Anemia	6/18
Lymphadenopathy	4/13
Normal cats	1/40

[a] FeLV antigen was not demonstrable in association with malignant tumors of man and of the dog.

instances these diseased cats were not immediately related to the infected normal animals identified serologically. This clearly points to spread of infection from cat to cat. The crucial point is that 6 of these serologically positive cats have since become leukemic. The

TABLE X

Occurrence of Demonstrable FeLV in the Peripheral Blood Cells of Normal Cats (Immunofluorescence Test)

	Number of FeLV + cats
Stray cats	0/67
Laboratory cat colonies	0/97
Cats from households without a history of feline leukemia or infectious peritonitis	0/33
Cats (mostly unrelated) from households with a history of feline leukemia or infectious peritonitis	44/181

conclusion is that although the cat leukemia virus genome is probably transmitted vertically, a majority of cases of leukemia in cats may in fact result from contact infection. This tells us that prophylactic procedures like vaccination are not necessarily contra-indicated because the viral genome is transmitted also via the gametes.

IV. IMMUNOBIOLOGICAL CONTROL OF CANCER

The facts discussed above, concerning the antigenic constitution of cell surfaces and the relation of viral genomes to host cells, bear on many aspects of biological research; but in the context of cancer they have one ultimate goal, and that is control of the disease in man. The last part of this talk will be devoted to some comments on how some of this information may be put to use in the treatment of cancer, and how it may be used to account for clinical observations that have not so far been adequately explained.

With all that is now known about antigens appearing in tumors, together with the many new methods of studying in detail the mechanisms of immune responses in general, both cellular and humoral, it is understandable that hopes are raised concerning the possibility of influencing the course of human cancer by immuno-logical methods (Klein, 1968; Alexander, 1970; Woodruff, 1972; Hellström et al., 1971; Mathé, 1971; Morton et al., 1971; Oettgen et al., 1971). But although it is topical to speak of immunotherapy as a fourth modality of cancer treatment, to be added to surgery, irradiation, and chemotherapy, it would be wrong to infer that there is at the moment any comparable scheme of immunotherapy with predictable benefit to the cancer patient. In general we have only hints of what might be expected in the future. Certainly it may soon be possible to think in terms of prophylactic vaccination, or mani-pulation of immune responses in favor of cellular vs. humoral immunity, or the transfer of immune resistance by means of antisera or immune cells or Lawrence's transfer factor, to mention some current ideas. But few people would care to estimate how much more detailed information from the laboratory will be necessary before such procedures can be realistically appraised in the clinic. Perhaps we should ask another question: Are there clinical observations which might be re-evaluated in the light of this new knowledge of tumor immunology, and drawn upon as guides to therapy? It is well known that there are reports, reaching back even to the last century, of unaccountable regression of tumors, occurring independently of therapy. A common factor in many of these cases was concurrent infection, usually bacterial. The first substantial study on the effects of bacteria or their products on the course of cancer was by Dr. W. B. Coley, a New York surgeon associated with Memorial Hospital (Nauts *et al.*, 1953). Those who have scrutinized Dr. Coley's records have little doubt that the bacterial products that came to be known as Coley's Toxins were in some instances highly effective. This form of therapy later fell into virtual disuse, no doubt in part because of high hopes raised by the introduction of radiotherapy, and afterward chemotherapy, which were more predictable and comprehensible, and whose mechanisms seemed more easily amenable to scientific inquiry.

Interest was not entirely extinguished, however. It was kept alive in the laboratory especially by Shear, who isolated a bacterial polysaccharide, now known to be endotoxin, which is a potent inhibitor of transplanted tumors in mice (Shear, 1944). Despite remarkable reports of induced regression of human tumors, Shear's polysaccharide was too toxic for adequate clinical assessment. Further ideas on the subject arose from another field, which came to be known as "nonspecific resistance." The key observation here is that treatment of mice with one of a number of microbial products raises the level of their resistance to unrelated bacterial infections (Rowley, 1955). Although there was a period when Properdin (Pillemer *et al.*, 1954) was suspected as the mediator of this enhanced resistance, the fact that these materials were found to activate the reticuloendothelial system (Thorbecke and Benacerraf, 1962) soon diverted interest in that direction. However, regardless of mechanism, these experiments prompted investigation of the activity of these agents on the growth of tumors (see "Role du Système Réticulo-Endothélial dans l'Immunité Antibactérienne et Antitumorale").

As an example of such results, Fig. 12 shows an experiment on the effect of prior injection of live BCG, an attenuated form of the tubercle bacillus, on the growth of a transplanted chemically induced tumor of inbred mice (Old *et al.*, 1961). All uninfected

Animal Number	Days Following Tumor Challenge			
	21	36	60	112

CONTROL

1				↑ 101
2				
3				↑ 98
4				
5				↑ 105
6				↑ 95
7				↑ 112
8				
9				
10				↑ 102

B.C.G. INFECTED

1				
2			Regressed	
3				
4			Regressed	
5	N.G.			
6				
7				
8			Regressed	
9				
10			Regressed	

controls died of progressive tumors. The tumors in the BCG-treated mice either regressed or grew at a much slower rate. This experiment, followed by many others of a similar kind, was performed in 1960. There were two major reasons why there was no immediate or direct clinical application at that time. First, agents like BCG were ineffective in mice unless given before tumor inoculation. Second, on the assumption that these effects have their basis in heightened immune responsiveness to tumor antigens, it seemed appropriate at the time first to gather more information about tumor antigens and immune responses to them. Now that the subject of tumor immunology is itself on a sounder footing, and with the assurance that the generality of human tumors are likely to be antigenic in some degree for their hosts, there is every reason to set about a thorough assessment of the prospects of what one might call immunobiological methods of treating cancer. The following is a brief summary of what we and our colleagues H. F. Oettgen, W. D. Hardy, Jr., R. Kassel, H. C. Nauts, E. A. Richards, T. Merigan, and R. Rogers are attempting in this area.

The various biological materials that have been shown to influence the growth of tumors seem to fall into 3 classes (Table XI), the prototypes being Bacillus Calmette-Guérin (BCG), endotoxin, and interferon. Treatment with materials like BCG, or fractions of BCG (Weiss *et al.*, 1966) generally are effective in mice only if given before the tumor, although in the guinea pig, direct inoculation of BCG into tumors has been seen to cause rejection of established transplants (Zbar *et al.*, 1971). These agents are known to increase immune responsiveness to a variety of antigens, including grafts of normal tissues (Balner *et al.*, 1962; Yashphe, 1971), and they can be counteracted by immunosuppressive measures. It seems likely that they affect the growth of antigenic tumors by raising the general level of immune responsiveness, and so are aptly termed immunopotentiators (as Sir Peter Medawar calls them). The next group is exemplified by endotoxin, the lipopolysaccharide component of gram-negative bacterial cell walls. In contrast to the BCG group,

FIG. 12. Influence of prior infection with BCG on the growth of a syngeneic transplanted sarcoma in inbred mice. The drawings indicate the relative size of the subcutaneous transplants. N.G., no growth; †, death on day stated.

TABLE XI

BIOLOGICAL MATERIALS THAT INFLUENCE THE GROWTH OF MOUSE TUMORS

	Inhibitory effect		
	When given before tumor transplant	On established tumor transplant	On primary AKR leukemias
I. BCG Zymosan Polysaccharides e.g., Lentinan Pachymaran	+	−	−
II. Endotoxin Lipid A, glycolipid Double-stranded RNA	−	+	+
III. Interferon Normal serum e.g., Horse Human	−	−	+

these agents have their most profound effect on *established* tumors. Their most dramatic manifestation is hemorrhagic necrosis of sub-cutaneous tumor masses, which has the hallmarks of what is known as a local Schwartzman reaction (Fig. 13). Hemorrhagic necrosis ensues within a few hours of endotoxin administration, and this is followed by total or partial tumor regression. While this regression is doubtless dependent on antigenicity and immune responsiveness, there is no evidence that hemorrhagic necrosis itself depends upon an immune response to the tumor; and in fact immunosuppressive measures do not prevent the occurrence of hemorrhagic necrosis in tumors. Agents that inhibit the Schwartzman reaction will in vary-ing degree inhibit hemorrhagic necrosis in tumors, but may not abrogate tumor regression. To determine whether the effect of endotoxin is directly upon the tumor, or whether it is mediated by factors released in the host by endotoxin, we have studied the reactivity of serum from nontumor-bearing mice treated with endotoxin. Figure 14 shows that serum from endotoxin-treated (nontumor-bearing) mice can itself induce hemorrhagic necrosis of

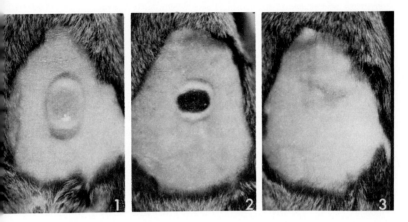

FIG. 13. The classic effect of endotoxin on a transplanted sarcoma; (1) A transplanted sarcoma growing in an untreated syngeneic inbred mouse. (2) The same sarcoma showing extensive hemorrhagic necrosis within a few hours of endotoxin administration. (3) Total tumor regression occurring several days later.

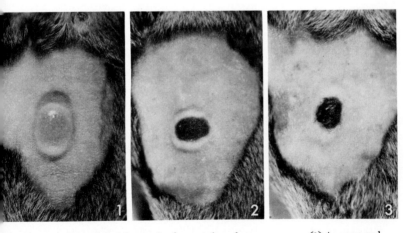

FIG. 14.   Serum-induced necrosis of a transplanted mouse sarcoma. (1) An untreated mouse. (2) A mouse treated with endotoxin. (3) A mouse that received serum from nontumorous mice; the serum-donor mice had been infected with Bacillus Calmette-Guérin and subsequently treated with endotoxin.

tumors in recipient mice. This serum-mediated effect is not due to residual endotoxin, first, because the reaction is both heightened and accelerated in comparison with primary administration of endotoxin, and second, because the amount of endotoxin needed to evoke such an active serum is lower than that needed to induce a corresponding degree of hemorrhagic necrosis.

A notable handicap of this second group of agents is their toxicity. That is why it is important to investigate methods of rendering them less toxic (see, e.g., Nowotny, 1969) or of identifying the mediator which is capable of transferring their effects without their toxicity.

Interferon, in the third category in Table XI, is of interest because several of the agents we have been discussing induce the host to produce interferon (Grossberg, 1972).

Interferon and interferon inducers are known to inhibit certain rodent tumors (Levy *et al.*, 1969; Gresser, 1970; "Symposium on Interferon and Host Response to Virus Infection"), and the question now being asked is whether interferon will have a place in the treatment of human cancer? Graff *et al.* (1970) discovered a dramatic effect of interferon on primary spontaneous leukemias of AKR mice. Massive resolution of leukemic nodes and spleen may occur within 24–48 hours of administration, microscopy showing cell death within as little as 2 hours. However, our recent and unexpected observations with Kassel and Richards, that normal sera from various sources can produce equally extensive resolution of primary AKR leukemias (Fig. 15), engenders caution as to what factor in the interferon preparations is really responsible for leukemia inhibition. The active substance in normal serum has at least some of the properties of a complement component, including inhibition by cobra venom factor, raising the possibility that the leukemia cells are sensitized by host antibody but that insufficiency of host complement prevents their destruction. Such remarkable regression of leukemic tissue is not restricted to the mouse: Cats with advanced lymphosarcoma treated with interferon-containing cat serum may show equally dramatic resolution of their disease (Fig. 16). It remains to be seen whether interferon or another cat serum factor such as complement is responsible.

The one factor common to all or most of these agents may be that their effectiveness depends in the last analysis on a specific immune

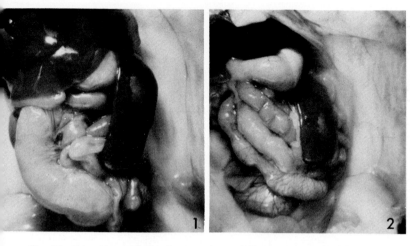

Fig. 15. Regression of leukemic tissue in an AKR mouse treated with normal serum. (1) Control: Untreated AKR mouse with advanced leukemia; note massive enlargement of liver, spleen, and mesenteric lymph nodes. (2) Matched leukemic AKR mouse treated with normal horse serum 48 hours previously. Liver, spleen, and mesenteric nodes are markedly reduced in size by comparison with control.

response of the host to the tumor. The relevant antigens, i.e., those involved in rejection, are at the cell surface, and so we come back once more to the central role of the cell surface in the study of cancer.

V. Conclusion

In conclusion, we must try to do justice to the title chosen for this lecture: "Current Enigmas in Cancer Research." Anyone who has worked in cancer research for even a short time could make up an impressive list of enigmas awaiting solution, and many who have never been engaged in cancer research have composed even longer ones. However, there is little reward in composing riddles that have no prospect of being solved at the present time. Some central and important questions are well known and appreciated. They include the following: How do cancers escape the consequences of their antigenicity; do they simply outpace the immune response? Can their antigens modulate? Are the tumors protected by blocking antibody?

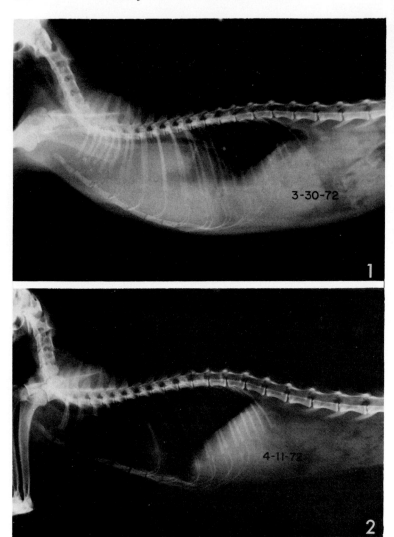

FIG. 16. A cat with advanced lymphosarcoma treated with interferon-containing cat serum (case of Drs. W. D. Hardy, Jr., and P. Hess). Radiographs taken (1) before

And again: Is there a single gene product, be it viral or cellular, that initiates and sustains the malignant phenotype? And does the ubiquity of leukemia virus genomes in mice indicate that the oncogenic RNA virus are not "true" viruses at all, in the sense of not having shared the same evolutionary history as the generality of viruses, but are in fact aberrant products of normal physiological processes carried on by cells? And so on.

The enigmas mentioned in concluding this lecture represent a few that are perhaps not so familiar, and which are not entirely inaccessible at the present time.

Map of Cell Surface Antigens: *Does this imply that cell interactions depend on codes of molecular patterning on the cell surface?* We are impressed by the possible significance of molecular patterning on the cell surface, which is indicated by the map of cell surface antigens. Does this sort of order in the cell surface hint at supramolecular codes that would underlie cell recognition and be essential to normal morphogenesis, being subject to aberrations leading to the invasion and metastasis characteristic of cancer?

Diversity of Distinctive Antigens on Chemically Induced Tumors: *Must such antigens be directly coded by genes? Or may they arise from defects in assembly of surface patterns which generate both new antigenicity and errors in cell interactions?* The recognition of molecular patterning suggests a possible alternative to genetic specification for the extreme diversity of antigens appearing on chemically induced tumors. We have assumed in the past that they must be coded genetically in the usual way, whether by a single gene subject to a great variety of mutations, or by a large series of genes whose products are not normally expressed on adult cells. But the possibility arises that errors in the assembly of cell surface components, not directly genetic in origin, might engender the surface abnormality that causes both defective cell recognition and altered antigenicity.

---

treatment, showing extensive obliteration of the thoracic cavity by a lymphoma; (2) 12 days later, after 5 days of treatment; the chest mass has almost totally disappeared.

312   LLOYD J. OLD AND EDWARD A. BOYSE

Antigenic Modulation: *Does this exemplify a general physiological mechanism for adaptive cellular changes initiated by signals from the cell surface?* Does the lability of certain cell surface components, notably TL, revealed by the phenomenon of antigenic modulation represent a more general physiological mechanism whereby cells respond to signals initiated by the union of cell surface receptors with complementary molecules?

Derepression of *Tla* Genes in Leukemia: *Is Tla an integrated (? defective?) viral genome, and is this chromosomal region indispensable for the malignant phenotype of TL⁺ leukemia cells?* The activation or derepression of genes at the *Tla* locus in leukemia is provocative in two respects. It has long been suspected that *Tla* might be an integrated viral genome, and the more recent finding that genes at the G_{IX} locus are also activated in leukemia cells enhances that idea. In any event the question whether this chromosomal region is indispensable for continued malignancy of TL⁺ leukemia cells is worth careful study.

Genetic Linkage of H-2:Tla:G_{IX}: *Does linkage group IX have a special role in leukemogenesis?* The similarities between the TL and G_{IX} systems, and the topographical evidence that TL and H-2 antigens are grouped together on the cell surface, all three loci being situated in linkage group IX, suggest that this whole linkage group may be specially related to leukopoiesis and leukomogenesis.

Inhibition of Tumors by "Immunobiological" Agents: *Is augmentation of an immune response, actual or potential, the common mechanism through which these agents act?* Finally, the last subject we dealt with was the influence of a number of diverse biological materials on the course of cancer. In relation to the clinical treatment of cancer this area may be the source of many rewarding problems for solution. But the central enigma here is whether in the last analysis these effects really are mediated by immunological factors, or whether their study may reveal wholly unexpected mechanisms of controlling cancer.

ACKNOWLEDGMENTS

We are indebted to Drs. T. Aoki, E. de Harven, and C. W. Stackpole for providing illustrations based on their work. Our own work was supported in part by NCI Grant CA 08748, and grants from the John A. Hartford Foundation, Inc., and the New York Cancer Research Institute, Inc.

REFERENCES

Aaronson, S. A., Hartley, J. W., and Todaro, G. J. (1969). *Proc. Nat. Acad. Sci. U.S.* **64**, 87.

Alexander, P. (1970). *Brit. Med. J.* **4**, 484.

Aoki, T., and Johnson, P. A. (1972). *J. Nat. Cancer Inst.* **49**, 183.

Aoki, T., and Takahashi, T. (1972). *J. Exp. Med.* **135**, 443.

Aoki, T., Boyse, E. A., and Old, L. J. (1968). *J. Nat. Cancer Inst.* **41**, 89.

Aoki, T., Hämmerling, U., de Harven, E., Boyse, E. A., and Old, L. J. (1969). *J. Exp. Med.* **130**, 979.

Aoki, T., Boyse, E. A., Old, L. J., de Harven, E., Hämmerling, U., and Wood, H. A. (1970). *Proc. Nat. Acad. Sci. U.S.* **65**, 569.

Balner, H., Old, L. J., and Clarke, D. A. (1962). *Soc. Exp. Biol. Med.* **109**, 58.

Barski, G. (1972). *Int. Rev. Exp. Pathol.* **9**, 151.

Boyse, E. A., and Old, L. J. (1969). *Annu. Rev. Genet.* **3**, 269.

Boyse, E. A., and Old, L. J. (1970). *In* "Immune Surveillance" (R. T. Smith and M. Landy, eds.), p. 5. Academic Press, New York.

Boyse, E. A., Stockert, E., and Old, L. J. (1967). *Proc. Nat. Acad. Sci. U.S.* **58**, 954.

Boyse, E. A., Old, L. J., and Stockert, E. (1968). *Proc. Nat. Acad. Sci. U.S.* **60**, 886.

Boyse, E. A., Stockert, E., Iritani, C. A., and Old, L. J. (1970). *Proc. Nat. Acad. Sci. U.S.* **65**, 993.

Boyse, E. A., Old, L. J., and Scheid, M. (1971). *Amer. J. Pathol.* **65**, 439.

Boyse, E. A., Old, L. J., and Stockert, E. (1972). *In* "RNA Viruses and Host Genome in Oncogenesis" (P. Emmelot and P. Bentvelzen, eds.), p. 171. North-Holland Publ., Amsterdam.

Davis, W. C. (1972). *Science* **175**, 1007.

Dulbecco, R. (1969). *Harvey Lect.* **63**, 33.

Fink, M. A., Sibal, L. R., and Plata, E. J. (1971). *J. Amer. Vet. Med. Ass.* **158**, 1070.

Frye, L. D., and Edidin, M. (1970). *J. Cell Sci.* **7**, 319.

Geering, G., Old, L. J., and Boyse, E. A. (1966). *J. Exp. Med.* **124**, 753.

Geering, G., Aoki, T., and Old, L. J. (1970). *Nature (London)* **226**, 265.

Gilden, R. V., and Oroszlan, S. (1972). *Proc. Nat. Acad. Sci. U.S.* **69**, 1021.

Gorer, P. A. (1956). *Advan. Cancer Res.* **4**, 149.

Graff, S., Kassel, R. L., and Kastner, O. (1970). *Trans. N.Y. Acad. Sci.* **32**, 545.

Gregoriades, A., and Old, L. J. (1969). *Virology* **37**, 189.

Gresser, I. (1970). *Int. Symp. Stand. Interferon Interferon Inducers, 1969, Symp. Ser. Immunobiol. Stand.* **14**, 209.

Gross, L. (1951). *Proc. Soc. Exp. Biol. Med.* **78**, 342.

Grossberg, S. E. (1972). *N. Engl. J. Med.* **287**, 122.

Hämmerling, U., Aoki, T., de Harven, E., Boyse, E. A., and Old, L. J. (1968). *J. Exp. Med.* **128**, 1461.

Hardy, W. D., Jr., Geering, G., Old, L. J., and de Harven, E. (1969). *Science* **166**, 1019.

Hardy, W. D., Jr., Geering, G., Old, L. J., de Harven, E., Brodey, R. S., and McDonough, S. K. (1970). *In* "Comparative Leukemia Research 1969" (R. M. Dutcher, ed.), p. 343. (*Bibl. Haematol.* **36**). Karger, Basel.

Hardy, W. D., Jr., Hirshaut, Y., and Hess, P. (1971). *In* "International Symposium, on Comparative Leukemia Research, Vth" (Sept. 13–17, 1971, Padova-Venice, Italy). Karger, Basel. In press.

Harris, H. (1970). "Cell Fusion." Harvard Univ. Press, Cambridge, Massachusetts.

Hellström, I., Hellström, K. E., Sjögren, H. O., and Warner, G. A. (1971). *Int. J. Cancer* **8**, 185.

Huebner, R. J. (1967). *Proc. Nat. Acad. Sci. U.S.* **58**, 835.

Huebner, R. J. (1970). *In* "Comparative Leukemia Research 1969" (R. M. Dutcher, ed.), p. 22. (Bibl. Haematol. **36**). Karger, Basel.

Huebner, R. J., and Todaro, G. J. (1969). *Proc. Nat. Acad. Sci. U.S.* **64**, 1087.

Huebner, R. J., Armstrong, D., Okuyan, M., Sarma, P. S., and Turner, H. C. (1964). *Proc. Nat. Acad. Sci. U.S.* **51**, 742.

Itakura, K., Hutton, J. J., Boyse, E. A., and Old, L. J. (1972). *Transplantation* **13**, 239.

Klein, E. (1968). *N.Y. State J. Med.* **68**, 900.

Klein, G. (1966). *Annu. Rev. Microbiol.* **20**, 223.

Klein, G. (1972). *Proc. Nat. Acad. Sci. U.S.* **69**, 1056.

Klein, G., and Klein, E. (1964). *Science* **145**, 1316.

Levy, H. B., Law, L. W., and Rabson, A. S. (1969). *Proc. Nat. Acad. Sci. U.S.* **62**, 357.

Lilly, F. (1970a). *In* "Comparative Leukemia Research 1969" (R. M. Dutcher, ed.), p. 213 (Bibl. Haematol. **36**). Karger, Basel.

Lilly, F. (1970b). *J. Nat. Cancer Inst.* **45**, 163.

Lilly, F., Boyse, E. A., and Old, L. J. (1964). *Lancet* **2**, 1207.

Lowy, D. R., Rowe, W. P., Teich, N., and Hartley, J. W. (1971). *Science* **174**, 155.

Mathé, G. (1971). *Advan. Cancer Res.* **14**, 1.

McDevitt, H. O., and Benacerraf, B. (1969). *Advan. Immunol.* **11**, 31.

Morton, D. L., Holmes, E. C., Eilber, F. R., and Wood, W. C. (1971). *Ann. Int. Med.* **74**, 587.

Nauts, H. C., Fowler, G. A., and Bogatko, F. H. (1953). *Acta Med. Scand.* **145**, Suppl. 276.

Nowinski, R. C., Old, L. J., Boyse, E. A., de Harven, E., and Geering, G. (1968). *Virology* **34**, 617.

Nowinski, R. C., Old, L. J., Sarkar, N. H., and Moore, D. H. (1970). *Virology* **42**, 1152.

Nowinski, R. C., Old, L. J., O'Donnell, P. V., and Sanders, F. K. (1971). *Nature (London) New Biol.* **230**, 282.

Nowotny, A. (1969). *Bacteriol. Rev.* **33**, 72.

Oettgen, H. F., Old, L. J., and Boyse, E. A. (1971). *Med. Clin. N. Amer.* **55**, 761.

Old, L. J., and Boyse, E. A. (1964). *Annu. Rev. Med.* **15**, 167.

Old, L. J., and Boyse, E. A. (1965). *Fed. Proc., Fed. Amer. Soc. Exp. Biol.* **24**, 1009.

Old, L. J., Benacerraf, B., Clarke, D. A., Carswell, E. A., and Stockert, E. (1961). *Cancer Res.* **21**, 1281.

Old, L. J., Boyse, E. A., and Stockert, E. (1965). *Cancer Res.* **25**, 813.

Old, L. J., Stockert, E., Boyse, E. A., and Kim, J. H. (1968). *J. Exp. Med.* **127**, 523.

Oroszlan, S., Huebner, R. J., and Gilden, R. V. (1971). *Proc. Nat. Acad. Sci. U.S.* **68**, 901.

Pasternak, G. (1967). *Nature (London)* **214**, 1364.

CURRENT ENIGMAS IN CANCER RESEARCH 315

Pillemer, L., Blum, L., Lepow, I. H., Ross, O. A., Todd, E. W., and Wardlaw, A. C. (1954). *Science* **120**, 279.

Pincus, T., Rowe, W. P., and Lilly, F. (1971). *J. Exp. Med.* **133**, 1234.

"RNA Viruses and Host Genome in Oncogenesis" (1972). Proceedings of a Conference held in Amsterdam, May 12–15, 1971 (P. Emmelot and P. Bentvelzen, eds.). North-Holland Publ., Amsterdam.

Raff, M. C. (1971). *Amer. J. Pathol.* **65**, 467.

"Role du Système Réticulo-Endothélial dans l'Immunité Antibactérienne et Anti-tumorale" (1953). B. N. Halpern, ed., No. 115. Éditions du Centre National de la Recherche Scientifique, Paris.

Rowe, W. P., and Hartley, J. W. (1972). *J. Exp. Med.* **136**, 1286.

Rowley, D. (1955). *Lancet* **1**, 232.

Rubin, H., Fanshier, L., Cornelius, A., and Hughes, W. F. (1962). *Virology* **17**, 143.

Sarma, P. S., Baskar, J. F., Huebner, R. J., Old, L. J., and Hardy, W. D., Jr. (1970). *In* "Comparative Leukemia Research 1969" (R. M. Deutcher, ed.), p. 368 (Bibl. Haematol. **36**). Karger, Basel.

Schäfer, W., Anderer, F. A., Bauer, H., and Pister, L. (1969). *Virology* **38**, 387.

Schäfer, W., Lange, V., Pister, L., Seifert, E., de Noronha, F., and Schmidt, F. W. (1970). *Z. Naturforsch. B* **25**, 1024.

Shear, M. J. (1944). *J. Nat. Cancer Inst.* **4**, 461.

Singer, S. J. (1959). *Nature (London)* **183**, 1523.

Smith, R. T., Klein, G., Klein, E., and Clifford, P. (1968). *In* "Advances in Trans-plantation" (*Int. Congr. Transplantation Soc. 1st, Paris, 1967*) p. 483. Williams & Wilkins, Baltimore, Maryland.

Snell, G. D. (1971). *Transplant. Proc.* **3**, 1133.

Stackpole, C. W., Aoki, T., Boyse, E. A., Old, L. J., Lumley-Frank, J., and de Harven, E. (1971). *Science* **172**, 472.

Steeves, R. A. (1968). *Cancer Res.* **28**, 338.

Stockert, E., Old, L. J., and Boyse, E. A. (1971). *J. Exp. Med.* **133**, 1334.

Stück, B., Old, L. J., and Boyse, E. A. (1964). *Proc. Nat. Acad. Sci. U.S.* **52**, 950.

"Symposium on Interferon and Host Response to Virus Infection" (1970). *Arch. Int. Med. Symp.* **126**, 49.

Takahashi, T. (1971). *Transplant. Proc.* **3**, 1217.

Thorbecke, G. J., and Benacerraf, B. (1962). *Progr. Allergy* **6**, 559.

Weiss, D. W., Bonhag, R. S., and Leslie, P. (1966). *J. Exp. Med.* **124**, 1039.

Woodruff, M. (1972). *Harvey Lect.* **66**, 161.

Yashphe, D. J. (1971). *Isr. J. Med. Sci.* **7**, 90.

Zbar, B., Bernstein, I. D., and Rapp, H. J. (1971). *J. Nat. Cancer Inst.* **46**, 831.

FORMER OFFICERS OF THE HARVEY SOCIETY

1905–1906

President: GRAHAM LUSK
Vice-President: SIMON FLEXNER
Treasurer: FREDERIC S. LEE
Secretary: GEORGE B. WALLACE

Council:
  C. A. HERTER
  S. J. MELTZER
  EDWARD K. DUNHAM

1906–1907

President: GRAHAM LUSK
Vice-President: SIMON FLEXNER
Treasurer: FREDERIC S. LEE
Secretary: GEORGE B. WALLACE

Council:
  C. A. HERTER
  S. J. MELTZER
  JAMES EWING

1907–1908

President: GRAHAM LUSK
Vice-President: JAMES EWING
Treasurer: EDWARD K. DUNHAM
Secretary: GEORGE B. WALLACE

Council:
  SIMON FLEXNER
  THEO. C. JANEWAY
  PHILIP H. HISS, JR.

1908–1909

President: JAMES EWING
Vice-President: SIMON FLEXNER
Treasurer: EDWARD K. DUNHAM
Secretary: FRANCIS C. WOOD

Council:
  GRAHAM LUSK
  S. J. MELTZER
  ADOLPH MEYER

1909–1910*

President: JAMES EWING
Vice-President: THEO. C. JANEWAY
Treasurer: EDWARD K. DUNHAM
Secretary: FRANCIS C. WOOD

Council:
  GRAHAM LUSK
  S. J. MELTZER
  W. J. GIES

1910–1911

President: SIMON FLEXNER
Vice-President: JOHN HOWLAND
Treasurer: EDWARD K. DUNHAM
Secretary: HAVEN EMERSON

Council:
  GRAHAM LUSK
  S. J. MELTZER
  JAMES EWING

---

* At the Annual Meeting of May 18, 1909, these officers were elected. In publishing the 1909–1910 volume their names were omitted, possibly because in that volume the custom of publishing the names of the incumbents of the current year was changed to publishing the names of the officers selected for the ensuing year.

1911–1912

President: S. J. MELTZER
Vice-President: FREDERIC S. LEE
Treasurer: EDWARD K. DUNHAM
Secretary: HAVEN EMERSON

Council:
  GRAHAM LUSK
  JAMES EWING
  SIMON FLEXNER

1912–1913

President: FREDERIC S. LEE
Vice-President: WM. H. PARK
Treasurer: EDWARD K. DUNHAM
Secretary: HAVEN EMERSON

Council:
  GRAHAM LUSK
  S. J. MELTZER
  WM. G. MACCALLUM

1913–1914

President: FREDERIC S. LEE
Vice-President: WM. G. MACCALLUM
Treasurer: EDWARD K. DUNHAM
Secretary: AUGUSTUS B. WADSWORTH

Council:
  GRAHAM LUSK
  WM. H. PARK
  GEORGE B. WALLACE

1914–1915

President: WM. G. MACCALLUM
Vice-President: RUFUS I. COLE
Treasurer: EDWARD K. DUNHAM
Secretary: JOHN A. MANDEL

Council:
  GRAHAM LUSK
  FREDERIC S. LEE
  W. T. LONGCOPE

1915–1916

President: GEORGE B. WALLACE*
Treasurer: EDWARD K. DUNHAM
Secretary: ROBERT A. LAMBERT

Council:
  GRAHAM LUSK
  RUFUS I. COLE
  NELLIS B. FOSTER

1916–1917

President: GEORGE B. WALLACE
Vice-President: RUFUS I. COLE
Treasurer: EDWARD K. DUNHAM
Secretary: ROBERT A. LAMBERT

Council:
  GRAHAM LUSK†
  W. T. LONGCOPE
  S. R. BENEDICT
  HANS ZINSSER

1917–1918

President: EDWARD K. DUNHAM
Vice-President: RUFUS I. COLE
Treasurer: F. H. PIKE
Secretary: A. M. PAPPENHEIMER

Council:
  GRAHAM LUSK
  GEORGE B. WALLACE
  FREDERIC S. LEE
  PEYTON ROUS

* Dr. William G. MacCallum resigned after election. On Doctor Lusk's motion Doctor George B. Wallace was made President—no Vice-President was appointed.

† Doctor Lusk was made Honorary permanent Counsellor.

1918–1919

President: GRAHAM LUSK
Vice-President: RUFUS I. COLE
Treasurer: F. H. PIKE
Secretary: K. M. VOGEL

Council:
  GRAHAM LUSK
  JAMES W. JOBLING
  FREDERIC S. LEE
  JOHN AUER

1919–1920

President: WARFIELD T. LONGCOPE
Vice-President: S. R. BENEDICT
Treasurer: F. H. PIKE
Secretary: K. M. VOGEL

Council:
  GRAHAM LUSK
  HANS ZINSSER
  FREDERIC S. LEE
  GEORGE B. WALLACE

1920–1921*

President: WARFIELD T. LONGCOPE
Vice-President: S. R. BENEDICT
Treasurer: A. M. PAPPENHEIMER
Secretary: HOMER F. SWIFT

Council:
  GRAHAM LUSK
  FREDERIC S. LEE
  HANS ZINSSER
  GEORGE B. WALLACE

1921–1922

President: RUFUS I. COLE
Vice-President: S. R. BENEDICT
Treasurer: A. M. PAPPENHEIMER
Secretary: HOMER F. SWIFT

Council:
  GRAHAM LUSK
  HANS ZINSSER
  H. C. JACKSON
  W. T. LONGCOPE

1922–1923

President: RUFUS I. COLE
Vice-President: HANS ZINSSER
Treasurer: CHARLES C. LIEB
Secretary: HOMER F. SWIFT

Council:
  GRAHAM LUSK
  W. T. LONGCOPE
  H. C. JACKSON
  S. R. BENEDICT

1923–1924

President: EUGENE F. DuBOIS
Vice-President: HOMER F. SWIFT
Treasurer: CHARLES C. LIEB
Secretary: GEORGE M. MACKENZIE

Council:
  GRAHAM LUSK
  ALPHONSE R. DOCHEZ
  DAVID MARINE
  PEYTON ROUS

---

* These officers were elected at the Annual Meeting of May 21, 1920 but were omitted in the publication of the 1919–1920 volume.

1924–1925

President: EUGENE F. DuBOIS
Vice-President: PEYTON ROUS
Treasurer: CHARLES C. LIEB
Secretary: GEORGE M. MACKENZIE

Council:
  GRAHAM LUSK
  RUFUS COLE
  HAVEN EMERSON
  WM. H. PARK

1925–1926

President: HOMER F. SWIFT
Vice-President: H. B. WILLIAMS
Treasurer: HAVEN EMERSON
Secretary: GEORGE M. MACKENZIE

Council:
  GRAHAM LUSK
  EUGENE F. DuBOIS
  WALTER W. PALMER
  H. D. SENIOR

1926–1927

President: WALTER W. PALMER
Vice-President: WM. H. PARK
Treasurer: HAVEN EMERSON
Secretary: GEORGE M. MACKENZIE

Council:
  GRAHAM LUSK
  HOMER F. SWIFT
  A. R. DOCHEZ
  ROBERT CHAMBERS

1927–1928

President: DONALD D. VAN SLYKE
Vice-President: JAMES W. JOBLING
Treasurer: HAVEN EMERSON
Secretary: CARL A. L. BINGER

Council:
  GRAHAM LUSK
  RUSSEL L. CECIL
  WARD J. MACNEAL
  DAVID MARINE

1928–1929

President: PEYTON ROUS
Vice-President: HORATIO B. WILLIAMS
Treasurer: HAVEN EMERSON
Secretary: PHILIP D. McMASTER

Council:
  GRAHAM LUSK
  ROBERT CHAMBERS
  ALFRED F. HESS
  H. D. SENIOR

1929–1930

President: G. CANBY ROBINSON
Vice-President: ALFRED F. HESS
Treasurer: HAVEN EMERSON
Secretary: DAYTON J. EDWARDS

Council:
  GRAHAM LUSK
  ALFRED E. COHN
  A. M. PAPPENHEIMER
  H. D. SENIOR

1930–1931

President: ALFRED E. COHN
Vice-President: J. G. HOPKINS
Treasurer: HAVEN EMERSON
Secretary: DAYTON J. EDWARDS

Council:
  GRAHAM LUSK
  O. T. AVERY
  A. M. PAPPENHEIMER
  S. R. DETWILER

1931–1932

President: J. W. JOBLING
Vice-President: HOMER W. SMITH
Treasurer: HAVEN EMERSON
Secretary: DAYTON J. EDWARDS

Council:
   GRAHAM LUSK
   S. R. DETWILER
   THOMAS M. RIVERS
   RANDOLPH WEST

1932–1933

President: ALFRED F. HESS
Vice-President: HAVEN EMERSON
Treasurer: THOMAS M. RIVERS
Secretary: EDGAR STILLMAN

Council:
   GRAHAM LUSK
   HANS T. CLARKE
   WALTER W. PALMER
   HOMER W. SMITH

1933–1934

President: ALFRED HESS*
Vice-President: ROBERT K. CANNAN
Treasurer: THOMAS M. RIVERS
Secretary: EDGAR STILLMAN

Council:
   STANLEY R. BENEDICT
   ROBERT F. LOEB
   WADE H. BROWN

1934–1935

President: ROBERT K. CANNAN
Vice-President: EUGENE L. OPIE
Treasurer: THOMAS M. RIVERS
Secretary: RANDOLPH H. WEST

Council:
   HERBERT S. GASSER
   B. S. OPPENHEIMER
   PHILIP E. SMITH

1935–1936

President: ROBERT K. CANNAN
Vice-President: EUGENE L. OPIE
Treasurer: THOMAS M. RIVERS
Secretary: RANDOLPH H. WEST

Council:
   ROBERT F. LOEB
   HOMER W. SMITH
   DAVID MARINE

1936–1937

President: EUGENE L. OPIE
Vice-President: PHILIP E. SMITH
Treasurer: THOMAS M. RIVERS
Secretary: McKEEN CATTELL

Council:
   GEORGE B. WALLACE
   MARTIN H. DAWSON
   JAMES B. MURPHY

1937–1938

President: EUGENE L. OPIE
Vice-President: PHILIP E. SMITH
Treasurer: THOMAS M. RIVERS
Secretary: McKEEN CATTELL

Council:
   GEORGE B. WALLACE
   MARTIN H. DAWSON
   HERBERT S. GASSER

* Dr. Hess died December 5, 1933.

1938–1939

President: PHILIP E. SMITH
Vice-President: HERBERT S. GASSER
Treasurer: KENNETH GOODNER
Secretary: MCKEEN CATTELL

Council:
  HANS T. CLARKE
  JAMES D. HARDY
  WILLIAM S. TILLETT

1939–1940

President: PHILIP E. SMITH
Vice-President: HERBERT S. GASSER
Treasurer: KENNETH GOODNER
Secretary: THOMAS FRANCIS, JR.

Council:
  HANS T. CLARKE
  N. CHANDLER FOOT
  WILLIAM S. TILLETT

1940–1941

President: HERBERT S. GASSER
Vice-President: HOMER W. SMITH
Treasurer: KENNETH GOODNER
Secretary: THOMAS FRANCIS, JR.

Council:
  N. CHANDLER FOOT
  VINCENT DU VIGNEAUD
  MICHAEL HEIDELBERGER

1941–1942

President: HERBERT S. GASSER
Vice-President: HOMER W. SMITH
Treasurer: KENNETH GOODNER
Secretary: JOSEPH C. HINSEY

Council:
  HARRY S. MUSTARD
  HAROLD G. WOLFF
  MICHAEL HEIDELBERGER

1942–1943

President: HANS T. CLARKE
Vice-President: THOMAS M. RIVERS
Treasurer: KENNETH GOODNER
Secretary: JOSEPH C. HINSEY

Council:
  ROBERT F. LOEB
  HAROLD G. WOLFF
  WILLIAM C. VON GLAHN

1943–1944

President: HANS T. CLARKE
Vice-President: THOMAS M. RIVERS
Treasurer: COLIN M. MACLEOD
Secretary: JOSEPH C. HINSEY

Council:
  ROBERT F. LOEB
  WILLIAM C. VON GLAHN
  WADE W. OLIVER

1944–1945

President: ROBERT CHAMBERS
Vice-President: VINCENT DU VIGNEAUD
Treasurer: COLIN M. MACLEOD
Secretary: JOSEPH C. HINSEY

Council:
  WADE W. OLIVER
  MICHAEL HEIDELBERGER
  PHILIP D. MCMASTER

1945–1946

President: ROBERT CHAMBERS
Vice-President: VINCENT DU VIGNEAUD
Treasurer: COLIN M. MACLEOD
Secretary: EDGAR G. MILLER, JR.

Council:
  PHILIP D. MCMASTER
  EARL T. ENGLE
  FRED W. STEWART

1946–1947

President: VINCENT DU VIGNEAUD
Vice-President: WADE W. OLIVER
Treasurer: COLIN M. MACLEOD
Secretary: EDGAR G. MILLER, JR.

Council:
    EARL T. ENGLE
    HAROLD G. WOLFF
    L. EMMETT HOLT, JR.

1947–1948

President: VINCENT DU VIGNEAUD
Vice-President: WADE W. OLIVER
Treasurer: HARRY B. VAN DYKE
Secretary: MACLYN MCCARTY

Council:
    PAUL KLEMPERER
    L. EMMETT HOLT, JR.
    HAROLD G. WOLFF

1948–1949

President: WADE W. OLIVER
Vice-President: ROBERT F. LOEB
Treasurer: HARRY B. VAN DYKE
Secretary: MACYLN MCCARTY

Council:
    PAUL KLEMPERER
    SEVERO OCHOA
    HAROLD L. TEMPLE

1949–1950

President: WADE W. OLIVER
Vice-President: ROBERT F. LOEB
Treasurer: JAMES B. HAMILTON
Secretary: MACLYN MCCARTY

Council:
    WILLIAM S. TILLETT
    SEVERO OCHOA
    HAROLD L. TEMPLE

1950–1951

President: ROBERT F. LOEB
Vice-President: MICHAEL HEIDELBERGER
Treasurer: JAMES B. HAMILTON
Secretary: LUDWIG W. EICHNA

Council:
    WILLIAM S. TILLETT
    A. M. PAPPENHEIMER, JR.
    DAVID P. BARR

1951–1952

President: RENÉ J. DUBOS
Vice-President: MICHAEL HEIDELBERGER
Treasurer: JAMES B. HAMILTON
Secretary: LUDWIG W. EICHNA

Council:
    DAVID P. BARR
    ROBERT F. PITTS
    A. M. PAPPENHEIMER, JR.

1952–1953

President: MICHAEL HEIDELBERGER
Vice-President: SEVERO OCHOA
Treasurer: CHANDLER McC. BROOKS
Secretary: HENRY D. LAUSON

Council:
    ROBERT F. PITTS
    JEAN OLIVER
    ALEXANDER B. GUTMAN

1953–1954

President: SEVERO OCHOA
Vice-President: DAVID P. BARR
Treasurer: CHANDLER McC. BROOKS
Secretary: HENRY D. LAUSON

Council:
    JEAN OLIVER
    ALEXANDER B. GUTMAN
    ROLLIN D. HOTCHKISS

1954–1955

President: DAVID P. BARR
Vice-President: COLIN M. MACLEOD
Treasurer: CHANDLER McC. BROOKS
Secretary: HENRY D. LAUSON

Council:
  ALEXANDER B. GUTMAN
  ROLLIN D. HOTCHKISS
  DAVID SHEMIN

1955–1956

President: COLIN M. MACLEOD
Vice-President: FRANK L. HORSFALL, JR.
Treasurer: CHANDLER McC. BROOKS
Secretary: RULON W. RAWSON

Council:
  ROLLIN D. HOTCHKISS
  DAVID SHEMIN
  ROBERT F. WATSON

1956–1957

President: FRANK L. HORSFALL, JR.
Vice-President: William S. TILLETT
Treasurer: CHANDLER McC. BROOKS
Secretary: RULON W. RAWSON

Council:
  DAVID SHEMIN
  ROBERT F. WATSON
  ABRAHAM WHITE

1957–1958

President: WILLIAM S. TILLETT
Vice-President: ROLLIN D. HOTCHKISS
Treasurer: CHANDLER McC. BROOKS
Secretary: H. SHERWOOD LAWRENCE

Council:
  ROBERT F. WATSON
  ABRAHAM WHITE
  JOHN V. TAGGART

1958–1959

President: ROLLIN D. HOTCHKISS
Vice-President: ANDRE COURNAND
Treasurer: CHANDLER McC. BROOKS
Secretary: H. SHERWOOD LAWRENCE

Council:
  ABRAHAM WHITE
  JOHN V. TAGGART
  WALSH McDERMOTT

1959–1960

President: ANDRE COURNAND
Vice-President: ROBERT F. PITTS
Treasurer: EDWARD J. HEHRE
Secretary: H. SHERWOOD LAWRENCE

Council:
  JOHN V. TAGGART
  WALSH McDERMOTT
  ROBERT F. FURCHGOTT

1960–1961

President: ROBERT F. PITTS
Vice-President: DICKINSON W. RICHARDS
Treasurer: EDWARD J. HEHRE
Secretary: ALEXANDER G. BEARN

Council:
  WALSH McDERMOTT
  ROBERT F. FURCHGOTT
  LUDWIG W. EICHNA

1961–1962

President: DICKINSON W. RICHARDS
Vice-President: PAUL WEISS
Treasurer: I. HERBERT SCHEINBERG
Secretary: ALEXANDER G. BEARN

Council:
  ROBERT F. FURCHGOTT
  LUDWIG W. EICHNA
  EFRAIM RACKER

1962–1963

President: PAUL WEISS
Vice-President: ALEXANDER B. GUTMAN
Treasurer: I. HERBERT SCHEINBERG
Secretary: ALEXANDER G. BEARN

Council:
  LUDWIG W. EICHNA
  EFRAIM RACKER
  ROGER L. GREIF

1963–1964

President: ALEXANDER B. GUTMAN
Vice-President: EDWARD L. TATUM
Treasurer: SAUL J. FARBER
Secretary: ALEXANDER G. BEARN

Council:
EFRAIM RACKER
ROGER L. GREIF
IRVING M. LONDON

1964–1965

President: EDWARD TATUM
Vice-President: CHANDLER McC. BROOKS
Treasurer: SAUL J. FARBER
Secretary: RALPH L. ENGLE, JR.

Council:
ROGER L. GREIF
LEWIS THOMAS
IRVING M. LONDON

1965–1966

President: CHANDLER McC. BROOKS
Vice-President: ABRAHAM WHITE
Treasurer: SAUL J. FARBER
Secretary: RALPH L. ENGLE, JR.

Council:
IRVING M. LONDON
LEWIS THOMAS
GEORGE K. HIRST

1966–1967

President: ABRAHAM WHITE
Vice-President: RACHMIEL LEVINE
Treasurer: SAUL J. FARBER
Secretary: RALPH L. ENGLE, JR.

Council:
LEWIS THOMAS
GEORGE K. HIRST
DAVID NACHMANSOHN

1967–1968

President: RACHMIEL LEVINE
Vice-President: SAUL J. FARBER
Treasurer: PAUL A. MARKS
Secretary: RALPH L. ENGLE, JR.

Council:
GEORGE K. HIRST
DAVID NACHMANSOHN
MARTIN SONENBERG

1968–1969

President: SAUL J. FARBER
Vice-President: JOHN V. TAGGART
Treasurer: PAUL A. MARKS
Secretary: ELLIOTT F. OSSERMAN

Council:
DAVID NACHMANSOHN
MARTIN SONENBERG
HOWARD EDER

1969–1970

President: JOHN V. TAGGART
Vice-President: BERNARD L. HORECKER
Treasurer: PAUL A. MARKS
Secretary: ELLIOTT F. OSSERMAN

Council:
MARTIN SONENBERG
HOWARD A. EDER
SAUL J. FARBER

1970–1971

President: BERNARD L. HORECKER
Vice-President: MACLYN McCARTY
Treasurer: EDWARD C. FRANKLIN
Secretary: ELLIOTT F. OSSERMAN

Council:
HOWARD A. EDER
SAUL J. FARBER
SOLOMON A. BERSON

CUMULATIVE AUTHOR INDEX*

* (h), honorary; (a), active; (d) deceased.
† Did not present lecture because of World War II.

Dr. Charles H. Rammelkamp, Jr., 1955–56 (h)
Dr. S. Walter Ranson, 1936–37 (d)
Dr. Kenneth B. Raper, 1961–62 (h)
Dr. Arnold R. Rich, 1946–47 (d)
Prof. Alfred N. Richards, 1920–21, 1934–35 (a)
Dr. Dickinson W. Richards, 1943–44 (a)
Prof. Theodore W. Richards, 1911–12 (d)
Dr. Curt P. Richter, 1942–43 (h)
Dr. D. Rittenberg, 1948–49 (d)
Dr. Thomas M. Rivers, 1933–34 (d)
Dr. William Robbins, 1942–43 (h)
Dr. O. H. Robertson, 1942–43 (d)
Prof. William C. Rose, 1934–35 (h)
Dr. M. J. Rosenau, 1908–09 (d)
Dr. F. J. W. Roughton, 1943–44 (h)
Dr. Peyton Rous, 1935–36 (d)
Dr. Harry Rubin, 1965–66 (h)
Prof. Max Rubner, 1912–13 (d)
Dr. John Runnstrom, 1950–51 (h)
Major Frederick F. Russell, 1912–13 (d)
Dr. F. R. Sabin, 1915–16 (d)
Dr. Wilbur A. Sawyer, 1934–35 (d)
Prof. E. A. Schafer, 1907–08 (d)
Dr. Harold A. Scheraga, 1967–68 (h)
Dr. Bela Schick, 1922–23 (h)
Dr. Oscar Schloss, 1924–25 (d)
Prof. Adolph Schmidt, 1913–14 (d)
Dr. Carl F. Schmidt, 1948–49 (h)
Dr. Francis O. Schmitt, 1944–45 (h)
Dr. Knut Schmidt-Neilsen, 1962–63 (h)
Dr. R. Schoeneheimer, 1936–37 (d)
Dr. P. F. Scholander, 1961–62 (h)
Dr. Nevin S. Scrimshaw, 1962–63 (h)
Dr. William H. Sebrell, 1943–44 (h)
Prof. W. T. Sedgwick, 1911–12 (d)
Dr. Walter Seegers, 1951–52 (h)
Dr. J. Edwin Seegmiller, 1969–70 (h)
Dr. Michael Sela, 1971–72 (h)
Dr. Philip A. Shaffer, 1922–23 (d)
Dr. James A. Shannon, 1945–46 (a)
Dr. David Shemin, 1954–55 (a)
Dr. Henry C. Sherman, 1917–19 (d)

Dr. Richard Shope, 1935–36 (d)
Dr. Ephraim Shorr, 1954–55 (d)
Dr. Robert L. Sinsheimer, 1968–69 (h)
Dr. E. C. Slater, 1970–71 (h)
Dr. G. Elliot Smith, 1930–31 (d)
Dr. Emil L. Smith, 1966–67 (h)
Dr. Homer W. Smith, 1939–40 (d)
Dr. Philip E. Smith, 1929–30 (d)
Prof. Theobald Smith, 1905–06 (d)
Dr. T. M. Sonneborn, 1948–49 (h)
Dr. S. P. L. Sorenson, 1924–25 (d)
Dr. Carl C. Speidel, 1940–41 (h)
Dr. Sol Spiegelman, 1968–69 (a)
Dr. Roger W. Sperry, 1966–67 (h)
Dr. William C. Stadie, 1941–42 (d)
Dr. Earl R. Stadtman, 1969–70 (h)
Dr. Roger Stanier, 1959–60 (h)
Dr. Wendell Stanley, 1937–38 (d)
Dr. Earnest H. Starling, 1907–08 (d)
Dr. Isaac Starr, 1946–47 (h)
Dr. William H. Stein, 1956–57 (a)
Dr. P. Stetson, 1927–28
Prof. George Stewart, 1912–13 (d)
Prof. Ch. Wardell Stiles, 1915–16 (d)
Dr. C. R. Stockard, 1921–22 (d)
Dr. Walter Straub, 1928–29 (h)
Dr. George L. Streeter, 1933–34 (d)
Dr. Jack L. Strominger, 1968–69 (h)
Dr. R. P. Strong, 1913–14 (d)
Prof. Earl W. Sutherland, Jr., 1961–62 (h)
Prof. Homer F. Swift, 1919–20 (d)
Dr. W. W. Swingle, 1931–32 (h)
Dr. V. P. Sydenstricker, 1942–43 (h)
Dr. Albert Szent-Gyorgyi, 1938–39 (h)
Dr. W. H. Taliaferro, 1931–32 (h)
Prof. Alonzo E. Taylor, 1907–08 (d)
Prof. W. S. Thayer, 1911–12 (d)
Dr. Hugo Theorell, 1965–66 (h)
Dr. Lewis Thomas, 1967–68 (a)
Dr. William S. Tillett, 1949–50 (a)
Dr. Arne Tiselius, 1939–40 (h)
Dr. A. R. Todd, 1951–52 (h)
Dr. Sidney Udenfriend, 1964–65 (a)
Colonel F. P. Underhill, 1917–19 (d)

ACTIVE MEMBERS

Dr. Liese L. Abel
Dr. Harold Abramson*
Dr. Ruth Gail Abramson
Dr. Harold N. Adel
Dr. Frederic J. Agate
Dr. Edward H. Ahrens
Dr. Philip Aisen
Dr. Salah Al-Askari
Dr. Anthony A. Albanese
Dr. Michael Harris Alderman
Dr. Benjamin Alexander
Dr. Robert Alexander
Dr. Emma Gates Allen
Dr. Fred H. Allen, Jr.
Dr. Jona Allerhand
Dr. Fred Allison, Jr.
Dr. Norman R. Alpert
Dr. Aaron A. Alter
Dr. Norman Altszuler
Dr. Burton M. Altura
Dr. J. Burns Amberson*
Dr. Richard P. Ames
Dr. Charles Anderson
Dr. Helen M. Anderson
Dr. Rubert S. Anderson*
Dr. Giuseppe A. Andres
Dr. Muriel M. Andrews
Dr. Alfred Angrist*
Dr. William Antopol*
Dr. Virginia Apgar
Dr. Henry Aranow, Jr.
Dr. Reginald M. Archibald
Dr. Irwin M. Arias
Dr. Donald Armstrong
Dr. Philip B. Armstrong*
Dr. Aaron Arnold
Dr. Robert B. Aronson
Dr. Paul W. Aschner*

Dr. Amir Askari
Dr. Muvaffak A. Atamer
Dr. Dana W. Atchley*
Dr. Kimball Chase Atwood
Dr. Joseph T. August
Dr. Peter A. M. Auld
Dr. Felice B. Aull
Dr. Robert Austrian
Dr. D. Robert Axelrod
Dr. Stephen M. Ayres
Dr. L. Fred Ayvazian
Dr. Henry A. Azar
Dr. Mortimer E. Bader
Dr. Richard A. Bader
Dr. George Baehr*
Dr. Silvio Baez
Dr. C. V. Bailey*
Dr. Robert D. Baird*
Mrs. Katherine J. Baker
Dr. Sulamita Balagura
Dr. David S. Baldwin
Dr. Horace S. Baldwin*
Dr. M. Earl Balis
Dr. S. Banerjee
Dr. Nils Ulrich Bang
Dr. Arthur Bank
Dr. Norman Bank
Dr. Alvan L. Barach*
Dr. Michael Barany
Dr. W. H. Barber*
Dr. Marion Barclay
Dr. S. B. Barker*
Dr. Lane Barksdale
Dr. Peter Barland
Dr. W. A. Barnes
Dr. Henry L. Barnett
Dr. Harry Baron
Dr. Howard Baron

* Life member.

Dr. Jeremiah A. Barondess
Dr. David P. Barr*
Dr. Bruce A. Barron
Dr. Guy T. Barry
Dr. Herbert J. Bartelstone
Dr. C. Andrew L. Bassett
Dr. Jeanne Bateman*
Dr. Jack R. Battisto
Dr. Stephen G. Baum
Dr. Leona Baumgartner*
Dr. Eliot F. Beach
Dr. Joseph W. Beard*
Dr. Alexander G. Bearn
Dr. Carl Becker
Dr. David Becker
Dr. E. Lovell Becker
Dr. Frederick F. Becker
Dr. William H. Becker
Dr. Paul B. Beeson
Dr. Jeannette Allen Behre
Dr. Richard E. Behrman
Dr. Sam M. Beiser
Dr. Julius Belford
Dr. A. L. Loomis Bell
Dr. Bertrand Bell
Dr. Fritz Karl Beller
Dr. Baruj Benacerraf
Dr. Morris Bender*
Dr. Aaron Bendich
Dr. Bernard Benjamin*
Dr. Bry Benjamin
Dr. Ivan L. Bennett
Dr. Thomas P. Bennett
Dr. Harvey L. Benovitz
Dr. Gordon Benson
Dr. Benjamin N. Berg*
Dr. Kåre Berg
Dr. Stanley S. Bergen
Dr. Adolph Berger
Dr. Eugene Y. Berger
Dr. Lawrence Berger
Dr. Ingemar Berggård
Dr. Edward H. Bergofsky
Dr. James Berkman

Dr. Alice R. Bernheim*
Dr. Alan W. Bernheimer
Dr. Harriet Bernheimer
Dr. Leslie Bernstein
Dr. Stanley Bernstein
Dr. Carl A. Berntsen
Dr. George Packer Berry*
Dr. Solomon A. Berson
Dr. John F. Bertles
Dr. Otto A. Bessey*
Dr. Joseph J. Betheil
Dr. Richard E. Bettigole
Dr. Margaret Bevans
Dr. Sherman Beychok
Dr. Edward Bien
Dr. John T. Bigger, Jr.
Dr. R. J. Bing
Dr. Carl A. L. Binger*
Dr. Francis Binkley
Dr. Robert M. Bird
Dr. LeClair Bissell
Dr. Mark W. Bitensky
Dr. Maurice M. Black
Dr. William A. Blanc
Dr. Kenneth C. Blanchard*
Dr. David H. Blankenhorn
Dr. Sheldon P. Blau
Dr. Richard W. Blide
Dr. Hubert Bloch
Dr. Konrad E. Bloch
Dr. Barry Bloom
Dr. Sidney Blumenthal
Dr. Oscar Bodansky*
Dr. Diethelm Boehme
Dr. Bruce I. Bogart
Dr. Victor Bokisch
Dr. Richard J. Bonforte
Dr. Roy W. Bonsnes
Dr. Robert M. Bookchin
Dr. Jaime Borrero
Dr. Max Bovarnick
Dr. John Z. Bowers
Dr. Barbara H. Bowman
Dr. Linn J. Boyd*

    * Life member.

Dr. Richard C. Bozian
Dr. Norman Brachfield
Dr. Stanley Bradley
Dr. Thomas B. Bradley
Dr. J. Leonard Brandt
Dr. Jo Anne Brasel
Dr. Goodwin Breinin
Dr. Esther Breslow
Dr. Robin Briehl
Dr. Stanley A. Briller
Dr. Anne E. Briscoe
Dr. William Briscoe
Dr. Susan Broder
Dr. Bernard Brodie
Dr. Felix Bronner
Dr. Chandler McC. Brooks
Dr. Dana C. Brooks
Dr. Vernon B. Brooks
Dr. D. E. S. Brown*
Dr. John Lyman Brown
Dr. Howard C. Bruenn*
Dr. Joseph Brumlik
Dr. J. Marion Bryant
Dr. J. Robert Buchanan
Dr. John L. Buchanan
Dr. Thomas M. Buchanan
Dr. Nancy M. Buckley
Dr. Joseph A. Buda
Dr. Elmer D. Bueker
Dr. George E. Burch
Dr. Joseph H. Burchenal
Dr. Dean Burk*
Dr. Edward R. Burka
Dr. E. A. Burkhardt*
Dr. John J. Burns
Dr. Earl O. Butcher*
Dr. Vincent P. Butler, Jr.
Dr. Joel N. Buxbaum
Dr. Roy Cacciaguida
Dr. Abbie Knowlton Calder
Dr. Peter T. B. Caldwell
Dr. Xenophon C. Callas
Dr. Berry Campbell
Dr. Virginia C. Canale

Dr. Robert E. Canfield
Dr. Paul Jude Cannon
Dr. Guilio L. Cantoni
Dr. Charles R. Cantor
Dr. Eric T. Carlson
Dr. Peter Wagner Carmel
Dr. Fred Carpenter
Dr. Malcolm B. Carpenter
Dr. Hugh J. Carroll
Dr. Steven Carson
Dr. Anne C. Carter
Dr. Sidney Carter
Dr. J. Casals-Ariet
Dr. Albert E. Casey*
Dr. William D. Cash
Dr. McKeen Cattell*
Dr. William Caveness
Dr. Peter P. Cervoni
Dr. R. W. Chambers
Dr. Philip C. Chan
Dr. W. Y. Chan
Dr. J. P. Chandler*
Dr. Merrill W. Chase*
Dr. Norman E. Chase
Dr. Herbert Chasis*
Dr. Theodore Chenkin
Dr. Norman L. Chernik
Dr. Shu Chien
Dr. C. Gardner Child
Dr. Francis P. Chinard
Dr. Purnell W. Choppin
Dr. Charles L. Christian
Dr. Ronald V. Christie*
Dr. Nicholas P. Christy
Dr. Jacob Churg
Dr. Louis J. Cizek
Dr. Duncan W. Clark
Dr. Delphine H. Clarke
Dr. Frank H. Clarke
Dr. Hans T. Clarke*
Dr. Albert Claude*
Dr. Hartwig Cleve
Dr. George O. Clifford
Dr. E. E. Cliffton

* Life member.

Dr. Leighton E. Cluff
Dr. Jaime B. Coelho
Dr. Bernard Cohen
Dr. Michael I. Cohen
Dr. Sidney Q. Cohlan
Dr. Mildred Cohn
Dr. Zanvil A. Cohn
Dr. Morton Coleman
Dr. Spencer L. Commerford
Dr. Richard M. Compans
Dr. Neal J. Conan, Jr.
Dr. Lawrence A. Cone
Dr. Stephen C. Connolly
Dr. James H. Conover
Dr. Jean L. Cook
Dr. John S. Cook
Dr. Stuart D. Cook
Dr. George Cooper
Dr. Norman S. Cooper
Dr. Jack M. Cooperman
Dr. W. M. Copenhaver*
Dr. George N. Cornell
Dr. George Corner*
Dr. Armand F. Cortese
Dr. Richard Costello
Dr. Lucien J. Cote
Dr. George Cotzias
Dr. Andre Cournand*
Dr. W. P. Covell*
Dr. David Cowen
Dr. Herold R. Cox*
Dr. Rody P. Cox
Dr. Francis N. Craig
Dr. Lyman C. Craig*
Dr. Elizabeth Crawford
Dr. Richard J. Cross
Dr. Dorothy J. Cunningham
Dr. Edward C. Curnen
Dr. Mary G. McCrea Curnen
Dr. T. J. Curphey*
Dr. Samuel W. Cushman
Dr. Samuel Dales
Dr. Marie Maynard Daly
Dr. Raymond Damadian

Dr. Joseph Dancis
Dr. Betty S. Danes
Dr. Farrington Daniels, Jr.
Dr. Isidore Danishepsky
Dr. R. C. Darling
Dr. James E. Darnell, Jr.
Dr. Fred M. Davenport
Dr. John David
Dr. Leo M. Davidoff*
Dr. Murray Davidson
Dr. Jean Davignon
Dr. Bernard D. Davis
Dr. Robert P. Davis
Dr. Emerson Day
Dr. Peter G. Dayton
Dr. Susan M. Deakins
Dr. Norman Deane
Dr. Robert H. De Bellis
Dr. Paul F. de Gara*
Dr. Thomas J. Degnan
Dr. A. C. DeGraff*
Dr. John E. Deitrick*
Dr. C. E. de la Chapelle*
Dr. Nicholas Delhias
Dr. R. J. Dellenback
Dr. Felix E. Demartini
Dr. Quentin B. Deming
Dr. Felix de Narvaez
Dr. Carolyn R. Denning
Dr. Miriam de Salegue
Dr. Ralph A. Deterling, Jr.
Dr. Wolf-Dietrich Dettbarn
Dr. Ingrith J. Deyrup
Dr. Leroy S. Dietrich
Dr. George W. Dietz, Jr.
Dr. Mario Di Girolamo
Dr. Alexander B. Dimich
Dr. Peter Dineen
Dr. J. R. Di Palma
Dr. Nicholas Di Salvo
Dr. P. A. Di Sant'Agnese
Dr. Zacharias Dische
Dr. Charles A. Doan*
Dr. William Dock*

* Life member.

Dr. Alvin M. Donnenfeld
Dr. Philip J. Dorman
Dr. Louis B. Dotti*
Dr. Joseph C. Dougherty
Dr. Gordon W. Douglas
Dr. Steven D. Douglas
Dr. Charles V. Dowling
Dr. Alan W. Downie*
Dr. Cora Downs*
Dr. Arnold Drapkin
Dr. Paul Dreizen
Dr. David T. Dresdale
Dr. William D. Drucker
Dr. René J. Dubos*
Dr. Allan Dumont
Dr. John H. Dunnington*
Dr. Vincent Du Vigneaud*
Dr. Murray Dworetzky
Dr. D. Dziewiatkowski
Dr. Harry Eagle
Dr. Lila W. Easley
Dr. Gerald M. Edelman
Dr. Chester M. Edelmann, Jr.
Dr. Howard A. Eder
Dr. Richard M. Effros
Dr. Hans J. Eggers
Dr. Kathryn H. Ehlers
Dr. Harold B. Eiber
Dr. Klaus Eichmann
Dr. Ludwig W. Eichna
Dr. Max Eisenberg
Dr. William J. Eisenmenger
Dr. Albert B. Eisenstein
Dr. Robert P. Eisinger
Dr. Borje Ejrup
Dr. Stuart D. Elliott
Dr. John T. Ellis
Dr. Rose-Ruth Tarr Ellison
Dr. Peter Elsbach
Dr. Samuel K. Elster
Dr. Charles A. Ely
Dr. Kendall Emerson, Jr.*
Dr. George Emmanuel
Dr. Morris Engelman

Dr. Mary Allen Engle
Dr. Ralph L. Engle, Jr.
Dr. Yale Enson
Dr. Leonard Epifano
Dr. Frederick H. Epstein
Dr. Joseph A. Epstein
Dr. Bernard F. Erlanger
Dr. Norman H. Ertel
Dr. Solomon Estren
Dr. Henry E. Evert
Dr. Elaine Eyster
Dr. John Fabianek
Dr. Stanley Fahn
Dr. Saul J. Farber
Dr. Mehdi Farhangi
Dr. Peter B. Farnsworth
Dr. John W. Farquhar
Dr. Lee E. Farr*
Dr. Don W. Fawcett
Dr. Martha E. Fedorko
Dr. Muriel F. Feigelson
Dr. Philip Feigelson
Dr. Maurice Feinstein
Dr. Daniel Feldman
Dr. Elaine B. Feldman
Dr. Colin Fell
Dr. Bernard N. Fields
Dr. Ronald R. Fieve
Dr. Laurence Finberg
Dr. Charles W. Findlay, Jr.
Dr. Bruno Fingerhut
Dr. Louis M. Fink
Dr. Stanley R. Finke
Dr. John T. Finkenstaedt
Dr. Edward E. Fischel
Dr. Arthur Fishberg*
Dr. Alfred P. Fishman
Dr. Patrick J. Fitzgerald
Dr. Martin FitzPatrick
Dr. Charles Flood*
Dr. Alfred Florman
Dr. Jordi Folch-Pi
Dr. Conrad T. O. Fong
Dr. Vincent Fontana

* Life member.

Dr. Frank W. Foote, Jr.
Dr. Joseph Fortner
Dr. Arthur C. Fox
Dr. Charles L. Fox, Jr.
Dr. Charles W. Frank
Dr. Harry Meyer Frankel
Dr. Edward C. Franklin
Dr. Andrew G. Frantz
Dr. Aaron D. Freedman
Dr. Alvin Freiman
Dr. Matthew Jay Freund
Dr. Richard H. Freyberg
Dr. Henry Clay Frick, II
Dr. Arnold J. Friedhof
Dr. Eli A. Friedman
Dr. S. Marvin Friedman
Dr. Charlotte Friend
Dr. George W. Frimpter
Dr. William Frisell
Dr. Harry Fritts
Dr. Joseph S. Fruton
Dr. Fritz F. Fuchs
Dr. George I. Fujimoto
Dr. Mildred Fulop
Dr. Robert F. Furchgott*
Dr. J. Furth*
Dr. Palmer H. Futcher
Dr. Jacques L. Gabrilove
Dr. Morton Galdston
Dr. Thomas F. Gallagher
Dr. Nicholas F. Gang
Dr. Henry Gans
Dr. G. Gail Gardner
Dr. Martin Gardy
Dr. Lawrence Gartner
Dr. Nancy E. Gary
Dr. Mario Gaudino
Dr. Malcolm Gefter
Dr. Walton B. Geiger
Dr. Jack Geller
Dr. Lester M. Geller
Dr. Dorothy S. Genghof
Dr. Donald Gerber
Dr. James L. German, III

Dr. Herbert Gershberg
Dr. Welton M. Gersony
Dr. E. C. Gerst
Dr. Menard Gertler
Dr. Melvin Gertner
Dr. Norman R. Gevirtz
Dr. Nimai Ghosh
Dr. Stanley Giannelli, Jr.
Dr. Lewis I. Gidez
Dr. Gerhard H. Giebisch
Dr. Harriet S. Gilbert
Dr. Helena Gilder
Dr. Alfred Gilman
Dr. Sid Gilman
Dr. Charles Gilvarg
Dr. H. Earl Ginn
Dr. Harold S. Ginsberg
Dr. Isaac F. Gittleman
Dr. Sheldon Glabman
Dr. Philip R. Glade
Dr. Warren Glaser
Dr. George B. Jerzy Glass
Dr. Vincent V. Glaviano
Dr. Frank Glenn*
Dr. Seymour M. Glick
Dr. Marvin L. Gliedman
Dr. David L. Globus
Dr. Martin J. Glynn, Jr.
Dr. David J. Gocke
Dr. Gabriel C. Godman
Dr. Walther F. Goebel*
Dr. Robert B. Golbey
Dr. Allen M. Gold
Dr. Harry Gold*
Dr. Burton Goldberg
Dr. Ross Golden*
Dr. Anna Goldfeder
Dr. Martin G. Goldner
Dr. Roberta M. Goldring
Dr. William Goldring*
Dr. Edward I. Goldsmith
Dr. Eli D. Goldsmith*
Dr. Jack Goldstein
Dr. Marvin H. Goldstein

* Life member.

Dr. Julius Golubow
Dr. Peter John Gomatos
Dr. Robert A. Good
Dr. Robert Goodhart
Dr. DeWitt S. Goodman
Dr. Laurance D. Goodwin
Dr. Norman L. Gootman
Dr. Albert S. Gordon
Dr. Alvin J. Gordon
Dr. Harry H. Gordon
Dr. Irving Gordon
Dr. Fred Gorstein
Dr. Emil Glaus Gotschlich
Dr. Eugene Gottfried
Dr. Dicran Goulian, Jr.
Dr. Arthur W. Grace*
Dr. Irving Graef*
Dr. William R. Grafe
Dr. Samuel Graff*
Dr. Frank A. Graig
Dr. Jose Luis Granda
Dr. Lester Grant
Dr. Arthur I. Grayzel
Dr. Jack Peter Green
Dr. Robert H. Green
Dr. Saul Green
Dr. Lowell M. Greenbaum
Dr. Elias L. Greene
Dr. Olga Greengard
Dr. Ezra M. Greenspan
Dr. Isidor Greenwald*
Dr. John R. Gregg
Dr. Gregory Gregariadis
Dr. John D. Gregory
Dr. Roger I. Greif
Dr. Ira Greifer
Dr. Arthur Grishman
Dr. David Grob
Dr. Howard S. Grob
Dr. Arthur P. Grollman
Dr. Milton M. Gross
Dr. Paul Gross*
Dr. Ruth T. Gross
Dr. Lionel Grossbard

Dr. Melvin Grumbach
Dr. Dezider Grunberger
Dr. Harry Grundfest*
Dr. Alan B. Gruskin
Dr. Richard S. Gubner
Dr. Peter Guida
Dr. Guido Guidotti
Dr. Stephen J. Gulotta
Dr. Alexander B. Gutman*
Dr. Sidney Gutstein
Dr. David V. Habif
Dr. Susan Jane Hadley
Dr. Wilbur D. Hagamen
Dr. Hanspaul Hagenmaier
Dr. Jack W. C. Hagstrom
Dr. Richard G. Hahn*
Dr. Seymour P. Halbert
Dr. David Hamerman
Dr. James B. Hamilton
Dr. Leonard Hamilton
Dr. Paul B. Hamilton
Dr. Warner S. Hammond
Dr. Chester W. Hampel*
Dr. Eugene S. Handler
Dr. Evelyn E. Handler
Dr. Leonard C. Harber
Dr. James D. Hardy*
Dr. Kendrick Hare*
Dr. Joseph Harkavy*
Dr. Peter Cahners Harpel
Dr. Albert H. Harris*
Dr. Ruth C. Harris
Dr. Benjamin Harrow*
Dr. Una Hart
Dr. Donald H. Harter
Dr. ReJane Harvey
Dr. Rudy Haschemeyer
Dr. George A. Hashim
Dr. Sam A. Hashim
Dr. George M. Hass*
Dr. William K. Hass
Dr. A. Baird Hastings*
Dr. A. Daniel Hauser
Dr. Teru Hayashi

* Life member.

Dr. Arthur H. Hayes
Dr. Richard M. Hays
Dr. Robert M. Heggie
Dr. Edward J. Hehre
Dr. Michael Heidelberger*
Dr. Henry Heinemann
Dr. William Carroll Heird
Dr. Leon Hellman
Dr. Milton Helpern
Dr. Lawrence Helson
Dr. Walter L. Henley
Dr. Philip H. Henneman
Dr. Victor Herbert
Dr. Robert M. Herbst
Dr. Morris Herman*
Dr. Frederic P. Herter
Dr. Robert B. Hiatt
Dr. Margaret Hilgartner
Dr. Charles H. Hill
Dr. James G. Hilton
Dr. Lawrence E. Hinkle, Jr.
Dr. Joseph C. Hinsey*
Dr. Christophe H. W. Hirs
Dr. Jacob Hirsch
Dr. James G. Hirsch
Dr. Jules Hirsch
Dr. Erich Hirschberg
Dr. Kurt Hirschhorn
Dr. George K. Hirst
Dr. Paul Hochstein
Dr. Paul F. A. Hoefer*
Dr. Thomas I. Hoen*
Dr. Joseph Hoffman
Dr. Lee Hoffman
Dr. Alan F. Hofmann
Dr. Frederick G. Hofmann
Dr. Duncan A. Holaday
Dr. Raymond F. Holden*
Dr. Charles S. Hollander
Dr. Vincent Hollander
Dr. J. H. Holmes
Dr. L. Emmett Holt, Jr.*
Dr. Erich Holtzman
Dr. Donald A. Holub

Dr. Edward W. Hook
Dr. Bernard L. Horecker
Dr. William H. Horner
Dr. Marshall S. Horwitz
Dr. Verne D. Hospelhorn
Dr. Rollin D. Hotchkiss
Dr. S. S. Hotta
Dr. Paul E. Howe*
Dr. Howard H. T. Hsu
Dr. Konrad Chang Hsu
Dr. Mon-Tuan Huang
Dr. William N. Hubbard, Jr.
Dr. L. E. Hummel*
Dr. George H. Humphreys*
Dr. Jerard Hurwitz
Dr. Dorris Hutchinson
Dr. Michale Iacobellis
Dr. Anthony R. Imondi
Dr. Henry D. Isenberg
Dr. Raymond S. Jackson
Dr. Richard W. Jackson*
Dr. Jerry C. Jacobs
Dr. Ernst R. Jaffe
Dr. Herbert Jaffe
Dr. S. Jakowska
Dr. George James
Dr. James D. Jamieson
Dr. Aaron Janoff
Dr. Alfonso H. Janoski
Dr. Henry D. Janowitz
Dr. Saul Jarcho*
Dr. Jamshid Javid
Dr. Norman B. Javitt
Dr. Graham H. Jeffries
Dr. Frode Jensen
Dr. Alan J. Johnson
Dr. Donald G. Johnson
Dr. Dorothy D. Johnson
Dr. Walter D. Johnson, Jr.
Dr. Barbara Johnston
Dr. Thomas Jones
Dr. Alan S. Josephson
Dr. Austin L. Joyner*
Dr. Elvin A. Kabat

* Life member.

Dr. Lawrence J. Kagen
Dr. Melvin Kahn
Dr. Alfred J. Kaltman
Dr. William Kammerer
Dr. Yoshinobu Kanno
Dr. Thomas G. Kantor
Dr. F. F. Kao
Dr. Barry H. Kaplan
Dr. David Kaplan
Dr. Attallah Kappas
Dr. Alan E. Kark
Dr. Arthur Karlin
Dr. Simon Karpatkin
Dr. Maxwell Karshan*
Dr. Arnold M. Katz
Dr. Michael Katz
Dr. Robert Katzman
Dr. M. Ralph Kaufmann
Dr. Seymour Kaufmann
Dr. Hans Kaunitz
Dr. Herbert J. Kayden
Dr. Donald Kaye
Dr. Gordon I. Kaye
Dr. B. H. Kean
Dr. Aaron Kellner
Dr. Muriel Kerr
Dr. Lee Kesner
Dr. Richard H. Kessler
Dr. Walter R. Kessler
Dr. Andre C. Kibrick*
Dr. John G. Kidd*
Dr. Edwin D. Kilbourne
Dr. Margaret Kilcoyne
Dr. Thomas Killip
Dr. Charles W. Kim
Dr. Anne C. Kimball
Dr. Daniel Kimberg
Dr. Thomas J. Kindt
Dr. Barry G. King*
Dr. Donald West King
Dr. Glenn C. King*
Dr. Mary Elizabeth King
Dr. Lawrence C. Kingsland, Jr.
Dr. John M. Kinney

Dr. Esben Kirk
Dr. D. M. Kirschenbaum
Dr. Bernard Klein
Dr. A. K. Kleinschmidt
Dr. Jerome L. Knittle
Dr. W. Eugene Knox
Dr. Joseph A. Kochen
Dr. Shaul Kochwa
Dr. Samuel Saburo Koide
Dr. Kiyomi Koizumi
Dr. M. J. Kopac*
Dr. Levy Kopelovich
Dr. Arthur Kornberg
Dr. Peter Kornfeld
Dr. Leonard Korngold
Dr. Irvin M. Korr
Dr. Nechama S. Kossower
Dr. Charles E. Kossmann
Dr. Arthur Kowalsky
Dr. O. Dhodanand Kowlessar
Dr. Philip Kozinn
Dr. Irwin H. Krakoff
Dr. Lawrence R. Krakoff
Dr. Benjamin Kramer*
Dr. Alvan Krasna
Dr. Stephen J. Kraus
Dr. Richard M. Krause
Dr. Norman Kretchmer
Dr. Howard P. Krieger
Dr. Isidore Krimsky
Dr. Robert A. Kritzler
Dr. Robert Schild Krooth
Dr. Stephen Krop
Dr. Saul Krugman
Dr. Edward J. Kuchinskas
Dr. Friedrich Kueppers
Dr. I. Newton Kugelmass*
Dr. William J. Kuhns
Dr. Henry G. Kunkel
Dr. Sherman Kupfer
Dr. Herbert S. Kupperman
Dr. Marvin Kuschner
Dr. Henn Kutt
Dr. David M. Kydd

* Life member.

Dr. John S. LaDue
Dr. Chun-Yen Lai
Dr. Michael Lamm
Dr. R. C. Lancefield*
Dr. Robert Landesman
Dr. M. Daniel Lane
Dr. William B. Langan
Dr. Gertrude Lange
Dr. Kurt Lange
Dr. Glen A. Langer
Dr. Philip Lanzkowsky
Dr. John H. Laragh
Dr. Daniel L. Larson
Dr. Etienne Y. Lasfargues
Dr. Sigmund E. Lasker
Dr. Richard P. Lasser
Dr. Raffaelle Lattes
Dr. John Lattimer
Dr. Henry D. Lauson
Dr. George I. Lavin*
Dr. Leroy S. Lavine
Dr. Claire Lawler
Dr. Christine Lawrence
Dr. H. S. Lawrence
Dr. Walter Lawrence, Jr.
Dr. Richard W. Lawton
Dr. Robert W. Leader
Dr. Stanley L. Lee
Dr. Sylvia Lee-Huang
Dr. Robert S. Lees
Dr. Albert M. Lefkovits
Dr. David Lehr
Dr. Gerard M. Lehrer
Miss Grace Leidy
Dr. Edgar Leifer
Dr. Louis Leiter
Dr. Edwin H. Lennette
Dr. E. Carwile LeRoy
Dr. Stephen H. Leslie
Dr. Gerson J. Lesnick
Dr. Harry Le Veen
Dr. Stanley M. Levenson
Dr. Arthur H. Levere
Dr. Richard D. Levere

Dr. Harold A. Levey
Dr. Robert Levi
Dr. Aaron R. Levin
Dr. Louis Levin
Dr. O. Robert Levine
Dr. Philip Levine*
Dr. Rachmiel Levine
Dr. Robert A. Levine
Dr. Cyrus Levinthal
Dr. Marvin F. Levitt
Dr. Barnet M. Levy
Dr. Harvey M. Levy
Dr. Lester Levy
Dr. Milton Levy*
Dr. Robert L. Levy*
Dr. Arthur Lewis
Dr. James L. Lewis
Dr. N. D. C. Lewis*
Dr. Allyn B. Ley
Dr. Koibong Li
Dr. Herbert C. Lichtman
Dr. Charles S. Lieber
Dr. Seymour Lieberman
Dr. Frederick M. Liebman
Dr. Martin R. Liebowitz
Dr. Fannie Liebson
Dr. Geoffrey C. Linder*
Dr. Alfred S. C. Ling
Dr. George Lipkin
Dr. Martin Lipkin
Dr. Fritz Lipmann*
Dr. M. B. Lipsett
Dr. Stephen D. Litwin
Dr. Teh-Yung Liu
Dr. Arthur Livermore
Dr. David P. C. Lloyd*
Dr. Joseph LoBue
Dr. Michael D. Lockshin
Dr. John N. Loeb
Dr. Robert F. Loeb*
Dr. Werner R. Loewenstein
Dr. Irving M. London
Dr. Morris London
Dr. L. G. Longsworth*

* Life member.

Dr. William F. Loomis
Dr. R. Lorente de Nó*
Dr. Donald B. Louria
Dr. Barbara W. Low
Dr. Jerome Lowenstein
Dr. Oliver H. Lowry
Dr. Bertram A. Lowy
Dr. Fred V. Lucas
Dr. Jean M. Lucas-Lenard
Dr. David J. L. Luck
Dr. E. Hugh Luckey
Dr. A. Leonard Luhby
Dr. Daniel S. Lukas
Dr. Clara J. Lynch*
Dr. Harold Lyons
Dr. George I. Lythcott
Dr. Ferdinand F. McAllister
Dr. Kenneth McAlpin*
Dr. Marsh McCall
Dr. W. S. McCann*
Dr. Kenneth S. McCarty
Dr. Maclyn McCarty
Dr. Walter S. McClellan*
Dr. Robert McClusky
Dr. David J. McConnell
Dr. James E. McCormack
Dr. W. W. McCrory
Dr. Donovan J. McCune*
Dr. Walsh McDermott
Dr. Fletcher McDowell
Dr. Currier McEwen*
Dr. Paul R. McHugh
Dr. Rawle McIntosh
Dr. Rustin McIntosh*
Dr. Cosmo G. MacKenzie*
Dr. John Macleod*
Dr. Philip D. McMaster*
Dr. Edmund F. McNally
Miss Helen McNamara
Dr. Charles K. McSherry
Dr. Thomas Maack
Dr. T. P. Magill*
Dr. Jacob V. Maizel, Jr.
Dr. Ole J. W. Malm

Dr. Benjamin Mandel
Dr. William M. Manger
Dr. Mart Mannik
Dr. James M. Manning
Dr. Wladyslaw Manski
Dr. Karl Maramorosch
Dr. Carlos Marchena
Dr. Aaron J. Marcus
Dr. Cyril Carlisle Marcus
Dr. Donald M. Marcus
Dr. Philip I. Marcus
Dr. Stewart L. Marcus
Dr. Morton Marks
Dr. Paul A. Marks
Dr. Donald J. Marsh
Dr. Douglas A. Marsland*
Dr. Daniel S. Martin
Dr. Richard L. Masland
Dr. Richard C. Mason
Dr. Arthur M. Master*
Dr. Edmund B. Masurovsky
Dr. James A. L. Mathers
Dr. Robert Matz
Dr. Paul H. Maurer
Dr. Evelyn A. Mauss
Dr. Morton H. Maxwell
Dr. Klaus Mayer
Dr. Aubre de L. Maynard
Dr. E. W. Maynert
Dr. Rajarshi Mazumder
Dr. Abraham Mazur
Dr. Valentino Mazzia
Dr. Edward Meilman
Dr. Gilbert W. Mellin
Dr. Robert B. Mellins
Dr. Ismael Mena
Dr. Walter Menaker
Dr. Milton Mendlowitz
Dr. Walter L. Mersheimer
Dr. Clarence G. Merskey
Dr. William Metcalf
Dr. Karl Meyer*
Dr. Leo M. Meyer
Dr. Alexander J. Michie

* Life member.

Dr. Catherine Michie
Dr. Gardner Middlebrook
Dr. G. Burroughs Mider*
Dr. Peter O. Milch
Dr. A. T. Milhorat*
Dr. David K. Miller*
Dr. Frederick Miller
Dr. Stephen J. Millian
Dr. C. Richard Minick
Dr. George S. Mirick
Dr. Alfred E. Mirsky*
Dr. William F. Mitty, Jr.
Dr. Walter Modell*
Dr. Carl Monder
Dr. William L. Money
Dr. Dan H. Moore
Dr. John A. Moore
Dr. Norman S. Moore*
Dr. Stanford Moore
Dr. Anatol G. Morell
Dr. Gilda Morillo-Cucci
Dr. Akiro Morishima
Dr. Robert S. Morison*
Dr. Thomas Quinlan Morris
Dr. Alan N. Morrison
Dr. Jane H. Morse
Dr. Stephen I. Morse
Dr. Norman Moscowitz
Dr. Michale W. Mosesson
Dr. Melvin L. Moss
Dr. Harry Most*
Dr. Isabel M. Mountain
Dr. Walter E. Mountcastle
Dr. Arden W. Moyer
Dr. Richard W. Moyer
Dr. R. S. Muckenfuss*
Dr. Stuart Mudd*
Dr. G. H. Mudge
Dr. John V. Mueller
Dr. Hans J. Müller-Eberhard
Dr. Ursula Müller-Eberhard
Dr. John H. Mulholland*
Dr. M. G. Mulinos*
Dr. Otto H. Muller

Dr. Equinn W. Munnell
Dr. Edward Muntwyler*
Dr. George E. Murphy
Dr. James S. Murphy
Dr. M. Lois Murphy
Dr. Carl Muschenheim*
Dr. W. P. Laird Myers
Dr. Martin S. Nachbar
Dr. Ralph L. Nachman
Dr. David D. Nachmansohn*
Dr. Gabriel G. Nahas
Dr. Tatsuji Namba
Dr. William Nastuk
Dr. Samuel Natelson
Dr. Gerald Nathenson
Dr. M. Nathenson
Dr. Stanley G. Nathenson
Dr. Clayton L. Natta
Dr. Enid A. Neidle
Dr. Norton Nelson
Dr. Harold C. Neu
Dr. Isaac Neuwirth*
Dr. Maria M. New
Dr. Walter Newman
Miss Eleanor B. Newton*
Dr. Shih-hsun Ngai
Dr. Warren W. Nichols
Dr. John F. Nicholson
Dr. John L. Nickerson*
Dr. Giorgio L. Nicolis
Dr. Julian Niemetz
Dr. Ross Nigrelli*
Dr. Jerome Nisselbaum
Dr. Charles Noback*
Dr. W. C. Noble*
Dr. M. R. Nocenti
Dr. Hymie L. Nossel
Dr. Richard Novick
Dr. Alex B. Novikoff
Dr. Victor Nussenzweig
Dr. Irwin Nydick
Dr. William B. Ober
Dr. Manuel Ochoa, Jr.
Dr. Severo Ochoa*

* Life member.

Dr. Michiko Okamoto
Dr. Arthur J. Okinaka
Dr. William M. O'Leary
Dr. Eng Bee Ong
Dr. Stanley Opler
Dr. Jack H. Oppenheimer
Dr. Peter Orahovats
Dr. Marian Orlowski
Dr. Ernest V. Orsi
Dr. Louis G. Ortega
Dr. Eduardo Orti
Dr. Priscilla J. Ortiz
Dr. Elliott F. Osserman
Dr. Elena I. R. Ottolenghi
Dr. Zoltan Ovary
Dr. M. D. Overholzer*
Dr. Norbert I. A. Overweg
Dr. Geraldine Pace
Dr. George H. Paff*
Dr. Irvine H. Page*
Dr. George Palade
Dr. Photini S. Papageorgiou
Dr. Paul S. Papavasiliou
Dr. George D. Pappas
Dr. A. M. Pappenheimer, Jr.
Dr. John R. Pappenheimer
Dr. E. M. Papper
Dr. Frank S. Parker
Dr. Raymond C. Parker*
Dr. Robert J. Parsons*
Dr. Pedro Pasik
Dr. Tauba Pasik
Dr. Pierluigi Patriarca
Dr. Philip Y. Patterson
Dr. Elsa Paulsen
Dr. Mary Ann Payne
Dr. O. H. Pearson
Dr. Edmund D. Pellegrino
Dr. Abraham Penner
Dr. James M. Perel
Dr. George A. Perera
Dr. Eli Perlman
Dr. Gertrude Perlmann
Dr. James H. Pert

Dr. Demetrius Pertsemlidis
Dr. Mary Petermann
Dr. Malcolm L. Peterson
Dr. Frederick S. Philips
Dr. Robert A. Philips*
Dr. Lennart Philipson
Dr. Emanuel T. Phillips
Dr. Mildred Phillips
Dr. Julia M. Phillips-Quagliata
Dr. E. Converse Pierce, II
Dr. John G. Pierce
Dr. Cynthia H. Pierce-Chase
Dr. Lou Ann Pilkington
Dr. Joseph B. Pincus
Dr. Johanna Pindyck
Dr. Kermit L. Pines
Dr. Margaret Pittman*
Dr. Robert F. Pitts*
Dr. Calvin F. Plimpton
Dr. Charles M. Plotz
Dr. Fred Plum
Dr. Norman H. Plummer*
Dr. Beatriz G. T. Pogo
Dr. Alan Paul Poland
Dr. Eric H. Pollaczek
Dr. Marcel W. Pons
Dr. Edwin A. Popenoe
Dr. J. W. Poppell
Dr. Hans Popper
Dr. Keith R. Porter
Dr. Jerome G. Porush
Dr. Jerome B. Posner
Dr. Joseph Post
Dr. Edward L. Pratt
Dr. Rudolf Preisig
Dr. John B. Price, Jr.
Dr. R. B. Pringle
Dr. Philip H. Prose
Dr. John F. Prudden
Dr. Lawrence Prutkin
Dr. Charles B. Pryles
Dr. Maynard E. Pullman
Dr. Dominick P. Purpura
Dr. Franco Quagliata

* Life member.

Dr. Paul G. Quie
Dr. Eder C. R. Quintao
Dr. S. Fred Rabiner
Dr. Michel Rabinovitch
Dr. Julian Rachele
Dr. Efraim Racker
Dr. Bertha Radar
Dr. C. A. Ragan, Jr.
Dr. Morris L. Rakieten*
Dr. Henry T. Randall
Dr. Helen M. Ranney
Dr. Felix T. Rapaport
Dr. Howard G. Rapaport
Dr. Fred Rapp
Dr. Maurice M. Rapport
Dr. Sarah Ratner*
Dr. Aaron R. Rausen
Dr. Rulon W. Rawson
Dr. Bronson S. Ray*
Dr. George G. Reader
Dr. Walter Redisch
Dr. Colvin Manuel Redman
Dr. S. Frank Redo
Dr. George Reed
Dr. Gabrielle H. Reem
Dr. Carl Reich
Dr. Edward Reich
Dr. Franz Reichsman
Dr. Christine Reilly
Dr. Joseph F. Reilly
Dr. Leopold Reiner
Dr. Donald J. Reis
Dr. Charlotte Ressler
Dr. Paul Reznikoff*
Dr. D. W. Richards*
Dr. Goetz W. Richter
Dr. Maurice N. Richter*
Dr. Ronald F. Rieder
Dr. Harold Rifkin
Dr. Robert R. Riggio
Dr. Walter F. Riker, Jr.
Dr. Conrad M. Riley
Dr. Vernon Riley
Dr. David Allen Ringle

Dr. Harris Ripps
Dr. Richard S. Rivlin
Dr. Elliott Robbins
Dr. William C. Robbins
Dr. Carleton W. Roberts
Dr. Jay Roberts
Dr. Kathleen E. Roberts
Dr. Richard B. Roberts
Dr. Alan G. Robinson
Dr. William G. Robinson
Dr. Dudley F. Rochester
Dr. Morris Rockstein
Dr. Muriel Roger
Dr. William M. Rogers*
Dr. Bernard Rogoff
Dr. Paul S. Roheim
Dr. Ida Pauline Rolf*
Dr. Walter S. Root*
Dr. Paul D. Rosahn*
Dr. Marie C. Rosati
Dr. Harry M. Rose*
Dr. Theodore Rosebury*
Dr. David M. Roseman
Dr. Gerald Rosen
Dr. John F. Rosen
Dr. Ora Rosen
Dr. Murray D. Rosenberg
Dr. Philip Rosenberg
Dr. Isadore Rosenfield
Dr. Herbert S. Rosenkranz
Dr. William S. Rosenthal
Dr. William Rosner
Dr. Herbert Ross
Dr. Alan B. Rothballer
Dr. Sidney Rothbard
Dr. Edmund O. Rothschild
Dr. M. A. Rothschild
Dr. J. Rotstein
Dr. Bruce Rowe
Dr. Lewis P. Rowland
Dr. Paul Royce
Dr. Albert L. Rubin
Dr. Benjamin A. Rubin
Dr. Ronald P. Rubin

* Life member.

Dr. Walter Rubin
Dr. Daniel Rudman
Dr. Maria A. Rudzinska
Dr. Paul Ruegeseggar
Dr. George D. Ruggieri
Dr. Mark G. Rush
Dr. Henry I. Russek
Dr. David D. Rutstein
Dr. David Sabatini
Dr. Stanley Walter Sajdera
Dr. Lester B. Salans
Dr. Gerald Salen
Dr. Lee Salk
Dr. Milton R. J. Salton
Dr. Paul Samuel
Dr. Herbert Samuels
Dr. Stanley Samuels
Dr. John Sandson
Dr. Jussi J. Saukkonen
Dr. Arthur Sawitsky
Dr. Philip N. Sawyer
Dr. Wilbur H. Sawyer
Dr. Brij Saxena
Dr. David Schachter
Dr. Russell W. Schaedler
Dr. Morris Schaeffer
Dr. Fenton Schaffner
Dr. Matthew D. Scharff
Dr. I. Herbert Scheinberg
Dr. Isaac Schenkein
Dr. Barbara M. Scher
Dr. Lawrence Scherr
Dr. Gerald Schiffman
Dr. Fred J. Schilling
Dr. E. B. Schlesinger
Dr. R. W. Schlesinger
Dr. Jeffrey Schlom
Dr. Willard C. Schmidt
Dr. Howard A. Schneider
Dr. J. B. Schorr
Dr. Henry A. Schroeder*
Dr. Ernest Schwartz
Dr. Gabriel Schwartz
Dr. Irving L. Schwartz

Dr. James H. Schwartz
Dr. Morton K. Schwartz
Dr. David Schwimmer
Dr. John J. Sciarra
Dr. T. F. McNair Scott*
Dr. John C. Scott-Baker
Dr. John Scudder*
Dr. Beatrice C. Seegal*
Dr. David Seegal*
Dr. Barry M. Segal
Dr. Sheldon J. Segal
Dr. George Seiden
Dr. Samuel Seifter
Dr. Stephen J. Seligman
Dr. Ewald Selkurt
Dr. Fabio Sereni
Dr. Aura E. Severinghaus*
Dr. Robert E. Shank
Dr. James A. Shannon*
Dr. Harvey C. Shapiro
Dr. Herman S. Shapiro
Dr. Lucille Shapiro
Dr. William R. Shapiro
Dr. Lewis Inman Sharp*
Dr. Joyce C. Shaver
Dr. Elliott Shaw
Dr. David Shemin
Dr. Paul Sherlock
Dr. Raymond Lionel Sherman
Dr. Sol Sherry
Dr. Maurice E. Shils
Dr. Bong-Sop Shim
Dr. W. C. Shoemaker
Dr. Sheppard Siegal
Dr. Charles D. Siegel
Dr. George Siegel
Dr. Morris Siegel*
Dr. Philip Siekevitz
Dr. Ernest B. Sigg
Dr. Selma Silagi
Dr. Robert Silber
Dr. Maximillian Silbermann*
Dr. Lous E. Siltzbach
Dr. Lawrence Silver

* Life member.

Dr. Richard T. Silver
Dr. Morris Silverman
Dr. William A. Silverman
Dr. Emanuel Silverstein
Dr. Martin E. Silverstein
Dr. Samuel C. Silverstein
Dr. Michael Simberkoff
Dr. Eric J. Simon
Dr. Norman Simon
Dr. Kai Lennart Simons
Dr. Joe L. Simpson
Dr. Melvin V. Simpson
Dr. Gregory Siskind
Dr. William R. Sistrom
Dr. Anneliese L. Sitarz
Dr. Vladimir P. Skipski
Dr. Lawrence E. Skogerson
Dr. Robert J. Slater
Dr. Paul Slotwiner
Dr. George K. Smelser
Dr. Carl Smith
Dr. Elizabeth M. Smithwick
Dr. I. Snapper*
Dr. Edna Sobel
Dr. Louis Soffer*
Dr. Richard Luber Soffer
Dr. Arthur Sohval
Dr. Leon Sokoloff
Dr. Samuel Solomon
Dr. Alex C. Solowey
Dr. Martin Sonenberg
Dr. Chull Sung Song
Dr. Sun K. Song
Dr. Chester M. Southam
Dr. Paul Spear
Dr. Abraham Spector
Dr. Francis Speer*
Dr. Robert Sisson Spiers
Dr. Frank C. Spencer
Dr. Sol Spiegelman
Dr. Morton Spivack
Dr. David Sprinson
Dr. Norton Spritz
Dr. Katherine Sprunt

Dr. P. R. Srinivasan
Dr. Frank G. Standaert
Dr. Neal H. Steigbigel
Dr. Richard M. Stein
Dr. William Stein
Dr. Philip R. Steinmetz
Dr. Herman Steinberg
Dr. Kurt H. Stenzel
Dr. Kenneth Sterling
Dr. Joseph R. Stern
Dr. Marvin Stern
Dr. Stephen Sternberg
Dr. Irmin Sternlieb
Dr. C. A. Stetson, Jr.
Dr. De Witt Stetten, Jr.
Dr. Fred W. Stewart*
Dr. Harold J. Stewart*
Dr. John M. Stewart
Dr. W. B. Stewart
Dr. Walter A. Stewart
Dr. C. Chester Stock
Dr. Walther Stoeckenius
Dr. Herbert Carl Stoerk
Dr. Peter E. Stokes
Dr. Daniel J. Stone
Dr. Fritz Streuli
Dr. William T. Stubenbord
Dr. Jackson H. Stuckey
Dr. Horace W. Stunkard*
Dr. John Y. Sugg*
Dr. W. James Sullivan
Dr. Martin I. Surks
Dr. Marcy Sussman
Dr. Emanuel Suter
Dr. Joseph G. Sweeting
Dr. Margaret Prince Sykes
Dr. Wlodzimierz Szer
Dr. Milton Tabachnick
Dr. John Taggart
Dr. Tadasu Takumaru
Dr. Igor Tamm
Dr. Donald F. Tapley
Dr. Suresh S. Tate
Dr. Edward Lawrie Tatum

* Life member.

Dr. Robert N. Taub
Dr. Harry Taube
Dr. Sheldon B. Taubman
Dr. Howard Taylor, Jr.*
Dr. Robert D. Terry
Dr. Gail A. Theis
Dr. Lewis Thomas
Dr. David D. Thompson
Dr. Gerald E. Thomson
Dr. Neils A. Thorn
Dr. David A. Tice
Dr. William S. Tillett*
Dr. Edward Tolstoi*
Dr. Helene W. Toolan
Dr. George L. Tritsch
Dr. Walter Troll
Dr. R. C. Truex
Dr. Orestes Tsolas
Dr. Ethel A. Tsutsui
Dr. Dan Tucker
Dr. Gerard M. Turino
Dr. Louis B. Turner
Dr. Robert A. Turner
Dr. Gray H. Twombly*
Dr. Sidney Udenfriend
Dr. Johnathan W. Uhr
Dr. John E. Ultmann
Dr. Paul N. Unger
Dr. Arthur Canfield Upton
Dr. Morton Urivetzky
Dr. Carlo Valenti
Dr. Fred Valentine
Dr. Parker Vanamee
Dr. William G. Van der Kloot
Dr. Mario Vassalle
Dr. Edward F. Vastola
Dr. Elliot S. Vesell
Dr. Carmine T. Vicale
Dr. Wolf Vishniac
Dr. F. Stephen Vogel
Dr. Henry J. Vogel
Dr. Mögens Volkert
Dr. Spyros M. Vratsanos
Dr. Irving H. Wagman

Dr. Bernard M. Wagner
Dr. Stanley Wallach
Dr. Lila A. Wallis
Dr. Roderich Walter
Dr. S. C. Wang
Dr. Lewis W. Wannamaker
Dr. George E. Wantz
Dr. Bettina Warburg*
Dr. Robert C. Warner
Dr. Louis R. Wasserman
Dr. Alice M. Waterhouse*
Dr. Robert F. Watson
Dr. Samuel Waxman
Dr. Annemarie Weber
Dr. Bruce Webster*
Dr. Rene Wegria
Dr. Richard Weil, III
Dr. Virginia L. Weimar
Dr. Herbert Weinfeld
Dr. I. Bernard Weinstein
Dr. Leonard H. Weinstein
Dr. Irwin M. Weinstock
Dr. John M. Weir
Dr. Harvey J. Weiss
Dr. Julius H. Weiss
Dr. Paul A. Weiss
Dr. Herbert Weissbach
Dr. Bernard Weissman
Dr. Norman Weissman
Dr. Gerald Weissmann
Mrs. Julia T. Weld*
Dr. Daniel Wellner
Dr. Gerhardt Werner
Dr. Sidney C. Werner*
Dr. Arthur R. Wertheim
Dr. W. Clarke Wescoe
Dr. C. D. West
Dr. Henry O. Wheeler
Dr. Frederick E. Wheelock
Dr. Abraham White
Dr. Abraham G. White
Dr. John C. Whitsell, II
Dr. Norman Wikler
Dr. Herbert B. Wilcox, Jr.

* Life member.

Dr. M. Henry Williams
Dr. John Wilson
Dr. Victor J. Wilson
Dr. Sidney J. Winawer
Dr. Erich E. Windhager
Dr. Myron Winick
Dr. Robert M. Winters
Dr. Evelyn M. Witkin
Dr. Jonathan Wittenberg
Dr. Herbert Wohl
Dr. Abner Wolf*
Dr. George A. Wolf
Dr. Julius Wolf
Dr. Robert L. Wolf
Dr. Stewart G. Wolf, Jr.
Dr. James A. Wolff
Dr. Harvey Wolinsky
Dr. Harrison F. Wood
Dr. Henry N. Wood
Dr. John A. Wood
Dr. John L. Wood
Dr. James M. Woodruff

Dr. Kenneth R. Woods
Dr. Melvin H. Worth, Jr.
Dr. Walter D. Wosilait
Dr. Irving S. Wright
Dr. Melvin D. Yahr
Dr. Sehchi Yasumura
Dr. Chester L. Yntema*
Dr. Tasai-Fan Yu
Dr. John B. Zabriskie
Dr. Ralph Zalusky
Dr. Esmail D. Zanjani
Dr. Vratislav Zbuzek
Dr. James E. Ziegler, Jr.
Dr. Arthur M. Zimmerman
Dr. Harry M. Zimmerman
Dr. Norton Zinder
Dr. Burton L. Zohman
Dr. Olga Zoneraich
Dr. Samuel Zoneraich
Dr. Joseph Zubin
Dr. Marjorie B. Zucker
Dr. Benjamin W. Zweifach

* Life member.

ASSOCIATE MEMBERS

Dr. A. F. Anderson*
Dr. John C. Baiardi
Dr. Charles Birnberg
Dr. A. Bookman*
Dr. Henry Colcher
Dr. George Craft
Dr. B. B. Crohn*
Dr. Aaron Feder
Dr. Saul Fisher
Dr. Lewis M. Fraad
Dr. Ralph Friedlander
Dr. William A. Gardner*
Dr. Herman Gladstone
Dr. Ephraim Glassmann
Dr. Henry P. Goldberg
Dr. Carlo E. S. Grossi
Dr. Connie M. Guion*
Dr. Bernard H. Hall
Dr. Louis Hausman*
Dr. George L. Kauer, Jr.
Dr. R. A. Kinsella*
Dr. Abraham M. Kleinman
Dr. Percy Klingenstein*
Dr. Michael Lake*
Dr. Louis Langman*
Dr. Hyman Levy
Dr. Marjorie Lewisohn

Dr. Asa L. Lincoln*
Dr. Edith M. Lincoln*
Dr. Julius Littman
Dr. Melville G. Magida
Dr. Kirby Martin*
Dr. Robert B. McKittrick
Dr. John A. P. Millett*
Dr. Hans W. Neuberg
Dr. Jean Papps
Dr. Francis M. Rackemann*
Dr. E. D. Rosenfeld
Dr. F. B. St. John*
Dr. B. J. Sanger*
Dr. Joseph Schattner
Dr. L. L. Shapiro*
Dr. M. DeForest Smith*
Dr. Hamilton Southworth
Dr. Roy C. Swingle
Dr. William A. Triebel
Dr. Harry E. Ungerleider*
Dr. Alfred Vogl
Dr. Jerome P. Webster*
Dr. Leo Weiner
Dr. Abner I. Weisman
Dr. Asher Winkelstein*
Dr. George A. Zak
Dr. Arthur Zitrin

* Life member.

DECEASED MEMBERS, FORMERLY ACTIVE AND ASSOCIATE

T. J. Abbott
Isidor Abrahamson
Mark H. Adams
Isaac Adler
David Adelersberg
Andrew J. Akelaitus
F. H. Albee
Harry L. Alexander
Samuel Alexander
F. M. Allen
Alf S. Alving
H. L. Amoss
Dorothy H. Anderson
W. B. Anderton
Wm. Dewitt Andrus
Herman Anfanger
W. Parker Anslow, Jr.
R. T. Atkins
Hugh Auchincloss
John Auer
J. Harold Austin
O. T. Avery
Halsey Bagg
Harold C. Bailey
Pearce Bailey
Eleanor DeF. Baldwin
Clarence G. Bandler
Bolton Bangs
W. Halsey Barker
F. H. Bartlett
Louis Bauman
W. W. Beattie
Carl Beck
William H. Beckman
Edwin Beer
Rhoda W. Benham
A. A. Berg
Max Bergmann
Charles M. Berry
Hermann M. Biggs

Francis G. Blake
N. R. Blatherwick
Ernest P. Boas
Aaron Bodansky
Charles F. Bolduan
Richard Walker Bolling
Ralph H. Boots
J. B. Borden
David Bovaird
Samuel Bradbury
Erwin Brand
A. Braslau
S. M. Brickner
Nathan E. Brill
J. J. Bronfenbrenner
Harlow Brooks
F. Tilden Brown
Samuel A. Brown
Wade H. Brown
Maurice Bruger
Joseph D. Bryant
Sue Buckingham
Jacob Buckstein
Leo Buerger
Henry G. Bugbee
Frederick C. Bullock
Jesse H. M. Bullowa
Joseph L. Bunim
Claude A. Burrett
Glenworth R. Butler
George F. Cahill
W. E. Caldwell
Wm. F. Campbell
Alexis Carrel
Herbert S. Carter
John R. Carty
L. Casamajor
Russell L. Cecil
William H. Chambers
Harry A. Charipper

352

John W. Churchman
F. Morris Class
A. F. Coca
Martin Cohen
Alfred E. Cohn
L. G. Cole
Rufus Cole
Charles F. Collins
Harvey S. Collins
Robert A. Cooke
Otis M. Cope
A. Curtis Corcoran
James A. Corscaden
Pol N. Coryllos
Frank Co-Tui
Edwin B. Cragin
Floyd M. Crandall
G. W. Crary
Glenn E. Cullen
John G. Curtis
Edward Cussler
H. D. Dakin
C. Darlington
William Darrach
Martin H. Dawson
Richard C. de Bodo
H. J. Devel, Jr.
Smith O. Dexter, Jr.
Henry D. Diamond
Joseph S. Diamond
Paul A. Dineen
Konrad Dobriner
Blake F. Donaldson
Edwin J. Doty
Henry Doubilet
W. K. Draper
Alexander Duane
E. F. DuBois
Theodore Dunham
C. B. Dunlap
F. Duran-Reynals
Walter H. Eddy
Wilhelm E. Ehrich
Max Einhorn
Robert Elman

C. A. Elsberg
W. J. Elser
A. Elywyn
Haven Emerson
Earl T. Engle
Albert A. Epstein
Lowell Ashton Erf
Samuel M. Evans
James Ewing
Gioacchino Failla
K. G. Falk
L. W. Famulener
Morris S. Fine
Maurice Fishberg
Simon Flexner
Austin Flint
Rolfe Floyd
Joseph E. Flynn
Ellen B. Foot
N. Chandler Foot
Joseph Fraenkel
Edward Francis
Thomas Francis, Jr.
Robert T. Frank
Virginia K. Frantz
Rowland G. Freeman
Webb Freundenthal
Wolff Freundenthal
E. D. Friedman
Lewis F. Frissell
H. Dawson Furniss
C. Z. Garside
Herbert S. Gasser
F. L. Gates
F. P. Gay
Samuel H. Geist
Bertram M. Gesner
H. R. Geyelin
William J. Gies
J. H. Globus
S. Goldschmidt
S. S. Goldwater
Kenneth Goodner
Frederick Goodridge
Malcolm Goodridge

N. W. Green
Harry S. N. Greene
Magnus I. Gregersen
Louise Gregory
Menas S. Gregory
Louis Gross
Emil Gruening
Frederick Gudernatsch
H. V. Guile
John H. Hall
John W. Hall
Robert H. Halsey
Franklin M. Hanger
Lawrence W. Hanlon
Meyer M. Harris
R. Stuart Hart
Frank Hartley
Robert A. Hatcher
Hans O. Haterius
H. A. Haubold
James A. Hawkins
Selig Hecht
George Heller
Carl M. Herget
W. W. Herrick
George J. Heuer
Howard H. Hines
Charles L. Hoagland
August Hoch
Eugene Hodenpyl
George M. Hogeboom
Arthur L. Holland
Franklin Hollander
A. W. Hollis
J. G. Hopkins
Henry Horn
Herbert I. Horowitz
Frank Horsfall, Jr.
Hubert S. Howe
Stephen Hudack
John H. Huddleston
F. B. Humphreys
H. M. Imboden
Moses L. Isaacs
Benjamin Jablons

Leopold Jaches
Holmes C. Jackson
Abraham Jacobi
Walter A. Jacobs
George W. Jacoby
A. G. Jacques
Joseph Jailer
Walter B. James
Edward G. Janeway
H. H. Janeway
James W. Jobling
Scott Johnson
William C. Johnson
Norman Jolliffe
Don R. Joseph
Louis Julianelle
Frederick Kammerer
David Karnofsky
Haig H. Kasabach
Ludwig Kast
Jacob Kaufmann
F. L. Keays
Foster Kennedy
Leo Kessel
Ben Witt Key
E. L. Keyes
George King
Francis P. Kinnicutt
D. B. Kirby
Stuart F. Kitchen
Herbert M. Klein
I. S. Kleiner
Paul Klemperer
Walter C. Klotz
Arnold Knapp
Hermann Knapp
Yale Kneeland, Jr.
Seymour Korkes
Arthur F. Kraetzer
Milton Lurie Kramer
Charles Krumwiede
L. O. Kunkel
Ann G. Kuttner
Raphael Kurzrok
William S. Ladd

ALBERT R. LAMB
ADRIAN V. S. LAMBERT
ALEXANDER LAMBERT
ROBERT A. LAMBERT
S. W. LAMBERT
ERNEST W. LAMPE
CARNEY LANDIS
GUSTAV LANGMANN
BURTON J. LEE
EGBERT LeFEVRA
E. S. L'ESPERANCE
P. A. LEVENE
MICHAEL LEVINE
SAM Z. LEVINE
CHARLES H. LEWIS
JACQUES M. LEWIS
EMAUEL LIBMAN
CHARLES C. LIEB
FRANK L. LIGENZOWSKI
WRAY LLOYD
JOHN S. LOCKWOOD
JACQUES LOEB
LEO LOEB
ROBERT O. LOEBEL
LEO LOEWE
ALFONSO A. LOMBARDI
PERRIN LONG
WARFIELD T. LONGCOPE
RAY R. LOSEY
ROSE LUBSCHEZ
SIGMUND LUSTGARTEN
JOHN D. LYTTLE
W. G. MacCALLUM
DUNCAN A. MacINNES
GEORGE M. MACKENZIE
THOMAS T. MACKIE
COLIN M. MacLEOD
WARD J. MacNEAL
F. B. MALLORY
A. R. MANDEL
JOHN A. MANDEL
F. S. MANDELBAUM
MORRIS MANGES
GEORGE MANNHEIMER
DAVID MARINE

W. B. MARPLE
WALTON MARTIN
HOWARD MASON
HUNTER McALPIN
CHARLES McBURNEY
GERTRUDE S. McCANN
W. S. McCANN
W. ROSS McCARTY
J. F. McGRATH
EARL B. McKINLEY
FRANKLIN C. McLEAN
GEORGE McNAUGHTON
EDWARD S. McSWEENY
FRANK S. MEARA
W. J. MEEK
VICTOR MELTZER
ADOLF MEYER
ALFRED MEYER
MICHAEL MICAILOVSKY
HENRY MILCH
EDGAR G. MILLER
GEORGE N. MILLER
SAMUEL CHARLES MILLER
H. C. MOLOY
ROBERT A. MOORE
C. V. MORRILL
A. V. MOSCHCOWITZ
ELI MOSCHCOWITZ
ABRAHAM MOSS
JOHN P. MUNN
J. R. MURLIN
JAMES B. MURPHY
CLAY RAY MURRAY
V. C. MYERS
JAMES F. NAGLE
JAMES NEILL
CARL NEUBERG
SELIAN NEUHOF
WALTER L. NILES
CHARLES V. NOBACK
JOSE F. NONIDEZ
VAN HORNE NORRIE
CHARLES NORRIS
JOHN H. NORTHROP
NATHANIEL READ NORTON

Francis W. O'Connor
Charles T. Olcott
Peter K. Olitsky
Eugene L. Opie
B. S. Oppenheimer
Hans Oppenheimer
Kermit E. Osserman
Sadao Otani
John Overman
Ralph S. Overman
Beryl H. Paige
Arthur Palmer
Walter W. Palmer
George W. Papanicolaou
A. M. Pappenheimer
William H. Park
Stewart Paton
John M. Pearce
Louise Pearce
Charles H. Peck
James Pedersen
E. J. Pellini
David Perla
E. Cooper Person
J. P. Peters
Frederick Peterson
Godfrey R. Pisek
Harry Plotz
Milton Plotz
G. R. Pogue
William M. Polk
Abou D. Pollack
F. L. Pollack
Sigmund Pollitzer
Nathaniel B. Potter
Thomas D. Price
T. M. Prudden
Edward Quintard
Geoffrey W. Rake
C. C. Ransom
Bret Ratner
George B. Ray
R. G. Reese
Jules Redish
Birdsey Renshaw
C. P. Rhoads

A. N. Richards
Henry B. Richardson
Oscar Riddle
Austen Fox Riggs
John L. Riker
Seymour Rinzler
David Rittenberg
Thomas M. Rivers
Andrew R. Robinson
Frank H. Robinson
Martin Rosenthal
Nathan Rosenthal
M. A. Rothschild
Peyton Rous
Wilfred F. Ruggiero
F. J. Ryan
George H. Ryder
Florence R. Sabin
Bernard Sachs
Wm. P. St. Lawrence
William A. Salant
T. W. Salmon
Benjamin Salzer
E. F. Sampson
Harold E. Santee
Wilbur A. Sawyer
Reginald H. Sayre
Herbert W. Schmitz
Rudolph Schoenheimer
Louis C. Schroeder
Herman Von W. Schulte
E. L. Scott
H. Shapiro
Harry H. Shapiro
George Y. Shinowara
Ephraim Shorr
Harold Shorr
William K. Simpson
M. J. Sittenfield
J. E. Smadel
A. Alexander Smith
Carl H. Smith
Homer W. Smith
R. Garfield Snyder
J. W. Stephenson
Kurt G. Stern

George D. Stewart
H. A. Stewart
E. G. Stillman
Ralph G. Stillman
L. A. Stimson
C. R. Stockard
George H. Stueck, Jr.
Arthur M. Sutherland
John E. Sutton
Paul C. Swenson
Homer F. Swift
Sam Switzer
Jerome T. Syverton
L. James Talbot
Sterling P. Taylor, Jr.
Oscar Teague
J. de Castro Teixeira
Edward E. Terrell
John S. Thacher
Allen M. Thomas
Giles W. Thomas
W. Hanna Thompson
Karl J. Thompson
Edgar W. Todd
Wisner R. Townsend
Theodore T. Tsaltas
James D. Trask, Jr.
H. F. Traut
Norman Treves
Folke Tudvad
Joseph C. Turner
Kenneth B. Turner
Cornelius J. Tyson
Edward Uhlenhuth
F. T. Van Beuren, Jr.
Philip Van Ingen
R. Van Santvoord
Donald D. Van Slyke
H. N. Vermilye
Karl Vogel
William C. Von Glahn
Harry Sobotka
F. P. Solley
H. J. Spencer
J. Bentley Squier, Jr.
W. C. Stadie

Norbert Stadtmüller
Henricus J. Stander
Daniel Stats
J. Murray Steele
Richard Stein
Antonio Stella
Augustus Wadsworth
Heinrich B. Waelsch
H. F. Walker
George B. Wallace
Wilbur Ward
James S. Waterman
Janet Watson
Leslie T. Webster
R. W. Webster
Webb W. Weeks
Richard Weil
Louis Weisfuse
Sara Welt
John R. West
Randolph West
George W. Wheeler
John M. Wheeler
J. S. Wheelwright
Daniel Widelock
Carl J. Wiggers
Herbert B. Wilcox
H. B. Williams
Armine T. Wilson
Margaret B. Wilson
Philip D. Wilson
Joseph E. Winters
Dan H. Witt
Harold G. Wolff
I. Ogden Woodruff
D. Wayne Woolley
Herman Wortis
S. Bernard Wortis
Arthur M. Wright
Jonathan Wright
Walter H. Wright
John H. Wyckoff
Frederick D. Zeman
H. F. L. Ziegel
Hans Zinsser